Guidelines for Clinical Practice

FROM DEVELOPMENT TO USE

MARILYN J. FIELD AND KATHLEEN N. LOHR, *Editors*

Committee on Clinical Practice Guidelines

Division of Health Care Services
INSTITUTE OF MEDICINE

D1526524

NATIONAL ACADEMY PRESS
Washington, D.C. 1992

National Academy Press • 2101 Constitution Avenue, N.W. • Washington, D.C. 20418

NOTICE: The project that is the subject of this report was approved by the Governing Board of the National Research Council, whose members are drawn from the councils of the National Academy of Sciences, the National Academy of Engineering, and the Institute of Medicine. The members of the committee responsible for the report were chosen for their special competences and with regard for appropriate balance.

This report has been reviewed by a group other than the authors according to procedures approved by a Report Review Committee consisting of members of the National Academy of Sciences, the National Academy of Engineering, and the Institute of Medicine.

The Institute of Medicine was chartered in 1970 by the National Academy of Sciences to enlist distinguished members of the appropriate professions in the examination of policy matters pertaining to the health of the public. In this, the Institute acts under both the Academy's 1863 congressional charter responsibility to be an adviser to the federal government and its own initiative in identifying issues of medical care, research, and education.

Support for this project was provided by the John A. Hartford Foundation of New York City and by the Agency for Health Care Policy and Research, U.S. Department of Health and Human Services, under Contract No. 282-90-0018. Additional funds were provided by the Blue Cross and Blue Shield Association, CIGNA Foundation, the Prudential Foundation, and the American College of Cardiology. The views presented are those of the Institute of Medicine Committee on Clinical Practice Guidelines and are not necessarily those of the funding organizations.

Library of Congress Cataloging-in-Publication Data

Institute of Medicine (U.S.). Committee on Clinical Practice
   Guidelines.
     Guidelines for clinical practice : from development to use /
   Committee on Clinical Practice Guidelines. Division of Health Care
   Services, Institute of Medicine ; Marilyn J. Field and Kathleen N.
   Lohr, eds.
      p. cm.
   Includes bibliographical references and index.
   ISBN 0-309-04589-4 (alk. paper)
    1. Medical care—Standards—United States. I. Field, Marilyn
Jane. II. Lohr, Kathleen N., 1941- . III. Title.
    [DNLM: 1. Clinical Medicine—standards—United States.
2. Delivery of Health Care—standards—United States. 3. Quality of
Health Care—standards—United States. W 84 AA1 I485g]
RA399.A3I56 1992
362.1'021873—dc20
DNLM/DLC
for Library of Congress   92-8613
                                               CIP

The serpent has been a symbol of long life, healing, and knowledge among almost all cultures and religions since the beginning of recorded history. The image adopted a a logotype by the Institute of Medicine is based on a relief carving from ancient Greece, now held by the Staatlichemuseen in Berlin.

Study Staff

HOLLY DAWKINS, Research Assistant
MOLLA S. DONALDSON, Senior Staff Officer
MARILYN J. FIELD, Study Director
KATHLEEN N. LOHR, Deputy Director, Division of Health Care Services
DONNA D. THOMPSON, Senior Project Assistant
KARL D. YORDY, Director, Division of Health Care Services

Acknowledgments

The Committee on Clinical Practice Guidelines and the study staff were assisted by many individuals and groups, most of whom we hope we have acknowledged here. The members of two groups—a health care liaison panel and a specialty society liaison program—are listed in Appendix C. That appendix also lists those who testified at a public hearing in December 1990.

This study benefited from the work of several other IOM projects. In particular, it builds on the work of the Committee to Advise the Public Health Service on Clinical Practice Guidelines, the Committee to Design a Strategy for Quality Review and Assurance in the Medicare Program, and the Committee on Utilization Management in the Private Sector.

The committee commissioned two papers that provided useful background and insights for this report. Gail Povar, M.D., of George Washington University prepared a thoughtful, in-depth examination of ethical issues; Frances Miller, J.D., of Boston University submitted an equally valuable overview of legal issues. The committee's understanding of inconsistencies among guidelines and of ways of identifying them was aided by the work performed by subcontractors Carmi Margolis, M.D., Lawrence Gottlieb, M.D., and their colleagues at the Harvard Community Health Plan and the Ben Gurion University of the Negev.

Initial directions for both this and the earlier project on guidelines were provided by a planning committee that met in November 1989. The meeting was chaired by Jerome H. Grossman, M.D.; the participants were Peter Bouxsein, J.D.; J. Jarrett Clinton, M.D.; Arthur J. Donovan, M.D.; David

M. Eddy, M.D., Ph.D.; Sheldon Greenfield, M.D.; Clark C. Havighurst, J.D.; Neil Hollander; Carmault B. Jackson, Jr., M.D.; John Kelly, M.D.; Marie Michnich, Dr.P.H., R.N.; Joel E. Miller; William H. Moncreif, Jr., M.D.; Charles E. Phelps, Ph.D.; William L. Roper, M.D.; Ralph Schaffarzick, M.D.; Richard S. Sharpe; Linda Johnson White; and Sally Hart Wilson, J.D.

Some of the substantive groundwork for the report's recommendation of attributes for review criteria was laid by an expert panel convened for the quality assurance project to consider desirable characteristics of quality-of-care indicators. That panel consisted of William A. Causey, M.D.; Arthur J. Donovan, M.D.; Leonard S. Driefus, M.D.; David M. Eddy, M.D., Ph.D.; Lesley Fishelman, M.D.; Sheldon Greenfield, M.D.; Robert J. Marder, M.D.; Jane L. Neumann, M.D.; Bruce Perry, M.D.; and Ralph Schaffarzick, M.D.

Among the many who provided the committee with important insights into the challenges of using practice guidelines are Brent James, M.D., and Alan Morris, M.D., of InterMountain Health Care; William Minogue, M.D., Elaine Campbell, Mark Smith, Jack Zimmerman, M.D., Stanley Deutsch, M.D., Robert Sherrick, M.D., and others at the George Washington University Hospital; Joanne Lynn, M.D., Rebecca Elon, M.D., Monica Koshuta, Mollie Sabol-Spencer, and others at the Washington Home and Hospice; Rob Johnson and James Herbert of Eastman Chemicals Company; James Mortimer of Midwest Business Group on Health; Dean Anderson of the Heritage National Health Plan; Paul Perlman, M.D., of Kingsport IPA; Paul Bishop, Ken Unger, Penny Romeo, Carol Gilreath, and others at Holston Valley Community Hospital and Indian Path Hospital in Kingsport, Tennessee; Sheldon Greenfield, M.D., Thomas Smith, M.D., Michael Goldberg, M.D., Deirdre Bigalow, Elizabeth Kantz, R.N., Tina Shapleigh, M.D., Karyl Woldrum, R.N., Paul Drew, M.D., and Cynthia Taft of the New England Medical Center; Dale Benson, M.D., and William Van Osdol, M.D., of the Community Health Network and Methodist Hospital of Indiana; Harvey Feigenbaum, M.D., at University Hospital of the Indiana University School of Medicine; and A. Alan Fischer, M.D., Indiana University School of Medicine.

Not known to us by name are the pediatricians and general surgeons in two focus groups organized for us under subcontract by Mathew Greenwald and Associates. We were assisted with the focus group of pediatricians by the American Academy of Pediatrics, in particular by Robert Sebring, Ph.D., and we discussed the other focus group with Paul Ebert, M.D., of the American College of Surgeons. In addition, to expand the insights available to us, we consulted with the American College of Physicians in developing formats that could be used both for this project's focus groups and for those the College was conducting as part of its evaluation of its Clinical Efficacy Assessment Project.

At the Agency for Health Care Policy and Research, many individuals helped keep us abreast of the activities and thinking of the organization: Kathleen McCormick, Ph.D., R.N.; Stephen King, M.D.; Kathleen Hastings, J.D.; Linda Demlo, Ph.D.; Margaret VanAmringe; Elaine Corrigan; and others. Project staff also attended the retreat organized by the agency to consider lessons learned from the first year of work on guidelines and participated in discussions of guidelines at conferences on medical liability and directions for health services research. Members of the IOM study committee were also in touch with members of the expert panels developing guidelines under AHCPR sponsorship. Marjorie Cahn of the new Center for Health Services Research Information at the National Library of Medicine helped in describing how the NLM will support the dissemination of guidelines.

Arnold Rosoff, J.D., and Eleanor Kinney, J.D., helped in sorting out the complexities of medical malpractice, and Edward David, M.D., J.D., answered many questions about the Maine Medical Liability Demonstration Project. At the American Medical Association, John Kelly, M.D., Margaret Toepp, Shirley Dodd, J.D., and others were unfailingly helpful. George Hripcsak, M.D., Robert Nease, Ph.D., and Douglas Owens, M.D., provided helpful discussions of ways of formatting practice guidelines. Robert Hayward, M.D., at the Johns Hopkins University, contributed a variety of insights into how medical schools might incorporate guidelines into the educational process. Harold Sox, Jr., M.D., and other members of the Clinical Efficacy Assessment Project of the American College of Physicians allowed us to see their process at work. Staff participation in the Harvard Community Health Plan seminar on guidelines development also provided important insights into the challenges of developing and formatting guidelines.

Very substantial assistance was provided to this project by several individuals who, at the request of specialty societies participating in our liaison program, reviewed the Provisional Instrument for Assessing Clinical Practice Guidelines. Some reviews were provided anonymously, but we can acknowledge the contributions of Hannan Bell, Ph.D.; Michael Greenberg, M.D.; Lester Rosen, M.D.; Thomas Harbin, M.D.; Andrew Schachat, M.D.; Harold Pincus, M.D.; Irene Feurer, M.S.Ed.; Richard A. Deyo, M.D.; David Hickham, M.D.; and William Golden, M.D. Betty King of the Internal Medicine Center to Advance Research and Education (IMCARE) secured more than 60 responses from an IMCARE task force. Anne-Marie Audet, M.D., contributed substantially to the initial draft of the instrument.

Contents

Guidelines for Clinical Practice

Summary

Guidelines for the provision of clinical care have been linked in recent years to almost every major problem and proposed solution on the American health policy agenda. Practice guidelines have been tied in some way, by some individual or organization, to costs, quality, access, patient empowerment, professional autonomy, medical liability, rationing, competition, benefit design, utilization variation, bureaucratic micromanagement of health care, and more. The concept has acted as a magnet for the hopes and frustrations of practitioners, patients, payers, researchers, and policymakers.

This recent surge of interest notwithstanding, guidelines are not new. Professional organizations have been developing guidelines for at least half a century, and recommendations about appropriate care can be found in ancient writings. What is new is the emphasis on systematic, evidence-based guidelines and the interest in processes, structures, and incentives that support the effective use and evaluation of such guidelines.

Given this history, the Institute of Medicine (IOM) study reported here had two objectives: first, to encourage constructive expectations for guidelines and, second, to promote the kind of care and rigor in their development, application, evaluation, and revision that would help such expectations to be realized. A committee of experts in clinical practice, health care policy and administration, health services research, and related fields met five times between June 1990 and September 1991 to develop this report.[1]

---

[1] Committee activities and sources of information included site visits, a public hearing, focus groups, commissioned papers, and published and unpublished literature. The committee was assisted by two liaison panels representing health care organizations and medical specialty societies.

1

The committee used as a starting point the 1990 IOM report, *Clinical Practice Guidelines: Directions for a New Program.* That report advised the Agency for Health Care Policy and Research (AHCPR) and its Forum for Quality and Effectiveness in Health Care on their responsibilities for guidelines.

Guidelines for clinical practice cannot realistically be viewed as *the* solution to the country's health care problems, in particular, the problem of escalating costs. Nevertheless, systematically developed, science-based guidelines can become part of the fabric of health care in this country, and they can serve as useful tools for many desirable changes. Their potential reach extends from improving the quality of clinical care (and its measurement) to helping reduce the financial costs of inappropriate, unnecessary, or dangerous care. Practice guidelines are among the building blocks for informed patient decisionmaking and rational social judgments about what care should be covered by public and private health benefit plans.

As tools and building blocks for positive change, guidelines need to be understood and encouraged in context. That context includes powerful economic interests; changing and sometimes conflicting attitudes about professional and patient autonomy; policymaking and implementing institutions that are intensely stressed and sometimes incapacitated; and scientific research that simultaneously expands both knowledge and uncertainty. Above all, the context includes the complex, intimate relationship between individual patients and practitioners who are trying to protect health, manage illness, and preserve dignity under conditions that range from routine to desperate.

WHAT ARE PRACTICE GUIDELINES?

As defined in the IOM's 1990 report, practice guidelines are "systematically developed statements to assist practitioner and patient decisions about appropriate health care for specific clinical circumstances." Medical review criteria, which are also discussed in this report, are "systematically developed statements that can be used to assess the appropriateness of specific health care decisions, services, and outcomes."

Practice guidelines focus, in the first instance, on assisting patients and practitioners in making decisions, but this defining characteristic does not and should not preclude their use for other purposes including quality improvement and payment policymaking. Conversely, medical review criteria and related tools emphasize the evaluation of health care decisions, actions, and outcomes, but they should and do build on guidelines and may in some cases be virtually identical.

Practice guidelines are not synonymous with the reimbursement or coverage policies of Medicare and other health insurance plans, which traditionally have excluded some items from coverage (for example, immunizations and blood products) for reasons unrelated to the appropriateness of the service. Policies for reimbursement and coverage certainly may be informed by practice guidelines, but the two should not be confused.

The potential users of clinical practice guidelines are diverse, and any single user of guidelines may employ them in various ways. Five major purposes for guidelines, which are not mutually exclusive, are (1) assisting clinical decisionmaking by patients and practitioners; (2) educating individuals or groups; (3) assessing and assuring the quality of care; (4) guiding allocation of resources for health care; and (5) reducing the risk of legal liability for negligent care. This report focuses on the primary users of guidelines: practitioners, patients and their families, and health care institutions. Other users include those payers, health benefit plans, and public policymakers and regulators who may use guidelines in making specific decisions about what health care to reimburse, cover, or encourage and in evaluating the decisions, actions, or performance of the primary users of guidelines.

WHY ARE POLICYMAKERS INTERESTED IN GUIDELINES?

Some would explain the interest in practice guidelines shown by legislators, regulators, and purchasers of health care (as contrasted with practitioners and patients) with a single phrase: out-of-control health care costs. Although the importance of costs as a stimulus for guidelines should not be understated, concerns about quality of care, risk management, and improved patient outcomes also figure prominently in the call for more and better practice guidelines.

Much of the interest in guidelines has been prompted by perceptions that higher health care expenditures have brought only marginal health benefits and that guidelines can help remedy this problem of "value." Virtually every major discussion of guidelines begins with a similar list of reasons for these perceptions: (1) wide variations in physician practice patterns and use of health services; (2) research indicating inappropriate use of many services; and (3) uncertainty about the health outcomes achieved by the use or nonuse of various services and procedures.

Whether the issue is unexplained variation, inappropriate care, or uncertain outcomes, many analysts come to similar conclusions. More research on outcomes and effectiveness of health care services is needed; more effort should be invested in using such research to formulate specific guidelines for clinical practice; more use of the resulting guidelines will help limit spending for health services.

How are guidelines to limit health care costs? How are they to increase the perceived value of health care spending? Implicitly or explicitly, the basic argument or hypothesis runs along these lines:

Scientific evidence and clinical judgment can be systematically combined to produce clinically valid, operational recommendations for appropriate care that can and will be used to persuade clinicians, patients, and others to change their practices in ways that lead to better health outcomes and lower health care costs.

At least six formidable—and often unrealistic—assumptions lie behind this model. First, a sufficient quantity and quality of scientific evidence exists to serve as a foundation for guidelines. Second, programs to develop guidelines will be organized, funded, and effectively managed to produce a considerable volume of valid, usable statements about appropriate care for clinically and financially significant health conditions or technologies. Third, substantial numbers of clinicians, patients, and others will have the opportunity, the support, and the incentives to read, understand, accept, and use these statements in ways that change patterns of clinical practice, health behavior, or payment for health care services in desired directions. Fourth, such changes will be broad and intense enough to improve health outcomes. Fifth, on balance, the entire body of guidelines as actually developed and used will lead to more cost-controlling than cost-increasing behavior on the part of providers and patients. Sixth, the body of guidelines will continually expand to cover new areas so that net rates of increase in health care costs and absolute levels of expenditures will be lower than they would otherwise be.

Again, these are formidable expectations. They outstrip current capacities with respect to the base of scientific knowledge, the translation of that science into usable practice guidelines, and the incentives and structures to encourage application of such guidelines. Even if the first four expectations stated above were to be fulfilled, the fifth and sixth expectations about the cost consequences of change are questionable. Some guidelines undoubtedly will save money by reducing the use of inappropriate or unnecessary services; some will increase expenditures by encouraging more use of underutilized services; and some will shift costs from one type of service to another or from one payer to another. The result should be better value, but the net impact on the rate of increase in total health care spending cannot be predicted with confidence, *even if* future priorities for guidelines development stress clinical conditions for which costly overuse of services is suspected.

In sum, guidelines for clinical practice are a promising but not a quick or sure strategy for improving and rationalizing the overall use of health services. The attention and resources now invested in guidelines could dissolve in the face of a collision between unrealistic hopes and limited immediate results. Persistent commitment over the long term is required from both policymakers and health care professionals.

GENERAL STRENGTHS AND WEAKNESSES OF CURRENT PRACTICE GUIDELINES ACTIVITIES

It is usually easier to spot problems than successes. The committee notes the limitations of current efforts to develop and use guidelines in a spirit of identifying opportunities for progress. It hopes that this attitude will help to encourage those interested in better development, use, and evaluation of guidelines. Ultimately, the committee is confident that the history of clinical practice guidelines will be a positive one.

What Are the Strong Points of Current Efforts?

A first strength of current efforts is their pluralism. The commitment of both public- and private-sector resources helps to protect guidelines efforts from real or perceived "capture" by narrow interests. The lack of a dominant model and the existence of multiple, diverse sponsors have encouraged innovation in methods and flexibility to accommodate different potential users. By fostering a wider range of development and implementation activities than would be prompted by less diverse sponsorship, pluralism may also facilitate wider understanding and acceptance of guidelines.

A second strength of the guidelines enterprise is simple enthusiasm. Policymakers have endorsed the undertaking, funding is increasing, and how-to-do-it conferences and similar products have been multiplying. Professional and specialty societies are clearly involved to a degree far beyond that observed two to five years ago. Processes for guidelines development are even seen as mechanisms for defining health insurance and benefit packages in ways that were rarely thought possible just a short time ago.

Third, guidelines are gaining credibility. Expectations about the rigor needed to develop sound guidelines are increasing, and processes for guideline development are beginning to be reshaped. Also growing is professional consensus on two scores: the outcomes of patient care must be more broadly defined and carefully appraised, and the appropriateness of both new and old services must be subjected to more objective, critical scrutiny.

A fourth strength is that researchers, clinicians, educators, and managers are being stimulated to consider how guidelines and other efforts to improve the quality and efficiency of health care can support and complement each other. These efforts include outcomes and effectiveness research, methods for strengthening informed patient decisionmaking, and both traditional and newer techniques for quality assessment and quality improvement.

The above strengths have not emerged from an overarching, deliberate plan. Rather, they are the result of a combination of deliberate steps (for example, the creation of a guidelines function in AHCPR) and the un-orchestrated accumulation of many separate organizational initiatives. Part of the message of this report is the dual need to understand and capitalize on these processes and to channel them to better match health care needs.

What Are the Limitations of Current Efforts?

Another part of the message of this report concerns the current limita-tions and weaknesses of efforts to develop and apply practice guidelines. Some of these drawbacks are the "downsides" of factors mentioned above. Others relate to more general problems inherent in the nation's health care system.

First, pluralism—the involvement of diverse groups in guidelines de-velopment—has negative as well as positive consequences. The limited resources for guideline development, use, evaluation, and improvement are inefficiently deployed. Development efforts are fragmented across groups with greatly varying goals, methods, and capacities, and cooperative efforts to develop guidelines that affect multiple specialties and practitioner types are still too atypical. Even when formal priorities have been established, actual selection of topics for guidelines development seems to be haphazard within organizations and thus across the entire system.

Second, the lack of quality control over methods and procedures is a particularly serious drawback of both national and local processes for de-veloping guidelines. Many national organizations involved actively in de-veloping guidelines and review criteria are moving to improve their programs, but weak procedures and products are common. Methods and procedures for local adaptation of national guidelines and for translation of guidelines into medical review criteria have not been thoroughly documented, but they certainly appear to be subject to equal or greater weaknesses. Potential users of guidelines and review criteria have no ready means to judge the soundness of materials produced by different groups with different approaches.

A third weakness is that efforts to evaluate the impact of practice guidelines have been limited. Despite widespread interest in guidelines as a tool for improving the quality and cost-effectiveness of care, virtually nothing is known about whether they can or do contribute to these goals.

IMPROVING THE DEVELOPMENT OF GUIDELINES

Although this committee intended to focus almost exclusively on the implementation of guidelines rather than on their development, it discov-ered that the application of guidelines was sufficiently dependent on certain characteristics of the development process that revisiting this subject be-came imperative. In doing so, the committee stressed several points. First, guidelines developers must do better in anticipating the needs and concerns of potential users and in building a case for their recommendations that users will find compelling. Second, for developers to do this, procedures and methods need improvement. Third, more attention should be paid to the identification and analysis of inconsistencies among guidelines and to the rationales and results of local processes to develop or adapt guidelines. The committee also questioned whether guidelines developers should be expected to take on even more demanding tasks by factoring cost-effectiveness into all their recommendations or by defining the minimum level and types of care that should be provided for all individuals.

Building a Compelling Case for Recommendations

Most guidelines fail to build a compelling case for the relevance, importance, and soundness of their recommendations. To varying degrees, practitioners, payers, risk managers, and those involved in quality assurance and improvement perceive that many guidelines fall short in their applicability to real-world circumstances and in their clarity and precision. In fundamental ways, they do not anticipate the needs of clinicians, patients, and programs to assure quality, control costs, and reduce medical liability.

One theme of this report is that the way clinical practice guidelines are developed can strongly affect their potential for effective use by practitioners, patients, and others. Those who devise guidelines must anticipate what will make the guidelines practical and credible. Thus, planning for successful implementation should begin with development and continue through cycles of revision and updating.

The IOM has specified desirable attributes of clinical practice guidelines and medical review criteria (Tables 1 and 2). Each attribute affects the likelihood that guidelines will be perceived as trustworthy and usable or the probability that they will, if used, help achieve desired health outcomes. For *practice guidelines*, four of the eight attributes relate to substantive content: validity, reliability, clinical applicability, and clinical flexibility. Four others relate to the process of guideline development or the presentation of guidelines: clarity, multidisciplinary process, scheduled review, and documentation. For *review criteria*, additional attributes are sensitivity, specificity, patient responsiveness, readability, minimum obtrusiveness, feasibility, computer compatibility, and appeals criteria.

This report emphasizes that every set of guidelines should be accompanied by (1) a statement of the strength of the evidence and the expert judgment behind the guidelines and (2) projections of the relevant health and cost outcomes of alternative courses of care. Assessments of relevant health outcomes will consider patient perceptions and preferences.

To the extent that guidelines move toward the characteristics outlined

TABLE 1   Desirable Attributes of Clinical Practice Guidelines

Attribute	Explanation
VALIDITY	Practice guidelines are valid if, when followed, they lead to the health and cost outcomes projected for them. A prospective assessment of validity will consider the substance and quality of the evidence cited, the means used to evaluate the evidence, and the relationship between the evidence and recommendations.
Strength of Evidence	Practice guidelines should be accompanied by descriptions of the strength of the evidence and the expert judgment behind them.
Estimated Outcomes	Practice guidelines should be accompanied by estimates of the health and cost outcomes expected from the interventions in question, compared with alternative practices. Assessments of relevant health outcomes will consider patient perceptions and preferences.
RELIABILITY/ REPRODUCIBILITY	Practice guidelines are reproducible and reliable (1) if—given the same evidence and methods for guidelines development—another set of experts produces essentially the same statements and (2) if—given the same clinical circumstances—the guidelines are interpreted and applied consistently by practitioners (or other appropriate parties).
CLINICAL APPLICABILITY	Practice guidelines should be as inclusive of appropriately defined patient populations as evidence and expert judgment permit, and they should explicitly state the population(s) to which statements apply.
CLINICAL FLEXIBILITY	Practice guidelines should identify the specifically known or generally expected exceptions to their recommendations and discuss how patient preferences are to be identified and considered.
CLARITY	Practice guidelines must use unambiguous language, define terms precisely, and use logical and easy-to-follow modes of presentation.
MULTIDISCIPLINARY PROCESS	Practice guidelines must be developed by a process that includes participation by representatives of key affected groups. Participation may include serving on panels that develop guidelines, providing evidence and viewpoints to the panels, and reviewing draft guidelines.
SCHEDULED REVIEW	Practice guidelines must include statements about when they should be reviewed to determine whether revisions are warranted, given new clinical evidence or professional consensus (or the lack of it).
DOCUMENTATION	The procedures followed in developing guidelines, the participants involved, the evidence used, the assumptions and rationales accepted, and the analytic methods employed must be meticulously documented and described.

TABLE 2 Desirable Attributes of Medical Review Criteria

Attribute	Explanation
SENSITIVITY	Review criteria are sensitive when it is highly likely that a case will be identified as deficient given that it really is deficient. (This assumes that a guideline or other source provides a "gold standard.")
SPECIFICITY	Review criteria are specific if it is highly likely that they will identify truly good care as such.
PATIENT RESPONSIVENESS	Review criteria should specifically identify a role for patient preferences or ensure that the process for using them allows for some consideration of patient preferences.
READABILITY	Review criteria should be presented in language and formats that can be read and understood by nonphysician reviewers, practitioners, and patients/consumers.
MINIMUM OBTRUSIVENESS	Review criteria and the process for applying them should minimize inappropriate direct interaction with and burdens on the treating practitioner or patient.
FEASIBILITY	The information required for review should be easily obtained from direct communication with providers, patients, records, and other sources, and the decision criteria should be easy to apply. Review criteria are accompanied by explicit instructions for their application and scoring.
COMPUTER COMPATIBILITY	Review criteria should be straightforward enough that they can be transformed readily into the computer-based protocols and similar formats that can make the review process more efficient for all involved parties.
APPEALS CRITERIA	Criteria should provide explicit guidance about the considerations to be taken into account when adverse review decisions are appealed by professionals or patients.

above, they will identify how compelling is the case for particular services or courses of care under particular clinical circumstances. They will distinguish care for which there is good scientific evidence, care for which there is good consensus but limited or no evidence, and care for which there is neither evidence nor consensus. Conclusions backed by scientific evidence are more compelling than those based on subjective judgments. To the degree that review criteria build on such guidelines and follow the attributes listed in Table 2, they will help those reviewing care to identify appropriate care more accurately.

In addition to following a careful analytic strategy in creating guidelines, developers should present their work to clinicians in ways that reflect the rigor of this approach and its emphasis on reasoning and critical analysis. Thus, the product of the process should not be perceived solely as information but more generally as an explication of the thinking processes that should be used in evaluating and applying that information. If guidelines are perceived only as information, they may very well be used (or rejected) as the "cookbooks" that many physicians decry. They will also not achieve their potential as educational tools.

In fact, few guidelines today provide any formal projections of health benefits and harms, any explicit treatment of patient preferences, or any estimates of the cost implications of their recommendations, certainly not in comparison with alternative practices. Most also lack explicit assessments of the strength of the evidence behind their recommendations. In addition, the educational opportunities implicit in guidelines cannot be fully exploited because the evidence and rationale for the guidelines are often not presented. Many of the future directions endorsed by this committee depend on better performance in these areas.

The committee recognizes that the development strategy recommended here is highly demanding and that some, perhaps most or all, guidelines will never fully achieve the ideal. It also recognizes the considerable gaps in empirical information about the natural history of many diseases and conditions, about health outcomes for many diagnostic or therapeutic interventions, and about the costs of providing those (or alternative) interventions. Nonetheless, if developers of practice guidelines make serious, persistent efforts in the directions recommended here, their products should become substantially more valuable and credible.

Procedural and Methodological Issues Needing Particular Attention

Although developers of guidelines have considerable room for improvement in the use of existing techniques, the methods for guidelines development are themselves in need of refinement. Given its emphasis on evidence, outcomes, and patient preferences and its concerns about the impact of guidelines on the quality and costs of health care, the committee focused on six questions of methodology:

1. means for setting priorities among topics for guidelines development;
2. procedures for securing thoughtful and useful statements of expert judgments;
3. methods for analyzing and rating scientific evidence;

4. techniques for improving knowledge of health outcomes and giving due importance to patient preferences;

5. methods for identifying and projecting the costs of alternative courses of care and comparing their cost-effectiveness; and

6. mechanisms for identifying and evaluating inconsistent or conflicting guidelines.

At the Interface Between Development and Use

The committee considered three subjects that arise at the interface between guidelines development and guidelines implementation: local adaptation of guidelines, inconsistent guidelines, and formatting and dissemination. In this context, the term *local* is used broadly to include multihospital systems, nationwide networks of HMOs, or other similar groups that may develop their own guidelines and modify those developed by others.

Local Adaptation of Guidelines

Some local adaptation of national guidelines is probably inevitable and may be useful, because even well-developed guidelines may have gaps and may not foresee significant local objectives or constraints. The process of adapting guidelines can also educate practitioners and serve as a ratifying mechanism that helps win acceptance.

Moreover, within a framework such as is offered by continuous quality improvement, empirical and incremental testing and modification of guidelines may well be appropriate (indeed, even necessary). Such testing may not conform to the highest standards of experimental research design, but it can provide a systematic, practical, and direct means of identifying where guidelines—as well as clinical practice—may need revision. Ideally, this kind of local but systematic information will become part of the broader evolutionary framework for guidelines development, revision, and improvement nationwide. To this end, the committee urges organizations that adapt guidelines to notify the originating group and explain the circumstances that led to their modifications.

Adaptation may also serve less benign purposes—for example, protecting professional habits and local customs for their own sake or guarding economic self-interest by endorsing unnecessary care or care that others could provide as well or more economically. Casual, "back-of-the-envelope" approaches to adaptation offer particular temptations and opportunities for such unacceptable behavior. Where carefully developed and documented "national" guidelines exist, local adaptation processes should provide explicit rationales that relate to specific, well-defined local conditions or objectives and that take notice of the strength of the case for the original guidelines.

Inconsistent Guidelines

Inconsistent guidelines appear to be unavoidable, even for groups looking at the same scientific evidence and using defensible expert-judgment procedures. Inconsistencies may worry or annoy clinicians, deter the use of sound guidelines, and undermine the credibility of guidelines generally. In some respects, however, inconsistent guidelines provide an opportunity as well as a problem. The opportunity resides in the process for identifying inconsistencies and for determining whether they should be tolerated, rejected, or reconciled. A disciplined approach to inconsistent guidelines would (1) strenuously seek areas of agreement, (2) make rationales for different recommendations explicit and susceptible to comparison with available evidence, (3) reject recommendations or options that conflict with available evidence, and (4) allow options to remain where a case can be made that evidence is inconclusive, professional consensus is split, and variation is unlikely to harm quality of care. In any event, the areas of disagreement point strongly to topics warranting further clinical research.

Formatting and Disseminating Guidelines

Finally, the work of guidelines developers typically extends to some activities beyond the formulation of statements about appropriate care, activities that shade into the work involved in guidelines implementation. One step is effective formatting—presenting guidelines in physical arrangements or media that can be readily understood and applied by practitioners, patients, or other intended groups. Another step is effective dissemination—delivering guidelines to the intended audiences in ways that promote the reception, understanding, acceptance, application, and positive impact of the guidelines. Effective dissemination presupposes effective formatting.

The issues relating to dissemination are many, and the committee did not explore them in depth. Certainly, dissemination alone will neither induce the use of the information being disseminated nor change behavior, and excessive distribution of information exacerbates information overload. The committee concluded that a recognition of these complexities and appropriate planning for dissemination are important components of what guideline *developers* should do in the future.

Going Further? Defining Cost-Effective and Minimum Levels of Care

This report recommends that every set of practice guidelines include information on the health and cost implications of alternative preventive, diagnostic, and management strategies for the clinical situation in question.

The rationale is that this information can help potential users, who must take financial and other resources into account, to better evaluate the potential consequences of different practices. Should guidelines developers go further? Specifically, should every set of guidelines include cost-effectiveness as an explicit criterion for judging or recommending what does or does not constitute appropriate care? Should guideline developers distinguish minimum, essential, or required levels of care in their products?

After much debate, the committee concluded that every set of guidelines need not be based on formal judgments of cost-effectiveness; sound guidelines for clinical practice can stand on rigorous assessments of clinical evidence and carefully derived expert judgment. In addition, the committee declined—with some dissent—to recommend that guidelines must include statements of what constitutes minimum or required care for particular clinical problems.

The committee did *not* say that conclusions and decisions based on cost-effectiveness should be or can be avoided. Governments, health benefit plans, health care providers, and others must make such judgments, although they may not always do so explicitly or rationally. However, committee members could not agree that guidelines developers were, in general and from a policy perspective, the right source of judgments about cost-effectiveness and minimum care. Indeed, several members feared that such judgments would complicate the resource decisions of managers, payers, and policymakers. Moreover, responsibilities for judging cost-effectiveness may be too expansive for individual guidelines panels or for organizations that face major challenges in following the path for guidelines development set forth in Chapters 1, 2, and 7 of the report.

The committee did recognize that some developers of guidelines may be technically, ethically, and politically positioned to make judgments about cost-effectiveness, particularly for some kinds of problems or when those who are developing guidelines are also the intended users. This report is not intended to forestall such recommendations.

In considering the issue of minimum, necessary, or required care, the committee noted troublesome inconsistency and confusion in terminology. For example, terms such as *medical necessity* and *basic benefits* are used in very different and even inconsistent ways that complicate and distort debates over important social issues. The committee's discussion underscored the substantial technical, administrative, ethical, and policy challenges involved in any effort to define what care is required, beneficial, unindicated, inappropriate, or harmful.

Doing More? Guidelines for Informed Patient Decisionmaking

With respect to informed patient decisionmaking, the committee concluded that guideline developers should do more. Good medical care requires shared decisionmaking by practitioners and patients. However, a commitment to shared decisionmaking does not in itself define what information should be provided to patients under different circumstances. Similarly, respect for patient preferences does not in itself answer all technical and policy questions about how to incorporate such preferences into the development or use of practice guidelines.

Two separate paths are suggested here to deal with some of the difficult practical and ethical questions related to patient decisionmaking and informed consent. The first path is the development of treatment- and condition-specific practice guidelines that identify the strength of the evidence behind statements about appropriate care and that estimate and assess outcomes in terms that *patients* perceive as relevant.

A second path for improving the conditions for informed patient decisionmaking is the development of general guidelines for patient information and consent. These guidelines would supplement condition- or treatment-specific practice guidelines, on the one hand, and legally oriented patient consent forms, on the other. Such "patient information guidelines" should be developed by a systematic process similar to that described for clinical practice guidelines. Once formulated, these guidelines would apply, unless specifically modified by condition-specific guidelines, to broad categories of patient care. Patient information guidelines would need to anticipate and specifically cover responsibilities and procedures appropriate for (a) different kinds of care for (b) different kinds of patients in (c) different delivery systems and settings, given (d) different levels of certainty about the benefits, risks, and costs of care.

ENSURING THE USE OF GOOD GUIDELINES

Even when specific, well-founded guidelines exist, their effective use by patients and practitioners will require a wide range of supportive conditions and organizations. As those involved in programs to manage quality, costs, and liability begin to rely on guidelines, these common uses will provide powerful support for their consistent application in actual clinical practice. In particular, the force of peer influence should not be underestimated.

Practitioner knowledge of guidelines and acceptance of their validity are key conditions for their successful application, but acceptance is not equivalent to behavioral change. As a practical matter, it may be better strategically or tactically to focus less on knowledge and acceptance and more on what changes behavior in desired directions. More than simple acceptance of a guideline's correctness may be required to overcome countervailing forces, in particular, information overload, habitual practice patterns, malpractice fears, and economic disincentives.

Quality Assurance and Improvement

Well-developed, scientifically based practice guidelines have an important role to play in assessing, assuring, and improving the quality of health care services provided in this country. Clear, specific guidelines and associated review criteria should help prevent or, alternatively, identify and remedy problems of overuse of care, underuse of care, and poor technical and interpersonal provision of care. Guidelines that have been accepted by those responsible for providing care, financing care, and monitoring care in the public interest are one means of bridging the chasm between internal and external quality assurance strategies.

With respect to models of continuous quality improvement, the committee urges that their focus on systems problems, strong customer-supplier relationships, improvement of average performance, and reduction of variation be more systematically and explicitly joined with an effort to apply and improve sound guidelines for clinical practice. Guidelines can support these and related quality assurance models in several ways.

First, to the extent that guidelines become more sensitive to patient preferences and participation in decisionmaking, they should improve patients' informed consent, their participation in decisionmaking and, ultimately, their satisfaction with both the processes and outcomes of care. Guidelines can also help identify important patient outcomes to incorporate in patient satisfaction surveys and other instruments designed to assess or improve performance. Second, guidelines and review criteria can play a role in identifying possible quality problems arising from underuse, overuse, or incompetent provision of care. They may be particularly useful in instances in which short-term health outcomes (those that are most readily employed) may not be good indicators of long-term results. Third, to the extent that guidelines identify how compelling is the evidence for certain clinical practices, they can help to determine priorities for improving or standardizing specific patterns of clinical care and to sort out competing claims for funding for biomedical and outcomes or effectiveness research. Fourth, participation by clinicians in the review, critique, and improvement of practice guidelines can help bring the science of medicine more forcefully into the planning, action, evaluation, and adjustment cycles required for quality assurance and improvement.

More specifically, the committee recommends the following:

• Guidelines, medical review criteria, and other evaluative tools should be used both to improve average performance and—as is still important—identify substandard performance;
• Inquiries into how individual practice patterns differ from average patterns should go beyond statistical analysis to consider relevant practice guidelines as benchmarks for performance;

• Both the statistical information from such analyses and the pertinent guidelines should be part of educational feedback on practice patterns;

• Evaluations of performance and outcome data should seek to determine the sources of poor outcomes and deviations from guidelines so that systems problems can be corrected and, if necessary, impaired individuals dealt with through training, counseling, limiting of privileges, or other appropriate mechanisms;[2]

• Evaluations of performance and outcomes data should be used to indicate or determine whether practice guidelines ought to be updated or revised;

• Developers of guidelines and health care institutions should convene educational conferences to acquaint practitioners with specific guidelines and provide an opportunity for them to discuss and plan setting-specific applications; and

• Institutional activities to develop or adapt guidelines or review criteria should aspire to meet the attributes for guidelines and for review criteria described in Tables 1 and 2.

Cost Management

On both philosophical and strategic grounds, this committee believes that thoughtfully designed and applied programs to encourage cost-effective use of health care have an important place in supporting the wider application of guidelines for clinical practice. Such programs are a clear market for guidelines and related materials that provide information on the cost-effectiveness of alternative ways of managing particular clinical problems.

Those who pay for health care services and their agents can use guidelines in various ways: (1) to help determine health insurance coverage and avoid payment for unnecessary or inappropriate care, (2) to aid in selecting or credentialing practitioners for participation in various health plans or institutions, and (3) to tailor other economic incentives to affect practitioner or patient behavior. Such approaches usually do not depend on a specific organized practice setting; that is, they can affect practitioners and patients in solo or group practice settings as well as those in larger organizational or institutional settings. Some approaches may be more or less confined to third-party payers whereas others may be shared by health care institutions, quality review programs, and others.

---

[2] The committee explicitly recognizes the need for protection of privacy and confidentiality as those concepts are understood in usual quality assurance terms (e.g., in actions of Medicare peer review organizations, state medical licensure boards, hospital quality assurance committees, and the like).

Programs that develop or employ review criteria to assess the appropriateness of care for specific patients should be guided by the attributes noted in Table 2 and should be supplemented by explicit efforts to monitor the quality and appropriateness of care. This recommendation applies to organizations that formulate or use criteria for retrospective review of care, that generate prospective preprocedure or preadmission criteria, and that engage in all manner of "review" between these two extremes. Review organizations of all sorts, if they follow these attributes, will perforce do certain things that should make their programs more effective, more palatable to practitioners, and less vulnerable to legal liability. They will make their review activities as manageable and as nonintrusive as possible for both patients and practitioners. They will make their review criteria available to practitioners and others. They will provide an explicit process for appealing negative decisions that is free from unreasonable complexity, delay, or other barriers.

It is the committee's hope that economic incentives and quality review mechanisms will, in the future, reduce the need for so-called micromanagement of professional and institutional behavior. External utilization review still may have a role in monitoring practice and targeting problem practices, but many payers will admit that they would prefer to rely more on effective self-regulation by practitioners and providers. Consistent with quality improvement principles, they can then stress education and feedback to physicians aimed at improving practice rather than punishing errors.

Risk Management and Medical Liability

Guidelines that are based on available scientific evidence and that are clear, specific, and developed by a reputable process should carry greater weight in malpractice decisionmaking than vague, nonspecific guidelines that lack documentation and careful reasoning. Guidelines that underscore their recommendations with reference to a strong foundation of scientific evidence should be particularly helpful.

Specific statutory recognition of guidelines, which is intended to provide legal protection to conforming clinicians, is desirable but premature. Acceptable legislation that provides immunity from liability would need to specify operational criteria for the organizations developing guidelines or particular criteria for guidelines themselves, or both. The criticisms directed at the variability and weaknesses of review criteria developed or adopted by Medicare PROs and carriers (and the fact that the criteria of the latter groups are often secret as well) made the committee reluctant to accept organizational imprimatur alone as a sufficient basis for a grant of immunity. Absent explicit procedures and standards for assessing the soundness of practice guidelines (as recommended in this report), the committee believes that giving formal legal stature to any guideline at this early stage may create more problems than it solves.

Information and Decision Support Systems

No existing information infrastructure can support the kind of effective, unobtrusive, easy application of guidelines envisioned by quality improvement models, future-oriented utilization management and cost-containment systems, and patient-centered care proposals. Clearly, however, information technologies are being developed that will make the application of guidelines much easier, particularly if other conditions support their use. For clinicians, creating user-friendly decision aids that relate information about specific patients to guidelines about classes of similar patients deserves greater emphasis and more effort.

The work of the National Library of Medicine and others to establish some capability of responding to user inquiries and dissemination needs related to guidelines should be encouraged. The committee also supports efforts of the library to expand its capacity to assist in guideline development through expansion of its Office for Health Services Research Information. In addition, the committee favors the translation and movement of guidelines into computerized decision aids of various sorts. It recommends, however, that those efforts conform to emerging computer industry standards to enable guidelines (however transformed) to be used on different types of computer-based equipment and systems.

A CRITICAL NEED: MEANS TO ASSESS THE SOUNDNESS OF GUIDELINES

This committee has strongly urged that processes for developing and revising guidelines be soundly based on science and expert clinical judgment *and* that guidelines should anticipate the needs of practitioners, patients, and many other interested parties. How can these groups determine whether different guidelines measure up to these expectations? The committee believes that one answer would be a mechanism for independent assessment of practice guidelines—a stance backed by many of the individuals and organizations consulted during this study.

The design and application of an assessment process will depend on many factors—ethical, political, economic, and organizational. Furthermore, such a process requires at least two basic program components. One is a practical and valid assessment instrument; the other is a feasible structure and process for applying that instrument.

Assessment Instrument

A major task of this committee was the development of a provisional instrument for assessing practice guidelines. The instrument (presented in full in Appendix B) is provisional because it requires more practical testing of its utility. It covers both the process used to develop a specific guidelines document and the substantive content of that document and its recommendations. In essence, the assessment instrument attempts to operationalize the attributes defined in Table 1. A major goal was an instrument that would not allow a set of scientifically invalid or questionable guidelines to receive a "good" rating based on process criteria alone. The committee believes the instrument will be useful as (1) an educational tool for those beginning to develop guidelines; (2) a self-assessment tool that developers of guidelines can use to check their work; and (3) a tool for external groups to use in judging whether a set of guidelines should or should not be recommended or adopted.

Assessment Organization

In considering recommendations about an assessment organization, the committee posed several questions. Is such an entity needed? What are the minimum conditions for its successful operation? Is there a reasonable probability that these conditions can be achieved?

The committee concluded that such an assessment organization could lead practitioners, patients, and others to the better guidelines from among the mixed lot now available and could generate several specific benefits. These benefits include: (1) firmer judgments about what care should be paid for under public and private health benefit programs; (2) better decisions about what information is necessary for informed patient decision-making; and (3) improved use of scientific evidence and expert judgment in malpractice cases and stronger assurance for practitioners that compliance with sound guidelines would reduce their exposure to medical liability.

The minimum conditions for the successful operation of an assessment organization were relatively easy to identify: effective demand for the product (that is, the assessments); integrity of process, participants, and assessments; and sufficiency and stability of effort and resources. The probability of achieving these conditions is less easy to determine. Nonetheless, the committee concluded that it could propose an approach to creating an assessment organization that was feasible. The four key elements of this approach are the following:

• **Governance.** Weighing the various pluses and minuses of governance options, the committee finally concluded that an assessment entity would best be organized as a private not-for-profit organization and that it should have a governing board drawn from a wide range of interested parties, both public and private. The entity must be apart from, but able to work with, all parties that have a stake in clinical practice guidelines. To forestall criticisms about objectivity and integrity, its board would develop clear procedures regarding bias, conflicts of interest, and other issues of accountability.

• **Products and focus.** The proposed assessment entity would have one primary product: periodic publication of assessments of guidelines issued by public and private organizations. A regular journal is an attractive option. Its articles or reports should combine the academic rigor of top professional journals with the user-oriented style of a publication like *Consumer Reports*. The latter journal has several attractive features. It compares similar-purpose products rather than reporting on products in isolation. It also uses graphics and other devices to great advantage to provide easy-to-assimilate information on the strengths, weaknesses, and characteristics of products. Finally, it explicitly recognizes that consumers have different preferences and situations that may lead them to different choices based on their own individual weighing of this information.

• **Funding.** Both public and private funding are desirable. This could be in the form of start-up monies, long-term core support, and special project grants. Of these, the long-term core financing is the most important. Additional financing could be obtained in several ways. One is to charge a substantial subscription for the products of the entity. The subscription response would provide an early test of market appeal and feasibility.

• **Credibility.** All of the features described above are intended to provide the assessment entity with initial and continuing credibility. One key objective should be the creation of a virtual "fail-safe" mechanism to prevent clinically flawed guidelines from receiving a generally favorable assessment. This may require a pretesting process. An important first step is for AHCPR to test the IOM's provisional assessment instrument and to compare the results with pretests of its guidelines. Another key to credibility is that the procedures used by the entity, the assessment instrument, and other tools be open and in the public domain.

The assessment organization should be oriented toward a broad set of potential users of guidelines. Nonetheless, its assessments should be *particularly* attuned to everyday clinical practice and sensitive to practitioners' reliance on their professional societies for guidance and support. Establishing a constructive relationship with these professional societies must be a priority for the organization.

RESEARCH AGENDA

In addition to proposing an assessment entity and identifying guidelines methodology issues in need of attention, the committee suggests a set of research activities aimed at guidelines development, implementation, and evaluation. They include three key areas: (1) testing and perhaps refining the provisional assessment instrument; (2) expanding research on the adoption and diffusion of medical innovations and information to consider whether, how, and why guidelines are adopted; and (3) evaluating the actual impact of clinical practice guidelines on what clinicians and patients do and on patients' health status. With respect to this last topic, "no-difference" results should be viewed as opportunities for further investigation rather than as dead ends; it is important to understand why particular guidelines have no impact.

More generally, the committee urges that recent investments in outcomes research and technology assessment be continued as a necessary part of the scientific support for clinical decisionmaking and guideline development. Such investment will also support better policy and management decisionmaking about how to allocate limited resources among alternative uses.

Finally, the committee notes that the clinical and health services research communities have an important role to play in smoothing the path from clinical research to better clinical practice and improved health outcomes. If more attention is paid to testing the effectiveness of procedures and patient management strategies in real-life settings rather than only assessing efficacy in highly controlled clinical trials, then developers of guidelines will be more likely to have a knowledge base with greater practical relevance. In turn, the more practitioners and institutions adopt the tools of outcomes management, the more information there will be to evaluate and revise guidelines.

FINAL NOTE: GUIDELINES AND HEALTH CARE REFORM

During its deliberations, the committee was quite conscious of the intense debates about broad health care reform and about the contributions that practice guidelines might make to workable reform. In the committee's view, reform is about two issues: access and cost. Politically, expansion of access is contingent on some sense that the rate of escalation in health care costs can be reduced. As noted already, the net impact of guidelines on costs cannot be predicted, and expectations in this area should not be too high. The committee also expressed reservations about cost containment strategies that would assign guideline developers the task of judging what care is worth paying for. It recommended instead that developers concentrate on providing the clinical information, judgments, and rationales on which policymakers, payers, managers, and others might base such decisions.

Some proposals for reform include provisions for cost containment that incorporate roles for clinical practice guidelines in defining or administering basic benefit packages, strengthening health plan competition and consumer choice, or restructuring malpractice decisionmaking. The specifics vary, but the basic ideas are that the reforms would do one or more of the following: override state benefit mandates, circumvent court-ordered coverage in individual cases, rewrite malpractice laws, reduce administrative costs through national or regional administrative and regulatory structures, and limit the coverage eligible for tax deductibility. These and other proposals for health care reform raise many questions that are beyond the scope of this committee's charge. Some reform proponents envision sweeping changes in the nation's health care delivery and financing systems that would certainly place guidelines in a framework of incentives for cost containment that is much different from what currently exists.

Some reforms—for example, those that foresee practice guidelines as the basis for defining a basic benefits package for all health insurance plans—would put a premium on the kinds of credible, accountable processes for developing and applying guidelines described in this report. The danger in such proposals is that the potential contributions guidelines have to make in improving the quality of health care and health outcomes may be lost in a perception that guidelines are to serve only cost-containment ends. The committee sees, therefore, both unprecedented opportunities for the clinical practice guidelines movement and exceptional challenges as well in the years ahead.

1

Introduction

Everywhere the old order changeth, and happy those who can change with it.

Sir William Osler, 1895

Guidelines for the provision of clinical care have been linked in recent years to almost every major problem and proposed solution on the American health policy agenda. Practice guidelines have been tied in some way, by some individual or organization, to costs, quality, access, patient empowerment, professional autonomy, medical liability, rationing, competition, benefit design, utilization variation, bureaucratic micromanagement of health care, and more. The concept has acted as a magnet for the hopes and frustrations of practitioners, patients, payers, researchers, and policymakers.

The broadest hopes of all parties are that practice guidelines will raise the quality of care and improve both the real and the perceived value obtained for health care spending. Beyond such widely held aspirations, individual groups differ in the emphasis they place on other narrower objectives. For example, administrators, regulators, and purchasers tend to stress cost control and reduced variation in practice patterns much more than physicians do. Practitioner groups tend to emphasize professionally developed guidelines as a means to maintain autonomy and to free professional decisionmaking from external micromanagement. Consumer and patient advocates focus on guidelines to inform patients' decisions, clarify patient preferences, and strengthen patient autonomy.

Each group that has positive objectives for practice guidelines also fears their misuse. Their fears are essentially the obverse of their hopes— less sensitivity to patient needs, poorer outcomes, increased costs, lower quality, reduced autonomy or "cookbook" medicine, more bureaucracy, and greater inequity in resource use. In particular, many physicians, especially those longer in practice, see guidelines as a challenge to clinical judgment and resist them as a threat to the most fundamental element of professional autonomy.

Recent public attention notwithstanding, guidelines are not new. Professional organizations have been developing guidelines for at least half a century, and recommendations about appropriate care can be found in ancient writings (Chassin, 1988). What is new is the emphasis on systematic, evidence-based guidelines and the interest in processes, structures, and incentives that support the effective use and evaluation of such guidelines.

Carefully developed guidelines for clinical practice can become part of the fabric of health care in this country and serve as important tools for many desirable changes. Their potential reach extends from improving the quality of clinical care (and its measurement) to helping to reduce the financial costs of inappropriate, unnecessary, or dangerous care. Practice guidelines are among the building blocks for informed patient decisionmaking and rational social judgments about what care should be covered by public and private health benefit plans.

To the extent that guidelines provide well-argued translations of scientific research and expert judgment framed as statements about appropriate care, they will be more readily accepted by many kinds of decisionmakers. Such acceptance in the domains of physician practice, health education, quality assurance, medical liability, cost management, and elsewhere will provide mutually reinforcing support for the application and improvement of practice guidelines. Guidelines are not the solution to the country's health care problems, but they do have a significant, useful role to play.

As tools and building blocks for positive change, guidelines need to be understood and encouraged in context. That context includes powerful economic interests; changing and sometimes conflicting attitudes about professional and patient autonomy; policymaking and implementing institutions that are intensely stressed and sometimes incapacitated; and scientific research that simultaneously expands both knowledge and uncertainty. Above all, the context in which guidelines will be used includes the complex, intimate relationship between individual patients and practitioners who are trying to protect health, manage illness, and preserve dignity under conditions that range from routine to desperate.

Also relevant are other strategies or forces for change that have their own challenges and uneven pace. Better clinical and outcomes research cannot produce results quickly, but the knowledge such studies generate will both strengthen guidelines over the longer term and build structures and processes for more constructive monitoring and feedback of information on performance to clinicians, managers, and others. Generational change, which obviously takes time, should lead to some greater acceptance of standardized, science-based guidelines as it brings to the fore practitioners, administrators, and patients who have been socialized in an era of growing resource constraints, oversight, and technological and organizational complexity. If new quality improvement models can be successfully applied and sustained, they may provide a more positive environment for evidence-based practice guidelines. Technological advances in information systems may help guidelines on all fronts—in development, application, evaluation, and revision. The pace and nature of developments in each of these areas will influence the content, acceptability, and impact of practice guidelines.

PURPOSE OF THE REPORT

The examination undertaken and reported here has had two objectives: first, to encourage constructive expectations for guidelines and, second, to promote the kind of care and rigor in their development, application, evaluation, and revision that will help such expectations be realized. The charge to the Institute of Medicine (IOM) study committee had three parts: (1) describe existing initiatives to develop, use, evaluate, and improve guidelines for clinical practice, (2) assess the strengths and limitations of these initiatives, and (3) based on these assessments, recommend a conceptual and practical framework for the future development, use, and evaluation of guidelines. This framework could include whatever new public and private institutional arrangements seemed to be needed and feasible.

The committee has built on the work of other groups including previous IOM committees. In particular, its starting point was the 1990 IOM report, *Clinical Practice Guidelines: Directions for a New Program* (IOM, 1990c). That report provided advice to the Agency for Health Care Policy and Research (AHCPR) and its Forum for Quality and Effectiveness in Health Care. Its recommendations focused on guideline development, stressing the need for (1) systematic, science-based processes for developing guidelines, (2) careful documentation of the assumptions, evidence, and rationale for recommendations, and (3) explicit projections of the health and cost outcomes expected from the use of particular services or procedures. (This report often draws on the earlier report without specific reference.)

To conduct this more comprehensive examination of practice guidelines, the IOM appointed a committee of experts in the spring of 1990. Appointments included experts in medical and nursing practice, clinical and health services research, research methodology and program evaluation, medical informatics, and health care policy, financing, and administration. Approximately half the committee participated in the first IOM project for AHCPR.

IOM staff organized and conducted five meetings of the committee between June 1990 and September 1991. Other study activities and sources of information included several staff, committee, and commissioned papers, a public hearing, site visits, and focus groups. In addition, the committee established a liaison panel representing major organizations involved in the development, use, and evaluation of practice guidelines. It also created a specialty society panel to assist communication with these groups. (See Appendix C for rosters of these panels.) This report was drafted, circulated to the committee for comment, revised, and then submitted for review in accordance with IOM and National Research Council (NRC) report review policies. The report was revised again based on the NRC review, and this document constitutes the committee's final report.

The primary audiences for this study are public and private policymakers, specialty society leaders, and managers of institutions or organizations that may support the application of practice guidelines. Others who are not likely to read an IOM report firsthand may nevertheless learn and benefit from the study as it is discussed in journals, conferences, and similar venues.

Throughout this report, implementation of practice guidelines is a particular focus. Policymakers, researchers, guidelines developers, and others have thus far paid more systematic attention to guidelines development than to guidelines implementation or evaluation. In contrast to that emphasis, in this document even the chapters on development of guidelines emphasize how the content of guidelines and the way they are developed may affect their use.

WHAT ARE PRACTICE GUIDELINES?

Definitions of Key Terms

Definitions for the word *guidelines* abound, as do other terms that different organizations or individuals prefer to use instead of guidelines (IOM, 1990c). Sometimes the term *practice guideline* serves as an umbrella label for practice standards, protocols, parameters, algorithms, and various other types of statements about appropriate clinical care; at other times, sharp distinctions are drawn. Debate about terminology reflects, in part, controversy and disagreement about the uses of guidelines and related materials.

This report, like its predecessor, uses the term *practice guideline*, largely because it is the term most generally used. For example, the 1989 legislation that created AHCPR and the Forum employed the term.[1] Prac-

---

[1] Two terms found in OBRA 89 (the Omnibus Budget Reconciliation Act of 1989)—standards of quality and performance measures—are not used here. The first term has quite different and even contradictory uses. The 1990 IOM report to AHCPR defined standards of quality as "authoritative statements of (1) minimum levels of acceptable performance or results, (2) excellent levels of performance or results, *or* (3) the range of acceptable performance or results." Statements described as standards should clearly indicate whether they articulate minimums, maximums, or ranges of quality. The term *performance measures* has no clear professional usage, and the 1990 report defined them provisionally as "methods or instruments to estimate or monitor the extent to which the actions of a health care practitioner or provider conform to medical review criteria and standards of quality."

tice guideline also will be the main entry term for the reference subject headings used by the National Library of Medicine to index the literature on health services research (Peri Schuyler, National Library of Medicine, personal communication, May 20, 1991).

As defined in the IOM's 1990 report, practice guidelines are "systematically developed statements to assist practitioner and patient decisions about appropriate health care for specific clinical circumstances."[2] Medical review criteria are "systematically developed statements that can be used to assess the appropriateness of specific health care decisions, services, and outcomes."

Practice guidelines focus, in the first instance, on assisting patients and practitioners in making decisions, but this defining characteristic does not and should not preclude their use for other purposes including quality assurance and payment policymaking. Conversely, medical review criteria and related tools emphasize the evaluation of health care decisions, actions, and outcomes, but they should and do build on guidelines and may in some cases be virtually identical.[3]

Practice guidelines are *not* synonymous with the reimbursement or coverage policies of Medicare and other health insurance plans, which traditionally have excluded some items from coverage (for example, immunizations and blood products) for reasons unrelated to the appropriateness of the service. Reimbursement and coverage policies certainly may be informed by practice guidelines, but this report attempts to distinguish between the two.

Although the IOM definition of clinical practice guidelines emphasizes those aimed at specific clinical problems such as diabetes, some apply to very broad ranges of clinical problems, patients, and services. For example, so-called universal precautions seek to control human immunodeficiency virus (HIV) and other infections by requiring that certain practices (such as using gloves and discarding needles in special containers) be followed for

---

[2] This report often refers, first, to "sets of guidelines," which present a series of statements about appropriate care and, second, to "guidelines documents," which may include short statements of recommendations, longer presentations summarizing methods and evidence, and very long documents describing methods, evidence, rationales, and other issues in great depth.

[3] One committee member strongly objected to the distinction between guidelines and review criteria, arguing that "there should not be one iota of difference between a good guideline intended for [practitioners] and a medical review criterion intended to assess care; they are different uses of the same clinical statement." The committee felt, on the whole, that distinguishing guidelines aimed at clinicians or patients from review criteria aimed at assessing care was useful even though the latter may and should draw on the former. In fact, given the importance accorded to quality assessment and cost containment objectives, some organizations may choose the development of review criteria as their starting point; however, the result may be statements that are presented in formats that are easy for review organizations to use but that are not readily employable by practitioners or patients.

all patients whether or not they are known to be infected. Guidelines for informed consent policies likewise apply quite generally. Broad guidelines, which are frequently adopted as institutional policies, sometimes in response to accreditation standards set by the Joint Commission on Accreditation of Healthcare Organizations or other bodies, may reflect difficult ethical, legal, and management issues as well as clinical concerns. Recent American Medical Association (AMA) guidelines on the use of "Do Not Resuscitate" orders are a case in point; they were issued by the AMA's Council on Ethical and Judicial Affairs (1991b). Later in this report, the committee recommends the development of general guidelines on information for patient decisionmaking.

A final note on terminology: the definitions of guidelines and review criteria refer to *appropriate care*, a term that also presents definitional problems. Sometimes it is used as a synonym for required care; at other times it seems to be viewed (consistent with dictionary usage) as care that is suitable or proper but not always necessary, absolutely required, or essential. For purposes of this report, appropriate care is conceptually defined as care for which "the expected health benefit [exceeds] the expected negative consequences by a sufficient margin" that the care is worth providing (Park et al., 1986, p. 6). (Concepts of necessary, appropriate, or minimum care resurface in Chapter 6.)

Terminological disagreements undoubtedly will continue, and rigid distinctions could sabotage some productive discussions. The field of clinical practice guidelines is still developing, and different terminology may prove more functional in the future.

Operationalizing this report's conceptual definition of guidelines is an exercise fraught with difficulties, both technical and normative. The general strategy urged in this report calls for developers of guidelines to state how compelling is the case for a particular course of care based on the strength of the evidence, the strength of professional judgment, and the importance of the benefits. If the case is clearly stated, others will have information and a model for evidence-based decisionmaking that they may use to reach different judgments.

Desirable Attributes of Guidelines

The above definitions attempt to identify essential characteristics and are not intended to describe the qualities that good practice guidelines and review criteria should have in every use to which they can be put. Thus, the first IOM committee on guidelines identified and discussed eight desirable attributes of guidelines for clinical practice. Chapter 5 of this report presents desirable attributes for medical review criteria. These two sets of attributes must be viewed as statements of aspirations, which are intended to encourage developers of guidelines and review criteria to improve their processes and products; they are not meant as vehicles for destructive criticism.

This committee has made one modification in the list of eight attributes proposed in 1990.[4] Under the attribute of validity, it adds that every set of guidelines should be accompanied by (1) a statement of the strength of the evidence and the expert judgment behind the guidelines and (2) projections of the relevant health and cost outcomes of alternative courses of care. Assessments of relevant health outcomes should consider patient perceptions and preferences. The attributes as amended are presented in Table 1-1.

The committee had two primary reasons for these amendments. First, those citing or using the first IOM report have tended to stress the formal list of attributes without mentioning the elements of validity that were identified in the accompanying text. Second, evidence, outcomes, and patient decisionmaking are emphasized in this second report, particularly in the discussion of ethics, costs, and informed consent; the amendments to the list of the attributes reflect this emphasis.

Four of the eight attributes relate to the content of guidelines: validity, reliability, clinical applicability, and clinical flexibility. Four others relate to the process of guideline development or the presentation of guidelines: clarity, multidisciplinary process, scheduled review, and documentation. Each affects the likelihood that guidelines will be perceived as credible and usable, and the probability that they will, if used, help achieve desired health outcomes. Collectively, these attributes tend to be what distinguishes systematically developed practice guidelines from general textbook knowledge, although the boundaries between these (and other) kinds of information or recommendations are not well defined. Because the IOM and AHCPR recognized that it would be useful but difficult to employ these attributes to assess practice guidelines, one objective of this study has been to develop a practical instrument to guide such assessments. The results are described in Chapter 8 and Appendix B.

Elements of Analysis

The above attributes imply a challenging analytic strategy for developers of practice guidelines that reflects a rigorous scientific process—"a rigorous and orderly asking and answering of questions," in the words of one reviewer of this report.[5] The components of such a strategy can be briefly summarized as

---

[4] The attributes are discussed at some length in Chapter 3 of the first IOM report, and readers are urged to consult that text for a fuller understanding of each attribute.

[5] More detailed discussions of analytic strategies and steps for developers of guidelines can be found in Eddy (1991c) and Woolf (1990a). Chapters 6 and 7 also comment further on some issues of analytic strategy.

TABLE 1-1 Desirable Attributes of Clinical Practice Guidelines

Attribute	Explanation
VALIDITY	Practice guidelines are valid if, when followed, they lead to the health and cost outcomes projected for them. A prospective assessment of validity will consider the substance and quality of the evidence cited, the means used to evaluate the evidence, and the relationship between the evidence and recommendations.
Strength of Evidence	Practice guidelines should be accompanied by descriptions of the strength of the evidence and the expert judgment behind them.
Estimated Outcomes	Practice guidelines should be accompanied by estimates of the health and cost outcomes expected from the interventions in question, compared with alternative practices. Assessments of relevant health outcomes will consider patient perceptions and preferences.
RELIABILITY/ REPRODUCIBILITY	Practice guidelines are reproducible and reliable (1) if—given the same evidence and methods for guidelines development—another set of experts produces essentially the same statements and (2) if—given the same clinical circumstances—the guidelines are interpreted and applied consistently by practitioners (or other appropriate parties).
CLINICAL APPLICABILITY	Practice guidelines should be as inclusive of appropriately defined patient populations as evidence and expert judgment permit, and they should explicitly state the population(s) to which statements apply.
CLINICAL FLEXIBILITY	Practice guidelines should identify the specifically known or generally expected exceptions to their recommendations and discuss how patient preferences are to be identified and considered.
CLARITY	Practice guidelines must use unambiguous language, define terms precisely, and use logical and easy-to-follow modes of presentation.
MULTIDISCIPLINARY PROCESS	Practice guidelines must be developed by a process that includes participation by representatives of key affected groups. Participation may include serving on panels that develop guidelines, providing evidence and viewpoints to the panels, and reviewing draft guidelines.
SCHEDULED REVIEW	Practice guidelines must include statements about when they should be reviewed to determine whether revisions are warranted, given new clinical evidence or professional consensus (or the lack of it).
DOCUMENTATION	The procedures followed in developing guidelines, the participants involved, the evidence used, the assumptions and rationales accepted, and the analytic methods employed must be meticulously documented and described.

- formulation of the problem (for example, the clinical condition to be considered, the key issues to be addressed, and the relevant alternative courses of care to be examined, which may include "watchful waiting");
- identification and assessment of the evidence from clinical trials, case-control studies, and other sources to determine where evidence is weak, missing, or in dispute;
- projection and comparison of health benefits and harms (including how they are perceived by patients) associated with alternative courses of care;
- projection of net costs associated with achieving the benefits of alternative courses of care;[6]
- judgment of the strength of the evidence (considering key areas of scientific uncertainty and theoretical dispute), the relative importance of the projected benefits and risks (again with patient perspectives considered), and—overall—how compelling is the case for particular interventions;
- formulation of clear statements about alternative courses of care, accompanied by full disclosure of the participants, methods, evidence, and criteria used to arrive at these statements; and
- review and critique of all these elements by methodologists, clinicians, and other relevant parties not involved in the original process.

This framework is only a brief summary of the strategy that is elaborated on at various points throughout the report. The analytic steps identified above can be managed by a single organization. Alternatively, different parties may contribute to the process. Today, for example, most professional societies do not consider costs or patient preferences. Others can add these steps later, although such additions will be more difficult if the initial work has not anticipated the questions to be asked in these later analyses.

In addition to following this analytic strategy in developing guidelines, developers should seek to present their work to clinicians in ways that reflect the rigor of this approach and its emphasis on reasoning and critical analysis. The product of the process should not be perceived solely as information but more broadly as an explication of the thinking processes that should be used in evaluating and applying that information. If guidelines are perceived only as information, they may very well be used (or rejected) as the "cookbooks" that many physicians decry.

---

[6] In addition, comparisons may usefully involve different clinical problems as well as different approaches to the same problem. For example, the cost-effectiveness of screening for hypertension ($16,280 per quality-adjusted life year—or QALY—for asymptomatic men aged 60) has been compared not only with other heart disease screening but also with treatment of heart disease (such as surgery for left main coronary artery disease, $4,500/QALY) and treatments for other problems (such as hospital hemodialysis for end-stage renal disease, $57,300/ QALY; Littenberg et al., 1991).

Guidelines presented to patients will necessarily be simpler than those presented to physicians, but they, too, should try to emphasize responsible decisionmaking and not just cut-and-dried advice or information. As guidelines are developed that are more sensitive to variations in patient preferences and the role of patients in making decisions, the initial formulation of guidelines is likely to make their translation into patient-usable forms easier. These initial formulations should clearly describe the possible outcomes of alternative management strategies in terms that are relevant to patients, discuss what is known about variations in patient preferences for different outcomes, and note points at which patient choices among alternatives should be requested.

The analytic framework presented above represents an ideal. Making progress toward this ideal will take time. Some, perhaps most or all, guidelines will not fully reach it. The committee recognizes this to be the case but, at the same time, emphasizes the importance of keeping the ideal in mind and making a serious and persistent effort to achieve it. In addition, the committee urges research methodologists and others to work to improve (and, when possible, simplify) the procedures and tools for analyzing evidence, reaching responsible group judgments, and otherwise arriving at sound recommendations for care (see Chapter 7 for further discussion).

State of the Evidence

In developing guidelines, conclusions backed by scientific evidence should take precedence over statements based on subjective judgments. When the empirical evidence has important limitations (as will typically be the case) or when experts reach conclusions that are not consistent with the evidence, the limits of the evidence should be clearly described and the rationale for departing from it should be explained. When expert judgment proceeds in the absence of direct empirical evidence about a particular clinical practice, the general scientific reasoning or normative (ethical, professional) principles supporting the expert judgments should be described. Statements about the importance of particular benefits and harms will reflect both empirical analyses and value judgments; Chapter 6 returns to this point.

For users of guidelines, this kind of argumentation, reasoning, and documentation can help in sorting out conflicting claims, considering how guidelines should or should not be adjusted to local circumstances, and independently evaluating the claims made for guidelines. That the relationship of evidence to recommendations cannot be taken for granted is illustrated by an analysis of recommendations on dietary cholesterol that found virtually all the cited references to be irrelevant or in conflict with the recommendations (Reiser, 1984; see also Eddy and Billings, 1988).

To the extent that guidelines move toward statements and arguments such as those outlined above, they will identify how compelling is the case for particular services or courses of care under particular clinical circumstances. They will distinguish care that is strongly or moderately supported (or contraindicated) by strong scientific evidence and consensus, care that is supported chiefly by consensus without any direct research backing, and care about which experts differ in the face of mixed or absent evidence. Along these lines, Eddy (1990e) has divided statements about appropriate care—what he calls practice policies—into three categories depending on the clarity of the evidence about outcomes and the importance of the outcomes to patients. When the case for a particular course of care is very strong, *standards* can be delineated for care that is to be provided or recommended to patients with only rare circumstances justifying exceptions. When the case is somewhat less compelling, *guidelines* (used by Eddy in a narrower sense than in this report) can be defined for courses of care to be provided or recommended in most cases but with more exceptions allowed than are warranted for standards. *Options* note that different courses exist and that evidence does not warrant specific recommendations.[7]

By the term *strong evidence*, the committee refers to (1) the characteristics of the evidence itself (for example, whether it shows a strong effect, no effect, an inconclusive effect, or something in between) and (2) the qualities of the process for generating that evidence. Formal hypothesis-testing processes range in strength from experimental to quasi-experimental to nonexperimental. However, a strong research design that is improperly executed may provide poorer evidence than a weaker but properly executed design. Single case reports and case series do not test hypotheses but do provide relatively weak forms of empirical evidence. Formal methods of generating expert consensus yield evidence of what clinicians believe about a particular form of care, based on their experience and their assessment of such evidence as does exist; statements of consensus may provide useful guidance but do not constitute clinical evidence as the term is used here. Problems involved in rating and combining evidence are revisited in Chapter 7.

Inevitably, given the state of scientific knowledge, many courses of care will not be supported by good evidence. Table 1-2 presents a purely hypothetical (but the committee believes plausible) illustration of how evidence and consensus might be distributed across the entire range of health care services. It is based on an example offered by one committee member

---

[7] In a similar vein, the American College of Cardiology has distinguished three broad classes of guidelines: (1) general agreement exists that the service/technology is appropriate; (2) general agreement exists that the service/technology is not appropriate; and (3) opinion is divergent (Dreifus, 1990).

TABLE 1-2   Hypothetical Distribution of Evidence
and Consensus for All Health Services and Patient
Management Strategies

Strength of Evidence	Strength of Consensus	Percentage of All Services
++	++	2
++	+	2
++	–	0
+	++	20
+	+	25
+	–	0
–	++	20
–	+	25
–	–	6

NOTE: ++ strong; + modest; - very weak or none.

as a means of clarifying the committee's understanding of the range of good science and evidence in today's world.

A guideline having strong evidence and strong consensus is the U.S. Preventive Services Task Force (USPSTF, 1989) recommendation that erythromycin ophthalmic ointment be used for all babies as soon as possible after birth to prevent gonococcal ophthalmia neonatorum infection.[8] In the category of little evidence but general consensus is the widely accepted, easily remembered blood "transfusion trigger" (hemoglobin levels of less than 10 grams per deciliter). There is no rigorous (and little nonrigorous) clinical research that evaluates patient outcomes for transfusions at this or other levels (Welch et al., 1991). Clearly, however, for a physician faced with a woman bleeding to death from a ruptured ectopic pregnancy or some similar emergency, the absence of research on specific thresholds for transfusion cannot be a counsel for inaction.[9]

---

[8]As rated using a scheme formulated by the USPSTF, the statement was based on evidence rated "I" (drawn from at least one properly designed randomized clinical trial) and strength of recommendations rated "A" (good evidence for the recommendation).

[9] The situation portrayed in Table 1-2 would be even more stark if the universe of care were defined in very detailed clinical terms. This point can be illustrated with one currently applied guideline for hysterectomy (Mark Chassin, Value Health Sciences, personal communication, September 19, 1991). This guideline (part of a larger set of guidelines) states that hysterectomy is inappropriate for women with all these characteristics: under age 30, no children, an expressed desire for no future pregnancy, mild dysfunctional bleeding (defined objectively and clinically), one dilatation and curettage in the previous 12 months, and no trial of hormone therapy. At this level of clinical detail, there are no outcome data, no functional status data indicating whether women experience the condition as impinging on their daily lives, no data on complications for this specific cohort of women, and no data on costs or even charges for care for this cohort.

Those who develop guidelines can highlight areas for which evidence exists, for which it is missing, and for which it is flawed. This process will identify specific holes in research—for example, the absence of work on appropriate intervals for blood pressure screening. It will also provide researchers and research funders with a helpful picture of the gaps in whole categories of research questions (for example, testing intervals in general).

Any discussion of the state of scientific evidence must also note the challenge posed by the rapid advance of clinical research (McGuire, 1990). Months of effort may be rendered largely or partly irrelevant by new information; for example, follow-up results may challenge earlier findings, or convincing findings from clinical trials may arise unexpectedly. This fact of life underscores the importance of processes for updating guidelines and for disseminating important contradictory research findings. However, constantly changing guidelines (based on changing data and consensus) are cited as one reason for an unsuccessful Swedish initiative to develop and apply practice guidelines in the 1970s (Little, 1990).

Inconsistent or Conflicting Guidelines

Guidelines are one means of clarifying acceptable and unacceptable variation in medical practice. Nevertheless, that clarification itself has limits that may lead different groups to different and even inconsistent guidelines. Weak evidence is still weak evidence, although the processes discussed in this report should allow the best use of whatever evidence is available. Moreover, differences of opinion (and, thus, differences in guidelines) can be expected about such matters as whether a research design flaw "matters" or whether differences in the results of two treatment alternatives are "clinically important" or only "statistically significant." In addition, individuals and groups will vary in their values and tolerance of risk. (For an interesting illustration of these factors at work in the debate over childhood cholesterol screening, see Newman et al., 1990 and Resnicow et al., 1991).

When evidence is limited or nonexistent, developers of guidelines have used different strategies for making recommendations (Hayward et al., 1991). Some offer recommendations; others do not. In any case, this committee calls for guidelines to explain the rationale for the presence or absence of a recommendation and to describe how compelling is the case for alternative approaches to particular clinical problems. Guidelines that do this can build a more credible and more powerful base for decisionmaking by patients, practitioners, and others. Ways of dealing with inconsistent or conflicting guidelines are discussed further in Chapter 7.

Types of Guidelines

Guidelines and medical review criteria can be categorized along many dimensions. As illustrated in Appendix A, guidelines and guidelines-like materials may vary in five main ways:

- **Clinical orientation.** Some guidelines deal with clinical conditions or problems (for example, throat infections in children), whereas others describe the indications for using procedures or services (for example, tonsillectomy).[10]
- **Clinical purpose.** Guidelines may address several broad kinds of health care interventions: (1) screening and primary prevention, (2) diagnosis, (3) treatment and management (including secondary prevention), and (4) rehabilitation.
- **Complexity.** Complexity is a function of many factors: the nature of the specific clinical conditions or technologies being dealt with; the extent and certainty of knowledge about the conditions or technologies; the options and interrelationships among options for managing the conditions; and the objectives, approaches, and skills of those developing the guidelines. As a case in point, the number of appropriateness criteria developed by researchers at the RAND Corporation ranges from 49 for cholecystectomy (Solomon et al., 1986) to 2,862 for colonoscopy (Kahn et al., 1986).
- **Format.** Format refers to how guidelines (particularly the statements about appropriate care rather than all the supporting documentation and rationales) are physically presented, whether in free text, through tables or other graphics, as algorithms, or by other means.
- **Intended users.** As noted elsewhere in this chapter and in this report, the sets of potential users are quite large and diverse; for purposes of the descriptions used in Appendix A, the main categories are "practitioners" and "patients."

WHY ARE POLICYMAKERS INTERESTED IN GUIDELINES?

Some would explain the interest in practice guidelines shown by legislators, regulators, and purchasers of health care (as opposed to that of practitioners and patients) with a single phrase: out-of-control health care costs. If, despite nearly two decades of intensifying efforts to contain spending, health care costs had not been increasing substantially faster than costs in other sectors, most of the recent legislation, conferences, and other activities to promote guidelines probably would not have happened despite the

---

[10] For further discussion of reasons for focusing research or guidelines on clinical conditions or specific technologies, see IOM (1989b, 1990j; 1992).

other concerns—most notably, quality improvement—that guidelines also address. Many interested parties may be disappointed if they think guidelines will not reduce costs (Bouxsein, 1988).

Although the importance of cost concerns as a stimulus for guidelines should not be understated, concerns about quality of care and risk management also figure prominently in the call for more and better practice guidelines. The attraction of guidelines also has had a political component. Guidelines were offered by and to physician groups as an acceptable, partial alternative to the specter of more stringent controls on Medicare payments for physician services (American Society of Internal Medicine [ASIM], 1989, 1990; Physician Payment Review Commission [PPRC], 1988, 1990; Kosterlitz, 1991). They were promoted as a selective approach that targets inappropriate or unnecessary care and relies on informed decisionmaking by practitioners and patients rather than by far-removed officials.

More specifically, the growing interest in guidelines has been prompted by perceptions, first, that higher health care expenditures have brought only marginal health benefits and, second, that guidelines can help remedy this problem of "value." Virtually every major discussion of guidelines begins with a similar list of reasons for these perceptions (PPRC, 1988, 1989; IOM, 1989a; Billings, 1990; Leape, 1990; Hammons, 1991). The discussion generally proceeds as follows.

• Research demonstrates major **variations in physician practice patterns and utilization of health services** (Wennberg and Gittelsohn, 1973, 1982; Wennberg, 1984, 1991; Chassin et al., 1986a, 1987; R.E. Brown et al., 1989). The lowest level of use may not be the right level, but the variations raise troubling questions about the justification for these variations and their accompanying costs.

• Other research indicates considerable **inappropriate use of many services** including laboratory tests, diagnostic and surgical procedures, prescription medications, and inpatient hospital admissions and days of care (Brook et al., 1986; Eisenberg, 1986; Lohr et al., 1986; Chassin et al., 1987; Foxman et al., 1987). Estimated inappropriate use of care for selected services ranges from 10 percent to more than 30 percent; estimates of associated unnecessary expenditures vary widely. Many of the services studied, however, have been those particularly suspected of overuse; even for these services, some degree of underuse may also exist.

• In addition, much health care is characterized by considerable **uncertainty about the health outcomes** achieved by the use or nonuse of various services and procedures (Office of Technology Assessment [OTA], 1978; Dersimonian et al., 1982; Eddy, 1984; Wennberg, 1984; Eddy and Billings, 1988; Roper and Hackbarth, 1988; Roper et al., 1988; Brook, 1989, 1990; IOM, 1989b, 1990a,b,e,f,h). Clinical research documenting the effectiveness of many services does not exist, particularly at the level of very specific patient circumstances; thus, the value received for spending on these services is likewise unknown.

Whether the issue is unexplained variation, inappropriate care, or uncertain outcomes, many analysts come to similar conclusions. More research on outcomes and effectiveness of health care services is needed; more work should be done, using such research, to formulate specific guidelines for clinical practice; and more use of the resulting guidelines will help limit health care spending.

How are guidelines to limit health care costs? How are they to increase the perceived value of health care spending? The basic argument or hypothesis runs along these lines:

Scientific evidence and clinical judgment can be systematically combined to produce clinically valid, operational recommendations for appropriate care that can and will be used to persuade clinicians, patients, and others to change their practices in ways that lead to better health outcomes and lower health care costs.

Six formidable and often unrealistic assumptions or expectations lie behind this partly explicit and partly implicit causal model.

• First, scientific evidence of sufficient quantity and quality exists to serve as a foundation for guidelines.

• Second, programs to develop guidelines will be organized, funded, and effectively managed to produce a considerable volume of valid, usable statements about appropriate care for clinically and financially significant health conditions or technologies.

• Third, substantial numbers of clinicians, patients, and others will have the opportunity, the support, and the incentives to read, understand, accept, and use these statements in ways that change patterns of clinical practice, health behavior, or payment for health care services in desired directions.

• Fourth, such changes will be broad and intense enough to improve health outcomes.

• Fifth, on balance, the entire body of guidelines as actually developed and used will lead to more cost-controlling than cost-increasing behavior on the part of providers.

• Sixth, the body of guidelines will continually expand to cover new areas so that net rates of increase in health care costs and absolute levels of expenditures will be lower than they would otherwise be.

Unfortunately, these six expectations outstrip current capacities in several respects. For many clinical conditions and services, the science base is limited, and even when it is reasonably satisfactory, clinicians and analysts may disagree in their interpretations of the evidence (recall Table 1-2). Developing guidelines based on systematic, evidence-based processes is expensive and time-consuming, and the volume of such efforts, though increasing, is still small in relation to the scope of clinical care. Moreover, despite the good intentions of many involved parties, much guideline development remains relatively unsystematic; the enterprise as a whole still lacks proven mechanisms for evaluating, improving, and targeting the development of guidelines. Psychological, economic, and other factors limit clinician and patient acceptance of and conformance with guidelines. Organizational systems for quality, cost, risk, and information management are not planned and structured to support awareness, acceptance, and use of credible practice guidelines. For the uninsured, underinsured, and others, indicated care may not be affordable or otherwise accessible.

Even if the first four of these expectations about the scope, quality, application, and health outcomes of guidelines were to be fulfilled, the committee regards as questionable the last two expectations about the cost consequences of change. As argued earlier, some guidelines undoubtedly will save money by reducing the use of inappropriate or unnecessary services; some will increase expenditures by encouraging more use of underutilized services; and some will shift costs from one type of service to another or from one payer to another. The net impact of guidelines on the rate of increase in total health care spending cannot be predicted with confidence, even if future priorities for guidelines development stress clinical conditions for which costly overuse of services is suspected.[11]

Furthermore, the current system of delivering and financing care does not have incentives for economy and efficiency that are strong and consistent enough to capitalize fully on the opportunities for cost control that some guidelines present. New technology and other factors also will continue to exert upward pressure on total costs, as will policies to improve access to care for the uninsured and other disadvantaged groups.

In sum, guidelines for clinical practice are a promising but not a quick or sure strategy for improving and rationalizing the use of health services. The attention and resources now invested in guidelines could dissolve in the face of a collision between unrealistic hopes and limited immediate results. For guidelines to fulfill their potential, persistent commitment over the long term is required from both policymakers and health care professionals.

---

[11] Besides costs, other relevant factors in selecting topics for guideline development include the potential for an assessment to change health outcomes, the amount of practice variation, the prevalence of a condition (or rate of use of a technology), and the burden of the illness (for example, quality-adjusted life expectancy).

WHO USES GUIDELINES AND FOR WHAT?

The potential users of clinical practice guidelines constitute a diverse group. This report focuses on the primary users of guidelines: practitioners, patients and families, and health care institutions. Other users include those payers, health benefit plans, and public policymakers and regulators who may use guidelines in making specific decisions about what health care to reimburse, cover, or encourage and in evaluating the decisions, actions, or performance of the primary users of guidelines. In addition, some individuals and organizations act, in a sense, as "conduits," facilitating or promoting the use of guidelines without directly applying them to make decisions. Examples of such users include educators of many sorts and science writers and journalists who may facilitate discussion and dissemination.

Any single user of guidelines may employ them in various ways, and any particular set of guidelines may need to be presented in different ways for different users and uses. Five major purposes for guidelines, which are not mutually exclusive, are

1. assisting clinical decisionmaking by patients and practitioners,
2. educating individuals or groups,
3. assessing and assuring the quality of care,
4. guiding allocation of resources for health care, and
5. reducing the risk of legal liability for negligent care.

The first and second uses may reflect a fairly straightforward application of guidelines; the third and fourth typically entail the translation of guidelines into medical review criteria and other evaluation tools. The fifth use may be a more indirect product of the other uses, although some guidelines have been developed with this use in mind.

The definition of guidelines used in this report highlights one crucial purpose: to assist individual practitioners and patients in making decisions about specific clinical problems. For example, a physician might use a guideline to assess medical management of a given condition versus expeditious surgical intervention before discussing risks, benefits, and options with the patient. Another physician might consult a guideline to determine the appropriate prescription medication to use, given that medical management of an illness is warranted. A patient may consult guidelines in deciding whether to seek specific screening services. A nurse might review a guideline in preparing a care plan for a homebound patient or nursing home resident; a nurse-practitioner might check a guideline, perhaps in the form of a protocol, to determine whether to treat a patient or refer the patient to a physician. These examples represent the central uses envisioned by most developers of guidelines.

Guidelines are also used for individual educational purposes. Physicians, nurses, and others may rely on guidelines to help patients and families understand clinical situations and available courses of action. Depending on the complexity of the guideline, its distribution, and patients' prior level of knowledge, patients might also use guidelines fairly directly in their own decisionmaking. In addition to individual educational uses, many guidelines are employed in continuing medical education, public health campaigns, and other organized programs to educate broad categories of professionals, patients, or others about appropriate health care or behavior.

To assess and improve the quality of health care, organizations and individuals may refer to practice guidelines (and review criteria) for several reasons: to structure organizational procedures, to guide equipment purchases and hiring decisions, and to set and implement priorities for monitoring, feedback, and other efforts to assess and improve performance. For example, health care plans may check their records to determine how successful their practitioners have been in immunizing children or screening adults for particular problems; depending on the results, they may then try to improve their reminder systems, patient education efforts, or other aspects of plan operation.

Given the hope of many that guidelines can help control health care costs, it is not surprising that individuals, health care organizations, and public and private payers refer to practice guidelines in making decisions about resource use and in attempting to influence the decisions of others. For example, practitioners and institutions at financial risk from their participation in capitated, per-case, or other non-cost-based payment schemes may employ guidelines and review criteria to identify wasteful patterns of care, avoid expensive purchases of equipment with few approved indications for use, and forestall inappropriate referrals to specialist consultants. Public and private payers may use practice guidelines or review criteria to help them make broad decisions about whether to cover particular services (for example, pancreas transplants) or to precertify the appropriateness of specific services for particular patients (such as carotid endarterectomy for asymptomatic individuals). To the extent that guidelines can be used to help rationalize the provision of health services, demands for explicit rationing of useful care may be avoided or minimized.

Specialty societies, health care institutions, malpractice insurers, and even legislators have become acutely interested in how guidelines and related review criteria may reduce the exposure of practitioners and institutions to malpractice liability. Such a use of guidelines, although worth noting in its own right, can also serve both quality- and cost-management goals. For example, less inappropriate or dangerous care should improve the processes and outcomes of care and reduce the number of malpractice claims and judgments, thereby reducing litigation and compensation costs.

BASIC PROPOSITIONS

This report offers six broad propositions about the current state and future role of clinical practice guidelines. First, practice guidelines can be (and are being) formulated and used now to improve the quality and value of health services. Even if limited in scope, they are a positive step.

Second, although guidelines development is not a firmly established enterprise with well-tested methods and procedures, efforts to develop practice guidelines are widespread, growing, and diverse. The movement is likely to remain pluralistic and perhaps in some ways even competitive—a circumstance that offers opportunity for growth and progress as well as some risk of confusion and contradiction.

Third, a major challenge for practice guidelines is better follow-through. To capitalize on sound guidelines that constructively anticipate practical problems faced in real clinical situations, practitioners, policymakers, and others need better strategies and processes to ensure that guidelines are effectively implemented.

Fourth, science can contribute more effectively to useful knowledge-based guidelines by devising research strategies to evaluate the effectiveness of emerging and existing services that better reflect the conditions of actual practice. The gap needs to be reduced between, on the one hand, clinical research conducted on homogeneous populations within carefully controlled settings and, on the other hand, effective knowledge for those providing health care to heterogeneous populations in diverse settings.

Fifth, although effectiveness research and clinical practice guidelines can inform action and contribute to basic ethical debates over what constitutes an appropriate distribution of resources or an appropriate structure for health care delivery, they cannnot resolve those debates. Decisions depend on many other factors including political judgments, cultural norms, economic calculations, and the power of affected interests.

Sixth, expectations that practice guidelines will help control total health care spending should be restrained. Wider application of guidelines aimed at currently overused services will likely reduce some spending. In other cases, spending will shift from inappropriate to more appropriate care. At the same time, guidelines that focus on currently underused services may stimulate increased expenditures, particularly if strategies to improve access for those who are not now adequately insured are successful. Collectively, the result undoubtedly will be better value but not guaranteed net savings—particularly given the health care system's lack of strong, consistent incentives for efficient and economical behavior by practitioners, patients, and others.

These caveats notwithstanding, clinical practice guidelines have real potential to help clarify the knowledge base for clinical practice and to improve the quality and effectiveness of medical care. Realization of that potential will depend on astute policymaking and steady management, as well as on sound scientific evidence and clinical judgments.

REPORT ORGANIZATION

The next chapter of this report discusses current efforts to develop clinical practice guidelines. The emphasis is on national activities; local development and adaptation of guidelines are considered later. As a prologue to later chapters, it begins by stressing that what happens during the development process will influence the probability of successfully implementing guidelines for clinical practice.

Chapter 3 provides an overview of guidelines implementation, including the various factors that shape decisions about implementation strategies and affect their application. In an attempt to bring to this report some sense of the real world in which guidelines are—and are not—used, the chapter uses several hypothetical case studies to illustrate various implementation issues.

Chapter 4 examines the societal context and the philosophical and strategic considerations that may influence efforts to bring guidelines into use. It also considers specifically the roles of education and of information and decision support systems. Chapter 5 then discusses how systems to manage quality, costs, medical liability, and information may support and be supported by clinical practice guidelines. It also proposes desirable attributes of medical review criteria.

Chapter 6 considers the pervasive issue of health care costs and some of the related ethical, political, and technical controversies about how guidelines should be developed and used. It includes an examination of issues in cost and cost-effectiveness analysis and consideration of informed consent and minimum standards of care.

Using the discussion in the preceding three chapters as a base, Chapter 7 returns to the procedures and methods for developing practice guidelines and reflects further on how guidelines developers can plan for effective implementation. This chapter also considers actions of local organizations in adapting national guidelines, problems of conflicting or inconsistent guidelines, and efforts to translate guidelines into medical review criteria.

In Chapter 8, the committee presents its views on the strengths and weaknesses of current efforts to develop and use clinical practice guidelines. It offers a research agenda and, more generally, proposes a framework for future development, use, evaluation, and improvement of clinical practice guidelines. A particular focus is strategies to assess the soundness of existing and future guidelines.

Several appendices help illustrate or elaborate on points raised in the text. Appendix A provides 16 diverse examples of guidelines and related materials. Appendix B presents a provisional instrument for assessing practice guidelines, a document that was reviewed independently of the report according to NRC procedures. Appendix C presents rosters of the committees and panels involved with or contributing to this study.

SUMMARY

The recent surge of interest in clinical practice guidelines was born of frustration about seemingly uncontrollable increases in health care expenditures combined with grave doubts about the real value of that increased spending. Very high expectations for what guidelines might do to control costs and improve the value or quality of care are, however, giving way to a more pragmatic appreciation of the potential and limitations of guidelines.

The challenge to this committee was to provide a constructive analysis of current efforts to develop, use, and evaluate guidelines and to propose a framework for the future that offers realistic potential for improving the caliber and effectiveness of these efforts. This chapter has provided definitions and a context for the description, analysis, and recommendations that follow.

2

Developing Clinical Practice Guidelines

Medicine . . . is mobile, and many of us get breathless not so much by trying to keep up with medical progress as by trying to avoid being run over by it.

Roger I. Lee, 1958

The rapid pace of development in biomedical science and technology can, on the one hand, make guidelines a useful aid to busy practitioners and, on the other hand, subject guidelines to rapid obsolescence. This reality underscores the importance of the review and updating process noted in Chapter 1.

More generally, the way clinical practice guidelines are developed can strongly affect their potential for effective use by practitioners, patients, and others. Thus, planning for successful implementation must begin with development and continue through cycles of revision and updating.

One theme underlying the attributes presented in the preceding chapter is that those who devise guidelines should anticipate what will make the guidelines practical and credible. Most obvious is that guidelines need to be specific, comprehensive, and flexible enough to be useful in everyday clinical practice. In addition, the logic, language, and symbols used in the guidelines should be unambiguous to intended users and easy to follow. Because practitioners and other potential users will want to know who developed the guidelines and how they did it, the development process and the participants in the process should be documented. Developers of guidelines should describe the strength of the evidence and the relative importance of the projected benefits and risks; they should also, in general, indicate how compelling is the case for particular interventions.

A multidisciplinary development process that includes all key groups will encourage acceptance of guidelines by the members of these groups— including patients and their surrogates. Inclusion in this sense need not be limited to representation in the group drafting the guidelines; it can extend to participation in hearings, reviews, pretests, and similar activities. Such an inclusive approach, although potentially requiring more time and funds, can help developers of guidelines better understand the situations in which guidelines may be applied.

The sense of this committee, therefore, is that planning for implementation and later evaluation of guidelines must take place during the development phase. What does or does not happen at the development stage may materially affect the success or failure of a set of guidelines, independent of the quality of the implementing efforts that follow. The examination of guidelines implementation in Chapters 3, 4, 5, and 6 underscores this point and leads to further discussion of guidelines development in Chapter 7.

The succeeding sections of this chapter first describe the major types of organizations involved in guidelines development in both the public and private sectors and then discuss how the enterprise is evolving. The chapter closes with a brief commentary on methods and costs of guideline development. For this overview, the study committee relied heavily on the published literature, its site visits, the public hearing, focus groups, and other study activities, as well as on its own expertise.

PLURALISM AND DIVERSITY IN GUIDELINES DEVELOPMENT

Systematic efforts to develop clinical practice guidelines have grown dramatically in recent years. Professional societies, public agencies, health care institutions, and researchers have become appreciably more active and visible in the guidelines arena (Woolf, 1990b; Kosterlitz, 1991); the field also has at least one regular newsletter, *Report on Medical Guidelines and Outcomes Research* (Robinson, 1991). According to the American Medical Association (AMA), 8 physicians organizations reported active involvement in developing guidelines before 1980; now, more than 50 organizations can report such activity (AMA, 1991a).[1] The creation in 1989 of the Agency for Health Care Policy and Research (AHCPR), and its Forum for Quality and Effectiveness in Health Care, provided new focus and visibility for public-sector activities. Insurers, health maintenance organizations (HMOs), and other private organizations have also become more active.

This pluralism of sponsorship reflects the breadth of interest in guidelines, the special concerns of different sponsors, and the varying outlooks on what topics warrant guideline development and by what methods (Audet

---

[1] The AMA publishes a *Directory of Practice Parameters* (AMA, 1991a); as of late 1991, it listed and cross-referenced 1,319 practice parameters developed by 45 U.S. organizations and provided information on how to obtain the actual parameters. The AMA also publishes quarterly updates of this directory, indicating newly completed and withdrawn guidelines.

et al., 1990). A recent General Accounting Office (GAO, 1991b) survey of medical specialty societies succinctly described this diversity: "No two medical specialty societies with whom we spoke have produced similar guidelines for similar reasons in a similar fashion" (p. 11). This observation applies broadly to the whole field of guidelines development.

The following overview of types of activities and trends illustrates some of the diversity of this undertaking without attempting to characterize the quality of specific activities in terms of the attributes identified in Chapter 1. The discussion, however, tends to slight less well-supported and less publicized efforts at guidelines development, which may be quite numerous and idiosyncratic to particular institutions; it also does not cover individuals working independently to develop guidelines, medical texts, and similar materials. As a consequence, this chapter risks implying that most efforts at guidelines development have the characteristics of the better-organized work described here. Such programs still appear to be atypical, although many organizations are attempting to improve their procedures and methods as discussed further in Chapter 7.[2] This chapter's discussion of the work of specific organizations does not imply endorsement.

PROFESSIONAL SOCIETIES AND RELATED ENTITIES

The last century has been marked by the development of professional medicine and by broad deference to its judgments, a deference that has been challenged in recent years. Although guidelines for clinical practice emerged initially as one sign of professional responsibility, the current acceleration of activity is a function both of the challenges to the profession and of the profession's responses.

Medicine is characterized by a wide array of professional organizations. Some are general in focus (most notably, the AMA), but most center on the medical specialties and subspecialties with which most physicians strongly identify. These "academies," "colleges," or "societies" often sponsor specialty-specific, peer-reviewed clinical journals that serve as a major source of information for physicians; a number of these organizations have added the development of practice guidelines to their agendas. Associations for health care professionals other than physicians—for example, the American Nurses Association (ANA) and the American Dental Association (ADA)—are also increasingly involved in guidelines efforts. Overall, professional societies are generally seen as having taken the lead in organized efforts to develop practice guidelines, thereby serving as an important, perhaps key,

---

[2] Readers interested in technical descriptions of current methods might examine the following: the AHCPR Forum manual developed to assist guidelines panels (Woolf, 1990a), the American College of Physicians procedure manual (ACP, 1986), and the introductory manual commissioned by the Council of Medical Specialty Societies (Eddy, 1991c).

source of authoritative communication to practitioners about what constitutes appropriate care. As illustrated below, the involvement of individual professional organizations varies both in scope and purpose.

How Are Professional Societies Involved?

Relatively formal specialty society activity in the area of guideline development appears to date back at least 50 years to the American Academy of Pediatrics (AAP) monograph on control of infectious diseases, first published in 1938 and now in its 22nd edition (AAP, 1991). Other organized efforts reaching back more than a decade include those of the American College of Obstetricians and Gynecologists (ACOG; beginning in 1959), the American Society of Anesthesiology (ASA; in 1968), the American College of Physicians (ACP; in 1976), and the American College of Radiology (ACR; in the 1970s).[3]

Some efforts related to guidelines are those of single-specialty societies; others are collaborative efforts. The ACP through its Clinical Efficacy Assessment Project has developed a particularly broad program that cuts across all facets of medical care and many medical specialties. Topics run from expensive and inexpensive diagnostic tests (e.g., magnetic resonance imaging and complete blood counts) to indications for surgery (e.g., carotid endarterectomy) to cardiac rehabilitation. Narrower in range and more typical is the work of the American Academy of Ophthalmology (AAO) to develop "preferred practice patterns" for comprehensive eye examinations and various disease specific topics (Sommer et al., 1990). In a broad-ranging look at a major medical problem, the American College of Cardiology (ACC) recently published a supplement to the *Journal of the American College of Cardiology* (ACC, 1989) based on a symposium covering quality- and cost-conscious cardiovascular care and the role of decision modeling.

In 1980, the ACC and the American Heart Association (AHA) together started a Task Force on Assessment of Diagnostic and Therapeutic Cardiovascular Procedures.[4] Work by this group on coronary artery bypass graft

---

[3] Space does not permit a complete listing of all the topics on which these specialty societies have developed guidelines in the past decade or so. As noted earlier, the AMA is now tracking such efforts as are some commercial firms. The *Medical Technology Assessment Directory* (IOM, 1988) provides a profile and complete list of assessment documents and guidelines produced by many groups. See also the February 1990 issue of the *Quality Review Bulletin* for detailed descriptions of selected specialty society programs.

[4] Among the ACC/AHA Task Force reports related to acute myocardial infarction (AMI) are guidelines on the following topics: ambulatory electrocardiography, percutaneous transluminal coronary angioplasty (see the excerpt in Appendix A), clinical use of cardiac radionuclide imaging, exercise testing, and permanent cardiac pacemaker implantation (IOM, 1990a). Some recent guidelines publications have discussed early management of patients with AMI (Gunnar et al., 1990).

surgery (Kirklin et al., 1991) is an instructive example of what can be accomplished by cooperative actions of specialty societies. To cite another example, the American College of Nuclear Physicians (ACNP) and the Society of Nuclear Medicine (SNM) may begin jointly to develop guidelines for nuclear medicine practitioners.

The AMA has spearheaded two broad, multiorganizational activities limited largely to physician groups. The first is a collaboration between the AMA and 14 national medical specialty societies known as the Specialty Society Partnership. The second is the Practice Parameters Forum comprising "all national medical specialty and state medical societies interested in participating . . . [in an activity] created for the purpose of facilitating the development, evaluation, and implementation of practice parameters" (AMA, 1990c, p. 16); the Forum numbers nearly 50 volunteer specialty and state medical societies. (The AMA prefers the term *practice parameters* to *practice guidelines.*)

In addition to playing a coordinating role, the AMA issues recommendations on specific clinical problems and technologies through its Diagnostic and Therapeutic Technology Assessment (DATTA) program and its Council on Scientific Affairs. The *Journal of the American Medical Association* has published a widely read and frequently cited series of articles on guidelines (Eddy, 1990a-j,l; 1991d,e). The organization also has issued a set of attributes to guide the development and assessment of practice guidelines (AMA, 1990a).

In the recent history of guideline development, the 1987 annual meeting of the Council of Medical Specialty Societies (CMSS) was a significant point (CMSS, 1987; Gschwend, 1990). Representatives of several societies that had taken a leading role in guideline development up to that time (for example, ACOG, ACR, ASA) debated the importance and risks of standard setting with representatives of many specialty groups that had not yet become involved. In summarizing the meeting, the president of the CMSS concluded that it is "the duty of specialty societies and physicians to lead in shaping quality guidelines" (CMSS, 1987, p. 71). The CMSS is also involved in coordination and training activities (Woolf, 1990b).

A 1988 conference sponsored by the congressional Physician Payment Review Commission (PPRC) provided further national focus by linking specialty society and other efforts to develop practice guidelines to a policy perspective that emphasized guidelines as one vehicle for rationalizing and controlling expenditures. AMA leadership in several areas has already been cited and also includes publication of a major paper (1990b) on legal implications of practice guidelines. That paper provided important reassurance to some groups that they would not be imprudently inviting legal problems by developing guidelines—as long as they followed objective procedures, focused on scientific and medical considerations, and exercised due care in formulating and updating their recommendations. (For commentaries on the AMA paper, see Miike, 1989; Brennan, 1990; Hall, 1990; and Havighurst, 1990b.)

The creation of the Society for Medical Decision Making in 1980 was a further important milestone for guidelines development, insofar as the society serves as a locus for experts in guideline and algorithm development and clinical decisionmaking to exchange information and share experiences. Some experts, in fact, regard the advanced medical decision analyses of this group as having provided the best advice about medical technologies and interventions in recent years. The field has published its own specialty journals (such as *The Journal of Medical Decision Making*) since the early 1980s.

An array of related professional initiatives, including certain kinds of textbooks and other publications, also deserve recognition. For example, the *Manual of Medical Therapeutics* (known colloquially as "The Washington Manual") from Washington University in St. Louis is a widely used pocket reference, now in its 29th edition. It is aimed at and used chiefly by house officers and others for assistance in how to perform diagnostic and other procedures, select correct therapeutic dosages for medications, and conduct other patient care activities. In that sense, it is more of a "how to do it" manual (for instance, how to perform a lumbar puncture) than a "whether to do it" guideline document (that is, whether it is appropriate to perform the lumbar puncture). Nonetheless, its popularity reflects intense interest, across the medical education and practice spectrum, in easy-to-use references and guidelines-like materials.

Several nonphysician professional associations are also engaged in guidelines development and related activities. Since the late 1960s, the American Nurses Association has developed standards of nursing practice and universal practice guidelines in consultation with specialty nursing organizations (ANA, 1990).[5] The American Dental Association recently developed its first practice guideline on the general-initial dental examination; the group is not planning a guideline for 1992 but may return to the effort in 1993.

Why Are Professional Societies Involved?

It is not surprising that professional societies are involved in guidelines development. In the GAO survey cited earlier (1991b), the 27 responding

---

[5] The American Nurses Association defines a standard as an "authoritative statement enunciated and promulgated by the profession by which the quality of practice, service, or education can be judged" (ANA, 1990, p. 4). It defines universal practice guidelines as "a process of client care management for nursing diagnoses with recommended interventions to accomplish desired client outcomes for a specific cluster of phenomena within a nursing specialty. These guidelines are established by research and/or professional consensus by practitioners in the specialty" (ANA, 1990, p. 5).

societies noted two primary reasons for involvement: (1) improving quality of care and (2) defending against outside forces. The second objective may cover efforts to reduce malpractice and its associated costs, to encourage greater uniformity in health insurance coverage and utilization review criteria, and to counter conflicting guidelines developed by other specialty societies.

Traditionally, the purposes and missions of specialty societies and professional organizations, whether or not they are explicitly stated, include fostering the provision of appropriate clinical care based on professional standards. In this vein, the American College of Preventive Medicine (ACPM) sees its role as "leadership in research, professional education, development of public policy, and enhancement of standards for preventive medicine" (ACPM, 1989, p. 56). This is surely not an atypical view, and it is entirely consistent with involvement in guidelines development. The AMA argues that physician organizations need to be involved in guideline development "to ensure that practice parameters are properly developed and that quality improvement, rather than cost containment, serves as the foundation for their development" (Kelly and Swartwout, 1990, p. 54).

Risk management—that is, the effort to lower or curb the number of events that might lead to malpractice litigation—is another possible goal of guidelines development. The American Society of Anesthesiology and the Risk Management Foundation at Harvard University have been particularly prominent in this arena (Holzer, 1990). Building on the work of anesthesiologists from the Harvard University-affiliated hospitals, the ASA recently developed "stricter standards intended for risk management activities, focusing on clinical practices that give rise to malpractice claims" (Pierce, 1990, p. 61). The lowering of malpractice insurance rates for physicians who agree to follow these anesthesia standards has attracted much interest among other specialty societies, although anesthesiologists themselves have noted that not all types of clinical practice lend themselves to this approach to risk management.[6] As discussed in Chapter 5, policymakers have also become interested in guidelines as one element in malpractice law reform.

In addition to professional societies, malpractice underwriters and self-insured physicians groups have themselves developed guidelines for practice, an effort that is sometimes characterized as a form of risk management (Holzer, 1990; Pierce, 1990).[7] For instance, the Doctors' Company in Santa Monica, California, produces for its member physicians a series called "Risk

---

[6] The anesthesia guideline that had the greatest influence in malpractice terms was a simple recommendation to use continuous oxygen saturation monitoring. The development of transcutaneous oxygen monitors played a significant role in the success of this guideline, which antedated the enormous increase in attention to guidelines at the end of the 1980s.

[7] For a broader discussion of risk management in this context, see Morlock and colleagues (1989) and Kapp (1990), as well as Chapter 5 of this volume.

Management Guidelines," which provides recommendations on diagnostic workups, treatment, clinical management, and practice management. One guideline on the evaluation of patients with chest pain, for example, makes recommendations about the taking of an appropriate medical history, the focus of the physical examination, and the proper use and interpretation of electrocardiograms.

Finally, some professional societies have tried to integrate concerns about quality with concerns about appropriate payment for physician services. For example, an explicit goal of the ACP Clinical Efficacy Assessment Project is to produce sound definitions of good medical practice that can contribute to a rational system of payment for medical care (White and Ball, 1990). Although in the past some parties have criticized the ACP for its explicit cooperation with third-party payers, the ACP maintains that "with the involvement of the professional societies, guidelines for payment have a far better chance to reflect appropriate medical practice" (White and Ball, 1990, p. 52). This broad policy perspective is also reflected in the college's recent decision to create a Center for Applied Research that will expand the ACP's involvement in both guidelines and outcomes research. (Appendix A includes an excerpt on the use of erythrocyte sedimentation rates from the organization's compendium *Common Diagnostic Tests*.)

PUBLIC AGENCIES

Government support for practice guidelines can serve two sets of aims: the broad goal of promoting the public health and welfare and the narrower ones of improving the quality and controlling the cost of government-funded health care programs. The activities described in the next section fall into both categories.

For the most part, guidelines development has been the domain of federal rather than state government, as described below.[8] The federal government has been involved in guidelines development in at least three distinct ways:

---

[8] States do get involved, however. The state of California, for example, requires patients who may undergo blood transfusion to receive a standardized explanation of risks, benefits, and options approved by the state Department of Health Services (an excerpt is included in Appendix A). "Guidelines" relating to AIDS prevention, tracing, reporting, and the like have been promulgated by virtually every state in the union. Many if not most state guidelines appear to start with guidelines published by federal agencies. To the extent that experimentation with health care reform takes place at the state rather than the federal level, activities in the states may become more prominent in coming years. A 1990 conference sponsored by the California Public Employees Retirement System and the Oregon Medicaid initiative described in Chapter 6 reflect state interest in defining basic health benefits using guidelines and similar materials as one basis for decisionmaking.

• directly convening and managing groups to develop practice guidelines (or similar statements of good clinical practice);

• funding the development of guidelines by other groups; and

• funding and conducting basic and applied research to strengthen the clinical knowledge base and the methodologic tools that support better guideline development.

U.S. Public Health Service

The major part of federal activity now occurs in the several agencies of the U.S. Public Health Service (PHS)—especially AHCPR and the National Institutes of Health (NIH). In addition, the Office of the Assistant Secretary for Health, through its program on health promotion and disease prevention, has had a major role in guidelines relating to screening and prevention. Other PHS agencies with related activities include the Food and Drug Administration (FDA) and the Centers for Disease Control (CDC). Some guideline-related activities for the Medicare program are also carried out under the auspices of the Health Care Financing Administration (HCFA).

Food and Drug Administration

Perhaps the earliest government entry into an activity similar to guideline development came with the assignment to FDA of responsibilities for the assessment of drugs (1938) and medical devices (1976). FDA activities involve both more and less than guidelines development as defined in Chapter 1. The agency engages in both technology assessment and formal regulation, and it has a defined but limited process for securing information on the use of drugs after they have been approved for marketing (postmarketing surveillance). FDA typically does not formally approve off-label uses of drugs (uses for indications other than those for which initial marketing approval was granted),[9] and the agency's assessments of safety and efficacy do not include comparisons with alternative therapies.

National Institutes of Health

A major example of the first government role cited above—direct government involvement in guidelines development or similar activities—is the Office of Medical Applications of Research (OMAR) at NIH, which has traditionally viewed its mission as knowledge building and dissemination.

---

[9] In a departure from its usual practices, FDA reviewed an ACP guideline on methotrexate for rheumatoid arthritis (then an off-label use of that pharmaceutical agent) that had been published in the *Annals of Internal Medicine*, and approved this use about six months later.

The NIH Consensus Development Conference Program, administered by OMAR in the Office of the NIH Director, was established in 1977 (Mullan and Jacoby, 1985; Perry, 1987, 1988; IOM, 1990d,g). Through a fairly stylized approach involving small expert panels and invited conference participants, the program develops what it calls consensus statements that it hopes will be useful to health care providers and the public alike.

These statements are not meant to be a primary source of data or detailed technical information; rather, the aim is to produce a document that will reflect the commonly held views of an expert panel that grasps the issues and examines relevant scientific information. Thus, consensus statements are expected to "help resolve the issue at hand, advance medical practice, and provide a clear, concise message for clinicians and the public" (OMAR, 1988, p. 2). A notable facet of the NIH consensus development effort has been its wide-ranging dissemination efforts.

Although some observers have asserted that the consensus statements are not guidelines (Jacoby, 1985), at least some OMAR-sponsored statements meet the IOM definition of guidelines ("systematically developed statements to guide practitioners and patients"). For example, the statement on the use of intravenous immunoglobulin (IVIG) discusses the safety, risks, effectiveness, and recommended regimens of IVIG for various clinical conditions and immunodeficiencies (NIH Consensus Conference, 1990).

Other parts of NIH also contribute to the guidelines scene. For example, the National Heart, Lung, and Blood Institute (NHLBI) has promulgated treatment guidelines in the cardiovascular field through its National Cholesterol Education Program for Adults and its National High Blood Pressure Education Program.

Centers for Disease Control

Another federal effort in direct development of guidelines is that of the Centers for Disease Control. Its approach tends to be decentralized; individual divisions develop guidelines using different procedures. Some use national committees, appointed by the Secretary of Health and Human Services; others appoint panels directly. By and large, however, guideline development involves a literature search followed by a consensus recommendation by the panel or working group (Steven Teutsch, Centers for Disease Control, personal communication, 1991). As examples of guidelines developed by CDC, those of the Immunizations Practices Advisory Committee are used by many state health organizations; they are published in the *Mortality and Morbidity Weekly Report* and as stand-alone documents. Another CDC publication, *The Prevention and Treatment of Complications of Diabetes Mellitus*, comes in a version for primary care practitioners and a version for patients.

Yet another example of the range of CDC publications is the annual report *Health Information for International Travel* from the CDC Division of Quarantine, which is updated biweekly with the "Summary of Health Information for International Travel" or "Blue Sheet." The scope of the publication is broad, covering such disparate topics as specific recommendations for vaccination and prophylaxis, geographical analysis of potential health hazards, motion sickness, cruise ship sanitation, and the possibility of anthrax contamination of goatskin products. (Appendix A contains an excerpt on vaccinations for pregnant women.) This publication is used by health departments, private practitioners, travel agencies, international airlines, and shipping companies.

Agency for Health Care Policy and Research

A hybrid public role—one that involves more than financial sponsorship but less than direct governmental promulgation of guidelines or review criteria—is exemplified by the role that the U.S. Congress mandated for the AHCPR Forum for Quality and Effectiveness in Health Care. The 1990 IOM report (IOM, 1990c) provides details on the early tasks assigned to AHCPR in the Omnibus Budget Reconciliation Act of 1989 (OBRA 89). The agency is to "arrange for"[10] the development and periodic review and updating of "clinically relevant guidelines that may be used by physicians, educators, and health care practitioners to assist in determining how diseases, disorders, and other health conditions can most effectively and appropriately be prevented, diagnosed, treated, and managed clinically." (Appendix A includes illustrative excerpts from the first guideline developed through this program.)

In addition, the Forum is also to arrange for the development of "standards of quality, performance measures, and medical review criteria through which health care providers and other appropriate entities may assess or review the provision of health care and assure the quality of such care." AHCPR has recently awarded a contract to the American Medical Review Research Center to translate three sets of guideline—on urinary incontinence, postsurgical pain management, and benign prostatic hypertrophy—into medical review criteria. Those criteria are to be applied by Medicare peer review organizations (PROs) to cases that have already been reviewed by PROs and are to be used in educational outreach programs. This project

---

[10]As explained by one individual intimately involved in the development of this legislation, the phrase "arrange for" is a key indicator of the "extent to which the legislation was structured to create a public-private enterprise with respect to guideline development. The Forum develops no guidelines; guidelines are not to be federal creations" (Peter Budetti, George Washington University School of Medicine, personal communication, July 13, 1990).

is discussed further in Chapter 5.[11] Thus, the Forum's broad objectives are to promote the development of instruments to assist clinical decisionmaking and to evaluate the quality of that decisionmaking and the resulting care.

OBRA 89 provided an option by which AHCPR could contract with others for guidelines development; exercising this option would perhaps signal greater emphasis on funding (and less on internal development). In fact, AHCPR moved in this direction in September 1991, awarding three contracts for guidelines for otitis media in children, congestive heart failure, and poststroke rehabilitation. The contractors are, respectively, a consortium headed by the American Academy of Pediatrics with subcontracts to the American Academy of Family Practice, the American Academy of Otolaryngology, and the Children's Hospital of Pittsburgh; the RAND Corporation; and the Center for Health Economics Research with a subcontract to the Harvard School of Public Health for the literature review and analysis.

The work for these contracts will be done in two phases. By the end of the first, 12-month phase the contractors are expected to produce a science-based, pilot-tested, peer-reviewed guidelines document; at that point AHCPR will determine whether the original contractor should continue with the second phase and translate the guidelines into medical review criteria and standards of quality. For both phases (phase 1 in parentheses), the funding ranges from just over $480,000 ($340,000) to just over $800,000 ($675,000).

This approach will leave the agency out of direct involvement in certain guideline development tasks, such as the review of the literature and of the scientific evidence. The Forum does expect, however, to exercise considerable oversight of the work (in view of the fact that the funding is awarded as a contract rather than a grant), especially in such matters as formation of the panels, details of the work plans, and the literature reports. The principal investigators for the three projects, who will not be the panel chairs, have been asked to follow the general precepts for guidelines panels laid out in the agency's interim manual (Woolf, 1990a), although they need not adhere to every detail.

AHCPR, through the Medical Treatment Effectiveness Program (MEDTEP) rather than the Forum, also sponsors a dozen or more Patient Outcomes Research Teams (PORTs), as authorized by Congress in 1989 (AHCPR, 1990).[12] A considerable fraction of AHCPR's annual budget (about $1

---

[11] In the early 1970s, AHCPR's predecessor, the National Center for Health Services Research and Development, sponsored the Experimental Medical Care Review Organization (EMCRO) program. Some EMCROs promulgated and acted on clear criteria for appropriate and inappropriate health care services. The efforts of the New Mexico EMCRO are probably the best known (Brook and Williams, 1976; Brook et al., 1978).

[12] A small unit in AHCPR—the Office of Health Technology Assessment (OHTA)—is responsible for responding to requests from HCFA for "technology assessments," chiefly of new

million per project per year) is devoted to these multiyear, multisite, and multidisciplinary research projects, which have several effectiveness and patient outcome objectives; guideline development is not an explicit or primary task. Their basic aim is to study the effectiveness of all (reasonable) approaches to care for patients with a specific clinical condition. Among the conditions being studied are those with large variations in clinical practices and outcomes, a criterion also used to set priorities for guidelines development. Each project includes a literature review and synthesis, an analysis of variations in medical practice and patient outcomes, a planned method of targeted dissemination of its findings concerning optimal approaches to patient management, and an evaluation of the impact of this dissemination effort. The latter two activities may involve the development of practice guidelines, although AHCPR and the projects do not necessarily label them as such (AHCPR, 1991). As with the guidelines effort itself, however, expectations that the PORTs (even at the collective levels of funding they now enjoy) will contribute to clear cost savings or significantly improved health care practices—at least in the short run—must be kept realistically cautious.

Other Public Agencies

Health Care Financing Administration

In the 1970s, HCFA-funded researchers associated with Boston University began to perform conceptual and methodological work on ways to measure the appropriateness of hospital use. This effort eventually led to the Appropriateness Evaluation Protocol and other tools that are still widely used in public and private quality assurance and utilization review programs (Gertman and Restuccia, 1981; Payne, 1987). In the 1980s, HCFA also helped fund the RAND Corporation's development of appropriateness criteria. These types of indicators, which have become one of the benchmark categories of medical review criteria, are discussed more fully in later sections of this chapter.

More recently, HCFA has also supported guideline development as part of its contracts with Medicare PROs. PROs are private physician-directed organizations funded by HCFA to perform a very specific scope of work as

---

or emerging technologies for which the other agencies must make insurance coverage (e.g., Medicare program) decisions. One aim of the OHTA is to amass information about the safety, efficacy, effectiveness, and other characteristics of certain technologies. However, to the degree that the OHTA literature review and conclusions constitute evidence or statements about appropriate (or inappropriate) use of a technology, they might be regarded as at least kin to guidelines being developed elsewhere. (The OHTA memo regarding reimbursement recommendations [yes or no] is not made public.)

defined nationally by the agency. One PRO responsibility has been to develop or adapt various kinds of guidelines or criteria for prospective (preadmission and preprocedure) utilization review efforts.[13]

In keeping with the legislative emphasis on "local" (regional or state) peer review, and in the face of a dearth of accepted national guidelines, the PROs generally have had and have exercised considerable discretion to create, adopt, or adapt review criteria. This has led to substantial state-to-state variation in review criteria as well as to criteria that are not based on much, if any, systematic analysis of the literature and that may be quite minimalist and liberal. All of these factors have played a role in the criticism leveled at past PRO utilization review criteria (Project Hope, 1987; IOM, 1990i [see especially vol. 2]; Kellie and Kelly, 1991; see also Chapter 5 of this report).

One way in which AHCPR and the PROs will be working together was noted earlier—the recently initiated project to develop medical review criteria. Another area in which the PRO program and AHCPR might link efforts is in the evolution of HCFA's so-called Uniform Clinical Data Set (UCDS; Krakauer, 1990; Krakauer and Bailey, 1991). The UCDS, which collects 1,600 data elements (typically about 250 to 400 per case), has between 3,000 and 4,000 algorithms governing how those clinical data from hospital inpatient records should be abstracted for various PRO review and data base purposes. It also includes 300 or more algorithms to identify potential cases of substandard care that may require review by a PRO physician advisor. Guidelines from AHCPR panels or other sources might be used to update and upgrade the UCDS algorithms, which date to the late 1980s. Whether such collaboration comes to pass, however, is a question for the future.

U.S. Preventive Services Task Force

Another example of a public-sector initiative involving substantial private leadership and participation is the U.S. Preventive Services Task Force (USPSTF). The initial objective of this four-year undertaking was "developing recommendations for clinicians on the appropriate use of preventive interventions, based on a systematic review of the evidence on clinical effectiveness" (USPSTF, 1989, p. xxi). The 20-person Task Force, commissioned in 1984 by the Department of Health and Human Services (DHHS), developed guidelines on 169 interventions and involved dozens of advisers, authors of background papers, and reviewers. (The guideline on screening

---

[13] The fourth scope of work for the Medicare PROs was released as this report was being prepared. Over objections from the PRO community, it proposed to abolish the prior-authorization tasks that the PROs have had for the past several years.

for low visual acuity in children appears in Appendix A.) The Task Force report states that "[r]ecommendations for or against performing these maneuvers should not be interpreted as standards of care but rather as statements regarding the quality of the supporting scientific evidence" (p. vii).[14]

Congressional Office of Technology Assessment

This discussion has focused on the federal executive branch. In the legislative branch, the Office of Technology Assessment (OTA) of the U.S. Congress conducts many studies related to health care technologies; their assessments are largely in the form of reviews of published literature and publicly available data. For instance, in 1990, OTA released *Preventive Health Services for Medicare Beneficiaries: Policy and Research Issues*, which compiles recommendations published by other groups concerning such topics as periodic health examinations. It also cites assessments of preventive services (e.g., screening for breast cancer, for other types of diseases such as cervical cancer or glaucoma, and for abnormally high levels of cholesterol; vaccines against pneumococcal pneumonia and certain types of influenza) that OTA has itself conducted. The findings and conclusions of these assessments are not guidelines in the typical sense of the term, but they may certainly be regarded as a form of guidance for appropriate use of services.

PRIVATE RESEARCH, PAYER, PROVIDER, AND OTHER GROUPS

Numerous other kinds of organizations have had some involvement in guidelines development. They include private research organizations, academic medical centers, staff- and group-model HMOs, hospitals and hospital systems, health associations, and payment-related organizations. The following discussion focuses on the relatively few such organizations that (1) have devoted considerable resources to systematic development of guidelines and (2) have reached out to a national audience with these guidelines. For the most part, the guidelines development activities of most hospitals, HMOs,

---

[14] The USPSTF used methods similar to those of the Canadian Task Force on the Periodic Health Examination, which was established in 1976 and issued its first monograph on 78 target conditions in 1979 (Canadian Task Force on the Periodic Health Examination, 1979). The Canadian group reconvened following that work and issued periodic updates in 1984, 1986, and 1988. The Canadian Task Force, following earlier work by Frame and Carlson (1975), analyzes and grades research on different services using a clinical-epidemiological approach. It has made, and continues to update, recommendations to the government that are used by the Canadian provinces to make decisions about the services to be included in the periodic health examination.

payers, and similar organizations are internally focused and not publicly available.

The research organization best known for its involvement in work on appropriate medical care is the RAND Corporation. Its Health Services Utilization Study began in the early 1980s with funding from a variety of sources: the Commonwealth Fund, the John A. Hartford Foundation, the Pew Memorial Trust, the Robert Wood Johnson Foundation, and HCFA (Chassin et al., 1986b). The project devised a formal (modified Delphi) consensus approach to the development of detailed "appropriateness criteria" (ratings of the appropriateness of up to several thousand separate indications for a given diagnostic or therapeutic procedure). The researchers created such indications for six medical and surgical procedures and conducted an extensive investigation of how variations in the per-capita rates of use of these procedures related to variations in their appropriateness for specific clinical problems; among the procedures studied were coronary artery bypass surgery and carotid endarterectomy (Winslow et al., 1988a, 1988b). (Appendix A contains an excerpt from RAND's publication on the latter procedure.)

Appropriateness criteria can be distinguished from guidelines (as understood in this report) because the criteria were not primarily designed to assist physician and patient decisionmaking; rather, they were to help evaluate the appropriateness of clinical decisions. RAND researchers have continued the appropriateness criteria endeavor in various ways (including projects overseas).[15] The approach has been adopted by at least one for-profit utilization management group (Value Health Sciences) that has contracts with a variety of private insurers and other health plans.

In 1990, the AMA, the RAND Corporation, and the Academic Medical Center Consortium (AMCC) signed a memorandum of agreement to cooperate in an initiative to develop appropriateness criteria and to convert them into practice guidelines (parameters) for everyday use by physicians. The original notion was that the AMCC and RAND would be responsible for conducting research to develop the criteria and for using them to evaluate cases at the individual medical centers. The AMA, through its Specialty Society Partnership and Practice Parameters Forum, would use the research results to facilitate the development and dissemination of practice guidelines. The four procedures that have been under study (and the sites of the principal investigators and administrators) are coronary artery bypass surgery (RAND); cataract surgery (University of Iowa); aortic aneurysm resection (Mayo Clinic); and carotid endarterectomy (Duke University).

To date, the Blue Cross and Blue Shield Association (BCBSA) is the

---

[15] However, as a contractor to AHCPR to develop guidelines on congestive heart failure, RAND will be employing different methods that are more in line with those followed by current AHCPR panels (David Hadorn, RAND Corporation, personal communication, October 9, 1991).

primary, and perhaps only, example of a private insurer that has invested considerable resources in both public guidelines aimed at a national physician audience and proprietary review criteria and other tools for use by local plans (Morris, 1987). Like government efforts, the BCBSA effort has proceeded on two fronts: primarily through funding of other organizations (what it calls a "catalyst role") and secondarily through direct BCBSA guidelines development. The former effort is based on several premises: subscribers (and all patients) are best served by affecting clinical practice positively through provider education rather than through retrospective review and possible claims denial; national medical organizations are a leading and appropriate source of guidance; and physicians will more readily accept such guidance when it is developed and provided by their representative medical organizations than when it is provided by an insurer (Morris, 1987).[16] BCBSA has also created the Technology Evaluation and Coverage program to provide proprietary information to Blue Cross and Blue Shield plans to use in making benefit coverage determinations.

Another interesting initiative is that being developed in Minnesota by more than 50 health care institutions and other organizations (Borbas et al., 1990; Catherine Borbas, Healthcare Education and Research Foundation, personal communication, December 31, 1991). Known as the Minnesota Clinical Comparison and Assessment Project (MCCAP), the project has developed guidelines on five conditions and procedures of interest to specific specialties. MCCAP "consensus panels" have convened to draft guidelines, which were then reviewed, revised, and disseminated to affected physicians. Data on physician performance are being collected, analyzed, and compared to the initial guidelines. MCCAP plans to rely as much as possible in future efforts on guidelines developed by national organizations, and it has already revised its locally developed guidelines to reflect and be consistent with new work by national specialty societies. It has gone beyond these national guidelines by developing outcome measures consistent with its data collection and analysis objectives.

Among the efforts of individual staff- and group-model HMOs in developing guidelines for their health care professionals, those of the Harvard Community Health Plan (HCHP) have received considerable attention (Gottlieb et al., 1990; Burda, 1991b). The HCHP Clinical Guidelines Program has invested substantial resources in the development of scientifically based clinical algorithms. Although a central objective of the program has been to develop algorithms to guide HCHP clinicians, it also has a major re-

---

[16] BCBSA independently considers the payment implications of the guidelines, but the transformation of guidelines into medical review criteria, if recommended, is undertaken primarily at the level of local plans, not at the central association level. Blue Shield of California has been particularly active in developing medical policies and has involved the public as well as professionals.

search and educational component aimed at teaching a national audience, through publications and training activities, how to develop and implement clinical algorithms. In particular, the program has attended to practical issues regarding guideline use in ambulatory care and in "continuous improvement" strategies for clinical care management. In addition, other HMO systems, such as U.S. HealthCare, United HealthCare, and Kaiser are involved in initiatives that include some role for guidelines. Some may begin to make such guidelines publicly available.

Finally, other types of private initiatives include various kinds of commercially sponsored publications. For example, Merck Sharp & Dohme Research Laboratories produces *The Merck Manual*, an extensive compendium of information about diagnosis and treatment (Berkow, 1982). Begun nearly a century ago, it has been designed to meet the information needs of medical students, practitioners, and other health professionals on a wide range of medical disorders and patient complaints and concerns. Although the information (contained in volumes that exceed 2,500 pages) is not presented as guidelines per se, the manual supplies commentary on the use, interpretation, and limitations of many common procedures and tests used in diagnosis and patient care management. Other such compendia are the *Physicians' Desk Reference* (which compiles, indexes, and cross-references information on prescription and nonprescription pharmaceuticals) and *Scientific American Medicine* (loose-leaf medical and surgical reference volumes that are periodically updated).

COSTS OF GUIDELINES DEVELOPMENT

Because evaluation of guidelines development eventually must consider the results of the process in relation to development and implementation costs, the committee tried to estimate the costs incurred in developing guidelines. This exercise turned out to be quite difficult, for three major reasons. First, many organizations had no cost estimates; the work was buried in the budgets of one or more organizational units. Second, some who had tried to estimate costs found a full description of costs so time-consuming that they abandoned the effort. Third, those cost estimates that were available were generally not comparable or comprehensive.

In some cases, guideline developers can cite direct costs for such items as travel, printing, meeting expenses, consultants, and other line items.[17] Few organizations, however, can report costs for staff support, general overhead,

---

[17] For example, the cost of developing appropriateness criteria, evidently counting staff time as well as other direct costs (including nominal honoraria to physician participants) but excluding related research activities, has been estimated at between $250,000 and $500,000 for each set of procedure-specific indicators.

and the value of volunteer efforts. For example, neither the USPSTF nor OMAR/NIH have good estimates of the *total* cost of their work to develop specific guidelines (Robinson, 1991; Steven Woolf, U.S. Public Health Service, personal communication, March 27, 1991). John Ferguson, the director of OMAR, estimates that each consensus conference costs about $82,000 in *direct* costs, but that estimate does not include staff or volunteer participant time (John Ferguson, National Institutes of Health, personal communication, 1991).

AHCPR expected to allocate $2 million in 1990 and $3 million in 1991 to guideline development. By the end of calendar year 1991, the agency probably will have three finished guidelines and half a dozen more at various stages of development. Exclusive of staff time, early costs for AHCPR panels appeared to run about $200,000 to $250,000 per panel; more recent estimates put the range between $350,000 and $800,000, depending on the complexity of the topic. The main variable in costs appears to be the number of questions the panel eventually elects to tackle and for which it must review the literature. AHCPR has been tracking some specific costs, such as those entailed in literature reviews, and has found considerable variation across its panels. Some of the variation in these direct costs is attributable to simple differences in the volume of clinical research from topic to topic; some of the variation also appears to be ascribable to differences in panel strategy, frugality, or ingenuity. For example, the depression guideline panel opted not to focus on a single type of depression but to look at a range of diagnostic categories within that broad rubric; the panel thus will produce a "family" of guidelines based on what may eventually total more than 90,000 abstracts from the clinical and research literatures.

The GAO survey of medical societies (1991b) found that the cost estimates provided by different groups varied substantially. The estimates, which excluded volunteer time, ranged from $5,000 to $130,000 per guideline or set of guidelines. One society estimated the value of volunteer time over a two-year period at more than $500,000. A recent directory of guidelines initiatives reported estimated costs per guideline from a few thousand dollars to more than $1 million (Robinson, 1991).

SUMMARY

Planning for successful implementation of guidelines begins with development. This chapter has described selected guidelines development efforts in both the public and private sectors as a means of highlighting how the enterprise is evolving. The pluralistic nature of guidelines becomes quite clear, thereby underscoring the utility of a firm understanding on the part of developers of the attributes of their processes *and* their eventual products. The diversity of developers, of the topics that are addressed, and of the guidelines that are produced are reflected especially in the methods used and in the costs; generally, costs for producing authoritative guidelines are higher than many experts originally anticipate, owing in large measure to the attention directed to a definitive review and analysis of the literature.

This report now moves on to issues of implementation. It returns, however, in Chapter 7 to reconsider development in the light of what has been learned about implementation and surrounding policy issues.

3

Implementing Guidelines: Overview and Illustrative Cases

It is getting to be harder to "run" a constitution than to frame one.
Woodrow Wilson, 1887

Difficult as it is to formulate guidelines, implementation is an even greater challenge. Viewed generally, implementation refers to the concrete activities and interventions undertaken to turn policies into desired results. In the context of guidelines, two overlapping but distinct implementation tasks can be distinguished. One is implementing a public or private program to develop and promote practice guidelines.[1] The other is implementing the guidelines themselves.

Implementation in this second sense involves the programs and activities that take guidelines out of the rather abstract phase of development and into the actual world of health care decisionmaking and action. This chapter provides an overview of implementation issues. Chapters 4 and 5 describe some specific programs and activities, focusing on those related to information systems, educational programs, quality assurance, health benefits management, and risk management and medical liability.

Guidelines implementation is a much more diffuse process than guidelines development. The time horizon extends from the near to the indefinite future; the number of involved parties multiplies; responsibilities blur; var-

---

[1] The Omnibus Budget Reconciliation Act of 1989 gave primary responsibility for establishing a public program to develop and promote practice guidelines to the Department of Health and Human Services, through the Agency for Health Care Policy and Research and its Forum for Quality and Effectiveness in Health Care. Necessary steps for implementing this program include hiring staff, developing a program agenda, letting contracts, convening and assisting expert panels, establishing an advisory council for AHCPR, and generally establishing and administering a broad, ongoing federal program.

ied local circumstances and priorities complicate decisionmaking and generate conflicting incentives; and actions become more difficult to track. These conditions make it hard to specify attributes of good implementation processes in the way that the first IOM report specified the attributes of good guidelines. They also help explain why efforts to implement guidelines and related kinds of recommendations have met with limited success to date (Eisenberg, 1986; Schroeder, 1987; Lomas et al., 1989, 1991).

GUIDELINES AND THE REAL WORLD

One challenging current reality surrounding the implementation of guidelines is that many potential users are either unaware of guidelines or view them as being of marginal utility in their day-to-day work. Hardly unique is the urban community hospital staff who responded to the committee's inquiry about a site visit to discuss the use of guidelines by saying that there was really nothing related to guidelines going on at their institution.

For practitioners, guidelines are just one element in a range of practical and interpersonal challenges of patient care and practice management. Further, the perceived salience of formal guidelines may be lessened by the likely tendency of clinicians to consider accepted, internalized guidelines as something other than guidelines; for example, schedules for well-baby care may be so deeply ingrained that they are simply no longer regarded as guidelines. Some practitioners may well resist guidelines as threats to their autonomy even when the source is a professional organization.

For senior health care executives, too, other issues come first: patients, staff, payers, suppliers, competitors, institutional survival—although not necessarily in that order. When these executives frame a vision of their institutions for the future and a management strategy to achieve that vision, guidelines are not likely to appear in mission statements and five-year plans.

For patients and their families, guidelines are even more remote. Few laypersons will know about formal efforts to develop clinical practice guidelines; even fewer will know of their initial products or be able to use them directly. The focus of guidelines for patients, therefore, is likely to be educational—for example, handbooks or brochures about proper care for a given ailment, appropriate preventive regimens, or when to seek professional health care and when to manage one's own care.

Keeping an overview of implementation reasonably compact but illuminating is difficult, given the scope and variety of implementation efforts, on the one hand, and the lack of systematic literature about the topic, on the other. Compared with the development of guidelines, implementation is not only harder to do but more difficult to describe and analyze. The complexity of the implementation task just in terms of potential users may be illustrated (perhaps overdramatically) by estimated numbers of those who may be involved in some aspect of implementation for some category of guidelines. In the United States alone, there are roughly

- 250 million patients and potential patients, differing in myriad ways;
- 500,000 physicians, 1.5 million nurses, and 160,000 dentists distributed across a large number of specialties and subspecialties;
- 6,000 hospitals and thousands of nursing homes, rehabilitation centers, and other health care institutions;
- faculties and students in 120 medical schools, 1,400 nursing education programs, 50 dental schools, and dozens of other training programs;
- 600 health maintenance organizations and independent practice associations, and hundreds of preferred provider networks, utilization management organizations, and similar entities;
- 54 Medicare peer review organizations with hundreds of involved peer reviewers;
- 6,000 to 10,000 attorneys specializing in health-related issues—even more if personal injury lawyers are included;
- 1,800 medical libraries; and
- untold numbers of state, federal, and private health care regulators or administrators as well as technical, lay, and clinical publications with direct or indirect educational purposes or intentions.[2]

To convey something of the realities of implementation in the absence of much documented description and analysis of actual experience, the committee has devised what it calls "synthetic case studies." They draw on the study's site visits, the diverse experience of the committee members and staff, the limited research and descriptive literature, and conversations with many individuals and groups.

Each of the six case studies presented in the next section is a mix of these sources, and none depicts any single organization or individual. The subjects of the case studies were developed to illustrate the perspectives and environment of individuals and organizations, practitioners and patients, and primary, secondary, and tertiary care settings.

The cases are intentionally simplified portraits designed to convey some, but by no means all, of the real and practical issues in the effective use of guidelines. They are not intended to portray uniformly flawless application of impeccable guidelines to achieve specifically desired results, nor can they provide the depth of description and analysis possible with true case studies. (The latter would undoubtedly be helpful and might be considered for funding by the government and other organizations interested in guide-

---

[2] Obviously, these are duplicated counts. Clinicians, for instance, can also be patients, "preferred providers," and faculty. No single set of guidelines is likely to involve all these parties in significant ways.

lines.) These composite cases attempt to show that guidelines can be more (or less) than adequate in meeting the needs of practitioners and patients, that intended users of guidelines vary in their willingness and ability to conform to guidelines, and that systems and incentives differ in the degree to which they support the application of guidelines. Nonetheless, the perceived relevance of guidelines is probably higher than "average" for the individuals and organizations represented in these case studies.

Two of these hypothetical case studies focus on ambulatory (office-based) care from the points of view of a physician and an administrator; two focus on inpatient hospital care (one large academic center, one small community hospital); one deals with nursing home and hospice care; and the final case study takes the point of view of a patient. Each case is preceded by several key words; these are intended as quick references to particular implementation issues that are raised by the case.

CASE STUDIES

Case Study 1: Small Internal Medicine Practice

KEY WORDS: patient needs, characteristics, and preferences; conflicts between perceived patient needs and guidelines; specificity and format of guidelines; utility of computer-based information and decision support systems; time constraints; hassle factor

Dr. Marcus practices in a typical setting: a small (in this case, five-person) fee-for-service internal medicine group in a middle-class suburb. Although she does not see guidelines as a major issue in her practice, Dr. Marcus can cite a number of them that she uses (for example, those related to preventive services, infectious disease, and pharmaceuticals). For more complex clinical problems, she thinks guidelines that include algorithms and flowcharts are the forms most likely to be precise enough to guide decisions.

When talking about guidelines, Dr. Marcus is adamant that the patient comes first—not the guideline. For example, one of her patients—a typical older patient—has high blood pressure, diabetes, asthma, a family history of stroke, and possible macular degeneration. Although guidelines for managing some of these conditions are precise, comprehensive, and relevant, most do not deal with the particular combination of clinical problems and preferences presented by this patient. It is clear to Dr. Marcus that judgment and experience, not arbitrary compliance with guidelines, are what this patient needs.

Dr. Marcus points out that the patient comes first not only in making judgments about what to do but in implementing those judgments. This is particularly true for office-based care because the patient, not the physician, has to carry out many steps in a specific course of treatment. Dr. Marcus and her partners audited selected preventive services for patients in their practice and learned that only 50 to 70 percent of their patients had, in fact, received the services that were recommended. In some cases, the patients simply did not accept the recommendations; in others, they failed to make return visits or to see referral physicians, despite follow-up calls and notes.

For example, Dr. Marcus has for several years urged one of her elderly patients to get a screening mammogram. When the patient was asked why she had not done so, she said she thought the examination would be painful but was finally planning to have one. The reason for her change of heart was that her neighbor had recently had a mammogram that had revealed a small cancerous tumor. Dr. Marcus's patient left the office with a mammography order form, specific advice about where she could obtain the mammogram in the building or elsewhere, and a friendly, concerned parting comment from Dr. Marcus that she would be looking for the radiologist's report. Dr. Marcus estimates the probability that she will eventually get such a report (that is, that this patient will have the mammogram) as not much better than 50/50.

Although Dr. Marcus sees both the value and the limitations of existing guidelines for physicians and patients, she is highly critical of the medical review criteria applied by third-party payers. She faces multiple, detailed, and often conflicting review criteria from different organizations. In fact, she often does not even know what criteria are being used. In addition, the language associated with Medicare and private insurer policies, which tends to be aimed at identifying "bad apples," is demoralizing, as is the "hassle factor" that arises in complying with the policies. The burden of paperwork and telephone calls is quite heavy, and Dr. Marcus's group has had to hire an extra person to help handle this workload in addition to the four clerical/data entry/support staff needed for patient records, receptionist duties, and so on. Dr. Marcus appreciates that some review organizations have made an effort to minimize the burdens on physician offices and to employ clinically knowledgeable reviewers and clinically respectable review criteria; unfortunately, other organizations are less well managed.

Dr. Marcus and her partners are atypical in that their group uses computers not only for administrative purposes but also for keeping patient clinical records and for alerting physicians to the need for certain follow-up tests and other activities. The system this group uses relies on software that was first developed in the mid-1970s; it was installed in this practice in the late 1970s. More guidelines for preventive services, diagnostic tests, and other topics could be programmed into this system's alerts and reminders, but Dr. Marcus says that priorities must first be set, because the number of services that could be provided with some marginal probability of benefit was virtually uncountable.

Although the practice has been committed to the creative use of computers, it has not yet invested in any on-line clinical information services. The partners feel that available systems do not allow quick enough reference to practice guidelines (while the patient is waiting) in an algorithmic or similarly accessible format. Currently, computers are most useful to the practice in organizing and retrieving information about individual patients.

Dr. Marcus still prefers well-known, hard-copy publications (such as the *Physicians' Desk Reference*) to most available on-line information systems. One of her partners does make limited, off-line use of some new software that helps him calculate objective risk assessments using models and formulas that he could not begin to keep in his head. At this time, however, these assessments are being applied only to a few patients.

Case Study 2: Managed Care Organization

KEY WORDS: local development and adaptation of guidelines; cost management; coverage policy; selective contracting; utilization and quality review; information feedback; patient education and incentives; sanctions

ColumbiaCare, or CC for short, is a 150,000-member health plan. It selectively contracts with physicians and hospitals and pays them on a negotiated basis that involves elements of capitation, per-case payment, discounts, and other payment methods. Its members must accept higher cost sharing if they use physicians or hospitals outside CC's panel of providers.

Dr. Potter, the plan's medical director, describes ColumbiaCare as an eager "market" for guidelines and review criteria. The plan uses medical review criteria and standards of quality in a variety of ways to influence clinical practice and to make decisions about what services to cover. When professional societies and other "suppliers" of guidelines and review criteria do not meet the plan's needs, Dr. Potter organizes expert panels and consultants to develop guidelines and review criteria for specific purposes.

For example, no completely acceptable guidelines were available to advise physicians on how best to diagnose and treat adolescent depression and related mental and emotional conditions. In particular, little consistent advice was available about when to refer marginally symptomatic patients to psychiatrists or clinical psychologists, or about when to manage patients in ambulatory versus inpatient settings. The issue was significant for three reasons: the membership comprises mainly families, so the plan covers a considerable number of adolescents; adolescent mental disorders are rising in prevalence; and the employers with which CC contracts were becoming alarmed at the proportion of expenditures for these conditions.

Consequently, Dr. Potter, with the assistance of experts at a nearby research firm, empaneled a group of clinicians (psychiatrists, psychiatric social workers, clinical psychologists, internists, and pediatricians) to examine the existing literature and to reach some consensus on appropriate indications for (1) referral from primary care to specialty care and (2) inpatient treatment. The guidelines will be implemented in several ways. First, CC will disseminate the guidelines (including a description of the development process and participants) through its monthly newsletter to practitioners and hospitals. Second, the inpatient indicators will be enforced (except for emergencies) through a preadmission review program. Third, the plan may require prospective member physicians or hospitals to agree to abide by the guidelines as a requirement for selection. Fourth, Dr. Potter hopes to get internal funds to evaluate whether referral and admission patterns change and whether expenditures are reduced. He has no plans at the moment, however, to monitor patient outcomes, although this is part of the organization's longer term planning.

Dr. Potter sees advantages in local practitioner involvement in guideline development. Even if local conditions may not require any changes from national guidelines, local development or adaptation work—participating physicians getting together and "chasing some rabbits," as Kentucky-raised Dr. Potter describes it—can be useful. If nothing more, it makes practitioners more comfortable with guidelines. Dr. Potter also says that the plan is willing to "shoot a few pigeons" (that is, sanction deviant practitioners) occasionally to show that guidelines are to be taken seriously. In general, however, the plan prefers not to take a punitive approach but to use guidelines as part of an information feedback process and as screens for selecting participating physicians.

Because appropriate use of established procedures and services, such as tonsillectomy and hysterectomy, often depends on a variety of patient-specific circumstances, Dr. Potter oversees an array of programs to review the appropriateness of care on a case-by-case basis. This process is contractually permitted under a provision that limits payment to care that is medically necessary. It includes prospective, concurrent, and retrospective review of care. The programs use medical review criteria based on both practice guidelines and statistical norms to screen, for example, hospital length of stay.

For preprocedure review, the plan uses a sophisticated system developed by a private company. That system is, in turn, based on detailed appropriateness criteria developed by a well-known research organization. Preprocedure review is viewed primarily as a cost-management tool that can also serve quality assurance objectives by deterring potentially harmful overuse or misuse of care. Dr. Potter insists that the actual review of individual care is based purely on clinical judgments, not cost.

For the most part, ColumbiaCare relies for hospital quality assurance on the processes required by the Joint Commission on Accreditation of Healthcare Organizations (JCAHO). It has also instituted a quality assurance program for its primary care physicians that, among other features, employs selected practice guidelines. Each year, the plan reviews a sample of medical records for each of its primary care groups to check conformance with two to five guidelines. Last year it considered the percentage of female patients over the age of 49 who were recommended for and who received mammography screening. In addition, the quality assurance program has adapted process-of-care criteria for the outpatient management of adult hypertension, both acute and chronic otitis media among children, and evaluation of abnormal uterine bleeding. These criteria have been distributed to participating physicians, who agree to periodic audits of their charts. The physicians receive reports on how their performance compares with that of their peers—for example, what percentage of the time they use an office-based procedure (endometrial sampling) versus an inpatient procedure (dilatation and curettage) to evaluate abnormal uterine bleeding. Whenever Dr. Potter sends these reports, he asks for suggestions about how the reports and criteria might be improved.

As part of its marketing and patient service strategy, ColumbiaCare provides health education and health promotion services (e.g., hotlines, brochures) that employ various clinical practice guidelines. Some employer-customers want to set up financial rewards (or penalties) for employees who pass (or fail) blood, urine, and other tests related to cholesterol levels, blood sugar levels, blood pressure, weight, and smoking. Dr. Potter has argued against this approach, believing that such programs are too intrusive a way of encouraging patient conformity to guidelines. Instead, he is working with employers to improve employer-based health education programs and to strengthen CC's own efforts, including patient-specific counseling by CC practitioners.

Case Study 3: Academic Medical Center Hospital

KEY WORDS: quality of care and continuous quality improvement; computer-based information and decision support systems; local adaptation of guidelines; practice variation; behavior change; economic incentives

University Medical Center Hospital (UMCH) is one of the relatively small number of sophisticated academic medical centers that have complex tertiary care cases, major clinical training responsibilities, and extensive clinical and health services research agendas. UMCH is also atypical in that it has officially adopted continuous quality improvement (CQI) as a management strategy. Dr. Pierce, vice president for quality improvement, has primary responsibility for overseeing implementation of the CQI initiative and has active support and reinforcement from the hospital's governing board and chief executive officer.

Consistent with CQI precepts, UMCH seeks to reduce unwarranted variations in key diagnostic and therapeutic processes and to instill a sense of practitioner and staff ownership of the processes and results. Outcomes management is a key strategic aim, and Dr. Pierce cites the argument that one cannot properly understand, measure, and manage patient outcomes until processes of care have been stabilized.

UMCH devotes considerable effort to identifying variations in care, determining their sources, and devising remedies where appropriate. Some of the variations can be traced to administrative problems. For instance, reports of radiological examinations performed on Saturdays and Sundays reach the appropriate physicians more slowly than examinations done on weekdays (and thus delay possible Sunday or Monday morning discharges). The reason is that, for months, the hospital has had fewer radiology technicians than it needs on weekends, in part because of indecision about salary increases, which has slowed advertising and recruitment efforts. On the clinical front, the hospital has been concerned about variations in physician practices. A particularly troublesome area has been blood transfusions: transfusion rates have varied from 0 to 70 percent of patients in some heart surgery categories. Efforts were made to determine outcomes associated with different practices and to identify clinical and administrative problems (e.g., inadequate blood retrieval procedures during surgery, long operating times, lack of explicit guidelines for blood use) that created or permitted unwarranted variations in care. Following the feedback of information on variations in blood retrieval rates and operating times and the establishment of guidelines for appropriate use of transfusions (including informed patient decisionmaking), the higher transfusion rates have begun to drop with no measured adverse effects on patients.

Although UMCH has invested substantial levels of resources in identifying administrative problems that lead to errors and practice variations, the institution has also devoted considerable effort to feeding back statistical information to physicians in ways that encourage more consistent practice without relying on punitive measures or embarrassment. As a case in point, when information showing the distribution of specific physician practices (e.g., days following major surgery before a patient is ambulated, preferences for certain kinds of antimicrobial agents, lengths of stay for particular conditions) is presented at medical staff meetings, the results for each physician are known to that physician but are blinded for the remainder of the group.

Sometimes the feedback is linked to practice guidelines ("benchmarking"), but at other times only the statistical information is provided.

Dr. Pierce expects to operate this feedback system indefinitely because he knows that practitioners often revert to old patterns of behavior once feedback is stopped. He also believes that clear, quickly available feedback on actual practice variations will change behavior more predictably, and sooner, than will simple dissemination of published guidelines.

In the feedback process for physicians, Dr. Pierce relies primarily on the structure offered by the medical staff meeting rather than on that of the hospital's quality assurance (QA) system. This decision is based on his observation that physicians look to their peers for guidance rather than to the administrative units of the hospital. The QA department is oriented mainly toward utilization review, risk management, and quality issues related to accreditation by JCAHO and external regulation by the state's Medicare peer review organization.

UMCH management views the future as an era of additional cost pressures on physicians; it believes that these pressures will take the form of resource-based relative value fee scales, selective contracting, and shared financial risk in the context of managed care systems. In recent years, Dr. Pierce has seen physicians become much more interested in information that will help them build a record of practice quality and efficiency that will attract invitations to participate in managed care plans and similar networks.

One of the keys to UMCH's quality improvement program is its very sophisticated computer-based information and decision support system, which not only provides a great deal of institutional data but also integrates a variety of practice guidelines in different formats. In describing UMCH's emphasis on this system, Dr. Pierce says that, as a practical matter, no one could work at the institution "without using the keyboard," although long-range plans are to introduce less cumbersome data-entry technologies, such as voice-recognition systems.

The current system's clinical applications are related to several features: the computer-based patient record; an integrated data base that permits timely aggregation of and access to essential patient data; pharmacy alerts for possible drug interactions; alerts about questionable or "red-flag" laboratory test results (such as out-of-range electrolyte levels); on-line quality assurance including automated screening, problem alerts, and reports; and clinical decision support involving various kinds of protocols and other tools. For example, ordering of parenteral hyperalimentation is controlled by a protocol that includes both default recommendations and restricted opportunity to depart from the protocol. For blood transfusion orders, the institution has—for the time being—made a deliberate choice against on-line constraints; specifically, the system does not at present reject physician orders when indications for possible transfusion are equivocal, but it does alert the physician to that information.

A few years ago, UMCH purchased protocols for certain kinds of hospital care from another institution; consistent with CQI philosophy, they were intended to provide benchmarks for performance. The medical staff did not accept these imported protocols, however, and they were subsequently abandoned. Dr. Pierce says the effort was probably unsuccessful because the protocols were externally created and were not accompanied by any explanation or rationale that could be evaluated by the UMCH staff. Now, protocols and guidelines from other organizations are consulted, but they are not adopted without the medical staff's explicit evaluation or, in some cases, modification and adaptation.

Case Study 4: Community Hospital

KEY WORDS: risk management and medical liability; management decisionmaking and follow-through; provider payment incentives; management of patient care; guideline content

Memorial Hospital is a 250-bed hospital serving a community of 58,000 and a large rural area around it. The hospital was facing substantial increases in its malpractice premiums, especially those related to anesthesiology. In response to this problem, Dr. Houlihan, a surgeon and chief of the medical staff, undertook with his anesthesiologist colleagues to learn more about the guidelines of the American Society for Anesthesiology (ASA) for different aspects of anesthesia care.

Having determined that these guidelines were being widely accepted throughout the state's hospital sector and were viewed favorably by malpractice insurers, Dr. Houlihan lobbied for their adoption to improve quality of care and to qualify the hospital and its anesthesiologists for lower malpractice premiums. Although in the past many of the medical staff had expressed a distinct lack of enthusiasm for practice guidelines, in this case they unanimously agreed to adopt the anesthesiology guidelines. They also appointed a subcommittee to work with hospital management on practical matters related to the selection of equipment and the establishment of institutional procedures and training programs. Simultaneously, the chairman of the board of the hospital appointed a subcommittee to undertake a special fund-raising effort to secure the funds necessary to quickly purchase the equipment needed to apply the anesthesiology guidelines. (The hospital administrator, however, would rather have used the money to acquire a magnetic resonance imaging machine because a competitor hospital in a nearby community had just ordered one.)

Memorial Hospital has a traditional utilization review and quality assurance department that bases most of its activities on retrospective reviews of samples of patient charts, which are judged against common "generic screens." However, Dr. Houlihan prevailed on the QA coordinator to institute a special, concurrent study of all adverse events related to the surgery and anesthesiology departments. Using before-and-after comparisons, they hope to be able to demonstrate a drop in the number and rate of adverse anesthesiology-related events. One of the hospital's QA analysts doubts that they will find enough events over a reasonable period of time to permit valid comparisons—but agrees it is worth a try.

As the anesthesiology efforts were gearing up, Dr. Houlihan and Ms. Johns, vice president for nursing, began to discuss how the hospital might develop or use practice guidelines of other sorts. One incentive for doing so is that Memorial Hospital is located in an "all-payer" state, meaning that hospital payments are regulated by a state agency that uses per-case reimbursements to hospitals, a method similar to Medicare's diagnosis-related groups. Dr. Houlihan and Ms. Johns hypothesized that "national" guidelines might be helpful in streamlining the care the hospital provides so that they do better financially under the state's payment scheme.

Through the nursing literature that she follows carefully, Ms. Johns began to learn more about various kinds of guidelines, including "critical pathways"—documents, often in the form of a matrix, that identify what major elements of care (e.g., ambulation, discontinuation of intravenous fluids or medications) should occur on which day of hospitalization to prepare patients for timely discharge. Development of these pathways does not appear to involve an explicit assessment of scientific evidence about appropriate care; rather, existing practice patterns (in this case, for both medical and nursing care) seemed to be the predominant source of information. Further, as Ms. Johns discovered, both consulting firms and other, similarly sized hospitals are also developing such pathways on their own.

To pursue this activity at Memorial Hospital, Dr. Houlihan and Ms. Johns have gone to the hospital's board of trustees. They saw this step as necessary because the pathways will be a new endeavor for medical and nursing staff at the hospital and because they believed that they needed the political backing of the board. A further reason for going to the board was that the acquisition of literature and similar materials would involve costs beyond those normally budgeted. Dr. Houlihan and Ms. Johns hope to start the clinical pathways effort coincidentally with the start of the hospital's next fiscal year.

Case Study 5: Nursing Home and Hospice

KEY WORDS: limited resources; regulation and interpretation of guidelines; local adaptation of guidelines

The Mapletown Home is a long-term care facility in a large metropolitan area. It also serves as an inpatient care unit for a local hospice program. It is a private, nonprofit, nonsectarian organization affiliated with University Hospital Medical Center (case study 3). About two-thirds of the home's patients are on Medicaid. The home has a long history and a considerable reputation in the area; it thus enjoys more-than-average support from philanthropic sources.

Despite the home's modest endowment and other private resources, Dr. Blake, the medical director, emphasizes how government reimbursement levels have directly limited patient care and patient choices. Furthermore, she notes, those levels have a somewhat pernicious indirect effect: once a "minimum" standard of care is set for a particular clinical problem, it quickly becomes a "ceiling" as well, and the institution's board of directors tends to question additional care or staffing levels based on patient need.

For example, to prevent pressure sores, the apparent options indicated by current research are a specially designed mattress, a specially designed bed, or frequent turning and nursing care. Regardless of what would be best for the patient, only the cheapest alternative—the mattress—is really possible. Dr. Blake stressed that exceptions to this and other similar policies that are made for the benefit of a particular individual bring "palpable and present trade-offs" in the care of the other residents.

Dr. Blake sees government as virtually incapable of treating guidelines as anything but rigidly applied regulations, noting that the nuances or variations that might be acceptable to guideline developers simply get lost in the insistence on conforming to rules. She cites, for example, regulations that severely circumscribe the use of physical and chemical restraints, which were promulgated following documented evidence of their widespread overuse. Although in complete agreement with the thrust of the new guidelines, Dr. Blake also points out that physical restraints may be required for some patients (for instance, those who are severely disturbed or demented) to permit use of a feeding tube or to prevent injury to themselves or to other patients. Yet the regulations, as presently interpreted and enforced by government surveyors, limit the use of restraints to such an extreme that for some patients the home has to choose between running the very great risk that they will hurt themselves (or others) and discharging them. Dr. Blake is distressed that more flexibility is not possible in taking account of the needs of all resident patients.

Dr. Blake described efforts at the Mapletown Home to develop guidelines—in this case, physician orders for pain control—adapted to the very special circumstances of hospice inpatients. The guidelines were developed empirically after observing the effects of different doses and combinations of medications on many different hospice patients. Compared with what the *Physicians' Desk Reference* indicates is appropriate for most clinical situations, these guidelines allow a much larger than usual range of pain-killing medications and dosages to *prevent* recurrent manageable pain. Once orders are initiated by a physician, they can be implemented within the specified ranges as needed by the hospice nursing staff. Physicians are not required to accept or use the guidelines, but if they do not, hospice nursing staff must telephone them to obtain authorization for *each* change in medication, dosage, timing, or route. Physicians thus have an incentive to accept the guideline, although most appear to have fully supported it from the beginning.

Case Study 6: Patient

KEY WORDS: human errors, incentives and disincentives, conflicting guidelines

Joan Chapman is 41 years of age and has no family history of breast cancer or other risk factors for this disease. She calls her gynecologist to make her yearly appointment for a breast and pelvic examination. When the receptionist learns that Ms. Chapman has not had a mammogram in the past two years (not since a baseline mammogram when she was 38), the receptionist asks that she schedule a mammogram so that the results can be sent before the physical examination.

Ms. Chapman arrives for her appointment to find that her gynecologist is ill but that his partner, Dr. Frank, can see her if she wishes. She agrees. After the history and physical examination, Dr. Frank is ready to leave the examining room and end the appointment when Ms. Chapman asks about the results of the mammogram. It becomes clear that Dr. Frank had not checked the file for the radiologist's report. The report describes a suspicious spot in the left breast and recommends that a second mammogram be done in six months—even though the radiologist thinks that the spot is probably just a lymph node. Ms. Chapman asks if this is really necessary. Dr. Frank responds that the practice is purchasing a unit during the next year and suggests that she simply obtain the second mammogram during her next annual visit to their offices.

At this point, Ms. Chapman decides to seek advice from the internist she is scheduled to see for another problem. He strongly recommends that the six-month follow-up films be obtained and urges Ms. Chapman to ask the radiologist to make sure the suspicious spot is not a large mole that he noted during his physical examination.

Ms. Chapman has the second mammogram, remembering to mention the mole. No one, however, remembers to obtain the baseline mammogram for purposes of comparison. While still at the radiology facility, Ms. Chapman is told that the findings are normal. Three days later she gets a call from her internist saying that the results indicate the need for follow-up biopsy. The internist, after hearing the conflicting information that has been given directly to his patient, checks with the radiologist's office and discovers that he has been sent an incorrect summary report. He calls Ms. Chapman back, straightens out the final results, and recommends that she get another routine mammogram in two years.

Motivated by this series of events, Ms. Chapman begins to read about mammography screening. She learns that different medical organizations have different guidelines for women in her age group and that many groups no longer recommend a baseline mammogram. She goes on to read some of the background literature and literature reviews on which the guidelines were based. She understands that the evidence of benefit for screening in her age group is weak and contradictory; she further grasps that some evidence suggests that cancers grow faster in younger women, so that a two-year (or even a one-year) screening interval may not be as useful for younger women as it is for older women in whom cancers grow more slowly.

Ms. Chapman does not know what to think about when to get another screening mammogram. Her indecision is a function of the conflicting guidelines, the apparently careless and possibly acquisitive behavior of Dr. Frank, the confusion surrounding the results of the follow-up mammogram, and the time and money involved. She also is somewhat annoyed that neither her gynecologist nor her internist mentioned any conflicting recommendations about screening for women her age, and she wonders about other kinds of screening tests she has always taken for granted. She is not prepared to complain to any of the involved physicians about what happened, but she now plans to see a gynecologist who a friend says is willing to explain options and discuss concerns.

GENERAL ISSUES IN IMPLEMENTATION

Factors Influencing the Effective Use of Guidelines

As these synthetic case studies illustrate, the attributes and context of specific guidelines, the characteristics of practitioners and patients, and other factors interact to influence whether and how guidelines are used. Those who develop and implement guidelines need to anticipate how such factors may influence the willingness and ability of individuals and organizations to make effective use of guidelines. Lomas and Haynes (1988) identify five crucial classes of factors: (1) patients and families, (2) practitioners, (3) provider institutions, (4) economics (as it affects practitioners and institutions), and (5) the environment. Interacting with these factors are characteristics of the guidelines themselves, as described in Chapter 2 and elsewhere.

Patient and family factors include most obviously the patient's health status and particular clinical problems, as well as the expectations, preferences, and knowledge about health care of the patient and his or her family. Age, gender, race or ethnicity, reading skills, income, residence, and similar demographic, social, and economic factors may also influence whether and how guidelines affect health care decisions, behaviors, and outcomes.

In the case study of the internal medicine practice, Dr. Marcus's elderly patient clearly feared mammography as painful and just as clearly was more impressed by her neighbor's personal experience than by her doctor's advice. In the nursing home case study, Dr. Blake sees the federal regulations barring physical and chemical constraints as rigid and insensitive to the trade-off (for a family, even if the patient is not aware of it) between a disturbed patient being physically restrained and that patient having to be discharged because of the danger he or she may pose to others. Ms. Chapman, the patient in the last case study, may be atypical in having the educational background and willingness to invest in her own examination of clinical research and practice guidelines related to mammography; she is probably not atypical in her reluctance to complain directly to her physician about some aspect of her care.

Practitioner factors also encompass such demographic and social characteristics as age, gender, and residence. Furthermore, the attitudes of practitioners toward the value of guidelines may be affected by the site and type of their professional training, their specialty affiliation, their association with academic medical centers, and the kinds of continuing education to which they are exposed. Other relevant variables include the type, size, and setting of their practices.

The physicians in the first and third case studies are representative of a cohort of practitioners who are comfortable with computers. In the community hospital case, Dr. Houlihan's experience as a surgeon and chief of the medical staff has most likely suggested to him the need for careful groundwork with the medical staff and the hospital board as part of his implementation strategy. At the academic center, Dr. Pierce had a lesson in medical staff sensitivity during his unsuccessful effort to import protocols from another institution. Drs. Marcus, Potter, and Pierce all reacted negatively to guidelines that were inadequate in scope, precision, or rationale.

Institutional factors include both cultural characteristics, such as management philosophy, objectives, and style of individual institutions, and their operational capacities, including the basic physical plant, equipment, personnel, information and monitoring systems and technologies, and quality-of-care and peer review structures and processes. Relationships with public or private multi-institutional systems may also affect how guidelines are identified and used.

In the case studies, the clinicians at University Hospital Medical Center, Memorial Hospital, and Mapletown Home work in worlds that offer quite different opportunities for the use of many kinds of practice guidelines. These opportunities are affected by the respective institutional missions and philosophies, governing structures, medical staff and other personnel, information systems, and other variables. At ColumbiaCare, Dr. Potter tries, for the most part, to emphasize cooperation and positive incentives and to make only limited explicit use of the organization's more regulatory or negative tools.

Economic factors that may affect potential users of guidelines include extent of insurance coverage, methods and levels of institutional or practitioner payment (e.g., fee for service, per case, capitated), other financial incentives or disincentives (e.g., for referral to specialist consultants), and provider ownership of related services (e.g., clinical laboratories, diagnostic testing facilities).

In the patient-centered case study, Ms. Chapman suspected, rightly or wrongly, that the gynecologist she saw was unduly motivated by economic considerations in recommending that she wait to have a follow-up mammogram until his practice had purchased the necessary equipment. On the other hand, Dr. Pierce at the community hospital and Dr. Potter at the managed care organization clearly view the financial incentives associated with managed care as supporting their efforts to implement guidelines. Dr. Blake just as clearly perceives the constrained economic environment in which Mapletown Home must operate as promoting a narrow application of guidelines and insensitivity to patient needs. Although generally receptive to clinical practice guidelines, Dr. Marcus has few kind words for the way they are used, misused, or not used by third-party payers.

Environmental factors include the prevalence and incidence of disease and illness, the composition and capability of the overall system of health care delivery, government regulations, the medical liability system, and the nature and extent of social consensus about matters affecting health care decisions and behaviors.

In the nursing home setting, exposure to detailed federal regulation and inspection in a resource-constrained and sometimes bleak environment has evidently left Dr. Blake suspicious that guidelines are vulnerable to public hysteria and regulatory intemperance. These kinds of public and private oversight—that is, regulation and inspection—may increase conformity to some kinds of guidelines but at the (perhaps considerable) cost of irritation and hostility. Although only touched on in the Memorial Hospital case, the medical liability system is clearly a noteworthy environmental variable.

Strategies to Encourage Effective Use of Guidelines

These six hypothetical cases barely begin to illustrate the diversity of strategies that might be used to encourage the effective use of guidelines and the considerations that might influence the choices made from among these strategies. The following discussion covers some of these considerations.

First, the particular *short- and long-term objectives* to be served by the implementation process will make some approaches more relevant than others. For example, an implementation strategy that is appropriate for quickly informing clinicians in private practice (like Dr. Marcus) about newly revised guidelines (as might be prompted by strong new research findings and expert consensus) is unlikely to be appropriate if the objective is to provide comprehensive, continuously accessible information to office-based physicians over the longer term. Further, implementation schemes that are suitable for either of the preceding situations are not likely to be suitable (at least not alone) for implementing guidelines that are intended to persuade patients (like those Dr. Marcus sees) to ask for and accept recommendations about important screening services or changes in lifestyle or personal habits.

Second, decisionmakers must assess the *expected effectiveness of alternative strategies* in achieving the objectives in question. As a case in point, if ColumbiaCare's objective is to reduce the rate of unnecessary repeat cesarean sections consistent with authoritative guidelines, then Dr. Potter is likely to consider the potential impact of several alternative ways of encouraging (and in some cases, enforcing) practitioner conformity with these guidelines. These methods might include provision of written information, education sessions using professional opinion leaders, feedback of comparative information on individual practice patterns, application of some form of utilization review, or perhaps reduction in the payment differential for vaginal delivery versus cesarean section. Lomas and colleagues (1991) tested the first three of these approaches and found the use of opinion leaders to be the most effective.

Third, the expected *benefits* of a particular strategy to promote the use of practice guidelines have to be *weighed against predicted costs and available resources*. Consider again an organization that is developing sets of guidelines for practitioners in private, office-based practice. To bring its guidelines to their attention, the organization might consider press conferences, direct mailings of announcements of guidelines or of the guidelines themselves, development of hard-copy, desk-top compendia of the guidelines (for example, something like the American Academy of Pediatrics' widely known "Red Book" [1991] on infectious diseases), and developmental support for computer-based interactive software. The costs of these and other kinds of implementation activities, singly or in combination, must be laid against both the likely results and the available resources.

Fourth, in assessing alternative means to encourage the use of practice guidelines, implementers must consider *the demands made on target users by different strategies and user receptivity and capacity to change*. For example, an organization considering implementation of a computer-based decision support system should take into account the benefits of user-friendly software and voice-recognition systems, which demand less of practitioners and patients than hard-to-use programs and keyboard entry systems. Recalling the first case study, Dr. Marcus found hard-copy guidelines more attractive than available on-line information systems. Similarly, the willingness to move on anesthesiology guidelines at Memorial Hospital despite general skepticism about guidelines illustrates the mixed picture of receptivity and resistance that doubtless prevails in the majority of settings.

A fifth issue is the *manageability of the tasks* for administrators or others responsible for implementing a strategy. Administrators face considerable challenges in putting into place viable programs for introducing and using guidelines and for evaluating their impact. Setting up and maintaining a system of financial incentives, for instance, involves both similar and different management tasks than installing and maintaining an information feedback system. The perceptions of Dr. Houlihan and Ms. Johns that they might need the backing of the hospital board, and the support of Dr. Pierce by the UMCH board and chief executive officer, highlight the financial and administrative exigencies of guidelines implementation.

Selecting the particular elements of an implementation plan plainly requires that these and other variables be carefully assessed. Inevitably, trade-offs will be required among some factors such as expected effectiveness and cost or manageability. In theory, these trade-offs may appear to be straightforward and easy to analyze; in the real world, they are unlikely to be so amenable to investigation or understanding. Little immediately relevant empirical research is available to guide decisions. The next chapters look further at supportive conditions for guideline implementation and at some organizational, legal, and policy aspects of implementation efforts. This context includes educational activities and information systems as well as structures and processes to assess and assure quality of care, to manage health care costs, and to reduce medical liability.

SUMMARY

This chapter has provided an overview of some factors that affect the implementation of clinical practice guidelines. Hypothetical case studies, based on situations encountered in study site visits, literature reviews, and other sources, illustrate the many ways guidelines may be employed and some real-world factors that may encourage or hamper guidelines implementation.

Among these factors are variables that relate mainly to patients—for instance, factors that motivate patients to follow or ignore professional advice (or guidelines) and activities relating to patient education and incentives. Also important are variables relating to practitioner behavior and decisionmaking in everyday practice: conflicts between perceived patient needs and guidelines, the hassle factor that confronts physicians in implementing guidelines, financial incentives and disincentives facing physicians in private practice, and the exigencies of day-by-day management of patient care. Several important elements cut across settings of care: administrative decisionmaking and follow-through; collaboration (or lack of it) across the main departments of an institutional provider; the role of top management; quality of care, quality assurance, and continuous quality improvement; risk management and liability; computer-based information and decision support systems; a myriad of elements relating to the local development, adaptation, and implementation of guidelines; and simple human error. External factors include the existence of conflicting guidelines, insurance benefit plans and coverage policies, requirements concerning preprocedure review, limited institutional or community resources, and local, state, and federal regulation.

Working models of the successful use of guidelines are not now abundant. Thus, opportunities to learn from one's peers, so common in other areas of health care management, seem to be rather scarce. This means that implementation is, in some respects, a challenge that must be met de novo by each health care organization. Until more practical experience with guidelines is available, discussions of implementation will necessarily be somewhat theoretical. The next two chapters consider how educational activities, information systems, and efforts to manage quality, costs, and liability may—in principle—support and be supported by guidelines for clinical practice.

4

Implementing Guidelines: Conditions and Strategies

It was not enough to produce satisfactory soap, it was also necessary to induce people to wash.

Joseph Schumpeter, 1939

Clinical practice guidelines may be meticulously developed, sound in content, clearly presented, and widely known, but they are without value if they are not successfully applied. Indeed, the resources consumed in producing and disseminating such guidelines are wasted if the guidelines are not employed to improve health or achieve other desired outcomes.

At the point of clinical decisionmaking, the key actors are patients and practitioners. Over time, guidelines can improve that decisionmaking by strengthening its science base, increasing its consistency across similar patients and problems, and explicitly identifying how compelling is the case for particular interventions. These steps require the projection and description of benefits and risks of alternative courses of care in terms relevant to patients.

However, even when specific, well-founded guidelines exist, patients and practitioners require a broad range of supportive conditions and organizations to secure their effective use. The creation and maintenance of these conditions will require resources and strong leadership by senior clinicians and managers.

This chapter begins by briefly examining the environment and the philosophical or strategic considerations that can shape how these conditions will be structured and how well they will function. The following sections consider how educational activities and computer-based information and decision support systems can encourage the application of guidelines. Chapter 5 discusses how quality, cost, and risk management systems may support and be supported by guidelines for clinical practice.

CONTEXT, PHILOSOPHIES, AND STRATEGIES

The context in which guidelines are to be implemented is important, involving as it does a cultural shift in American society. The nation is moving away from a tradition of substantial deference to professional judgment and discretion toward more structured support and accountability for such judgment. This shift takes visible and sometimes controversial form when guidelines for clinical practice move from the development to the application stage, especially when application is backed by formal organizational structures and procedures and by forceful incentives.

The ways in which practice guidelines can and do operate as instruments for professional support and accountability are affected by the dynamics of a health care system that is changing and evolving, very often with no particular regard for practice guidelines. These complex, ongoing changes involve such fundamental matters as

- how medical care is organized and monitored
- how health benefits are provided to individuals and groups
- how practitioners and providers are paid
- how patient preferences are treated
- how information is recorded, manipulated, and retrieved.

These changes may both support and undermine practice guidelines. Although policymakers may try to anticipate and avoid mismatched incentives, those managing the health care system inevitably will be left to deal with inconsistencies or conflicts, such as payment systems that reward overuse of care and guidelines that are intended to discourage such excess.

In addition, guidelines are affected by the conduct of clinical research—its scope, priorities, and methods. Clinical and health services researchers can play an important role in making guidelines more applicable to operating environments. In particular, if researchers pay more attention than they have in the past to testing the effectiveness of procedures and patient management strategies in real settings as well as in highly controlled clinical trials, developers of guidelines are likely to have a knowledge base with greater practical relevance to practitioners and others. In turn, the greater the number of practitioners and institutions that adopt the outcomes management tools developed by health services researchers, the greater the body of information that will be available to evaluate and revise guidelines to make them still more useful in achieving desired outcomes. Overall, the influence on behavior of the varied and complex operational environments in which guidelines are to be applied cannot be stressed too much.

Practitioner knowledge of guidelines and acceptance of their validity are key conditions for their successful application, but acceptance is not equivalent to change. Thus, as a practical matter, it may be better strategically or tactically to focus less on knowledge and acceptance and more on what changes behavior in desired directions (Schroeder, 1987; Lomas et al., 1989, 1991). The rationale for this position is that guidelines may be resisted or, if accepted, fail to motivate change, given strong countervailing forces—in particular, habitual practice patterns, malpractice fears, economic disincentives, information overload, and fear of diminished professional autonomy.[1] Eisenberg (1985, 1986) has discussed six sets of activities required for successful alteration of physician practice patterns—education, feedback, participation, administrative changes, incentives, and penalties— and advised that a combined strategy is most likely to be effective.

Proposals to change behavior generally reflect a mix of philosophical, strategic, and tactical considerations. For example, discussions of the relative importance of regulatory oversight versus market incentives typically reveal philosophical positions as well as practical views about how to achieve particular goals. Likewise, controversy about proposals to motivate individual conformance with dietary and other health promotion guidelines by charging higher insurance premiums or creating other penalties for noncompliers typically reflects disagreements about both what is fair and what is likely to work. In fact, money and fear figure in many behavioral change strategies (especially for practitioners), although proponents of change may downplay this fact in public statements.

Furthermore, many attitudinal and "socialization" barriers stand in the way of behavioral change for traditionally educated physicians and, by implication, other health care professionals as well. These obstacles include the tension between professional autonomy and accountability for the quality of care rendered, processes of recruitment, training and socialization of members of the medical profession, and their preference for informal rather than formal quality assurance interventions (Donabedian, 1991). External barriers include the alienating effect (from the physician's perspective) of formal quality assurance efforts that emphasize identification of individual malfeasance and the near-total unfamiliarity of physicians and other clinical professionals with the concepts, methods, and tools of quality assurance or quality improvement. Among the approaches for overcoming these barriers and changing professional behavior are educational interventions, supportive organizational adaptations, directives, and incentives and disincentives of various sorts. Cutting across these factors are variables such as level of institutional resources and the commitment and competence of senior managerial and clinical leaders.

The next section of this chapter discusses education and then turns to

---

[1] One anonymous reviewer of this report argued that physician resistance to guidelines was part of a more general resistance to making clinical practice and judgment more regular, and that clinical judgment remains the "inner rampart" of physician autonomy.

information and decision support systems. Both are foundations on which to build the quality, risk, and cost-management strategies discussed in the next chapter. The discussion of educational strategies is intentionally brief. The committee judged that its efforts were better spent in focusing on strategies that had been less widely discussed. This lack of emphasis should not be taken to imply lack of importance.

EDUCATION

Education constitutes both a use of guidelines in itself and an essential component of quality assurance, risk management, and most other strategies for the effective application of guidelines. In medical school, residency, and continuing medical education, weaving guidelines into the fabric of educational processes is an important step in weaving guidelines into the fabric of medical practice. At this time, however, incorporation of guidelines into medical education is little documented and still subject to considerable debate (Darby, 1991b). In continuing medical education programs, specialty societies may organize sessions related to practice guidelines they have promulgated.

In medical education, the recommendations contained in a set of guidelines may be less important than the literature reviews, descriptions of analytic processes, rationales, and other materials that should accompany them. Guidelines that provide thorough analyses of evidence, projections of benefits and harms for alternative courses of care, and clear rationales for statements about appropriate care offer a powerful teaching tool, more powerful in some cases than textbooks that lack such documentation and such demonstration of the processes of scientific reasoning.

Greenfield, for example, argues that such guidelines can be "hypereducational" in exposing students to physiopathology, pharmacology, literature review, and the translation of information into practice (Darby, 1991b). Exposure to specific guidelines combined with explicit training in how to assess them (and, for that matter, how to assess medical texts) provides opportunities to hone critical faculties in ways that can benefit clinicians throughout their professional careers. To this end, the Johns Hopkins University Program for Medical Technology and Practice Assessment is developing a curriculum to teach physicians such assessment skills (Robert Hayward, Johns Hopkins Medical Institutions, personal communication, 1991; Ackerman and Nash, 1991). As the revision and updating of guidelines become more systematic and as the opportunities for more-or-less instant electronic communication are more fully realized, some guidelines may become, in essence, the textbooks of tomorrow.

Current initiatives to improve the assessment of medical competence and performance should be another stimulus to integrate guidelines into practice throughout a professional's career (Nuckolls, 1990; Langsley, 1991). Board certification, which follows residency training and examinations administered by the boards, is a statement about physician qualifications at the time of certification, not about continuing competence over the long run of practice. Some medical specialty boards (notably family practice but increasingly others such as internal medicine) have begun to issue time-limited board certification; after 10 years, or some other designated period, the physician needs to reapply for certification. The recertification process administered by the American Board of Family Practice includes a review of office records using performance criteria that apparently are not based on formal practice guidelines but that could be (Langsley, 1991). Some groups, such as the American Board of Internal Medicine, have been considering a role for clinical practice guidelines in establishing criteria either for recertification or for eligibility to apply for recertification, but close links between guidelines and board certification or recertification almost certainly lie well into the future.

For patients, too, corresponding avenues exist for lifetime learning about healthful behavior and problem-oriented decisionmaking. Guidelines-related information can be incorporated in school, employment-related, insurer-based, and other health education activities; a long, albeit not uniformly successful, tradition of such education already exists as a foundation for these efforts. For example, health educators recognize that many patients or consumers—perhaps one in five—lack important reading skills. When the American College of Obstetricians and Gynecologists developed a magazine for parents or prospective parents who might not be able to use its existing publication, it quickly received requests for 700,000 copies; it had expected to distribute 500,000 copies over three years (Rovner, 1991).

The American Cancer Society (ACS) has employed a different simplifying strategy in some of its materials. To attract attention and help embed key information in individual memory, the ACS (1990) uses a simple mnemonic device that highlights the first letters of each of the seven warning signs for cancer to spell C-A-U-T-I-O-N.

- Change in bowel or bladder habits
- A sore that does not heal
- Unusual bleeding or discharge
- Thickening or lump in breast or elsewhere
- Indigestion or difficulty in swallowing
- Obvious change in wart or mole
- Nagging cough or hoarseness

Educational strategies for both professionals and laypersons can help build a foundation for specific quality assurance, risk management, and similar programs. Unfortunately, the appeal of educational strategies appears to be offset by uneven and sometimes discouraging information about their impact and cost-effectiveness (see, for example, Eisenberg, 1986). The continuing challenge is to make this most commonly used approach for changing behavior more consistently productive.

Many individuals and organizations are trying to meet this challenge, building on extensive behavioral research and practical experience (Eisenberg, 1986; Chassin, 1988; Kanouse and Jacoby, 1988; Green, 1991; Siu and Mittman, 1991). The Agency for Health Care Policy and Research (AHCPR), in particular, is committed to an extensive dissemination and education effort to support the guidelines it is developing (AHCPR, 1991).

One important feature of educational strategies such as those cited above is their diversity. Education can be

- informal or formal
- impersonal or personal
- one-way or interactive
- isolated or connected to ongoing relationships
- knowledge oriented or change oriented
- sponsored by individuals or organizations of varying credibility.

The most prominent educational strategies for practitioners focus on relatively formal, organized activities. These activities include medical school, graduate medical education, and continuing education courses that tend to be impersonal and involve only one-way communication. Computer or other self-teaching modules, on the other hand, are impersonal but can be interactive.

Research on the impact of different educational strategies indicates that personal, interactive strategies tend to be more influential in changing practitioner behavior than are more formal or indirect approaches (Avorn and Soumerai, 1983; Eisenberg, 1986; Chassin, 1988; Soumerai and Avorn, 1990; Siu and Mittman, 1991). Programs undertaken by respected authorities in the context of ongoing organizational relationships are also effective, and sometimes the involvement of respected leaders may be the key to success or failure of efforts to modify the clinical practice. Small group education, individualized "academic detailing," and operations-level feedback of information on practice patterns are personal, interactive strategies with both formal and informal aspects.[2] All of these activities can vary in the degree to which they go beyond knowledge building to stress behavioral change.

Adequate evaluation of strategies for change requires that benefits be

---

[2] For example, Avorn and Soumerai (1983) and Soumerai and Avorn (1990) describe academic detailing as including interviews to establish baseline knowledge and motivation associated with a practice; programs focused on specific categories of physicians and their opinion leaders; clearly stated educational and behavioral objectives; sponsorship by a respected organization; use of authoritative and unbiased information and concise graphic materials, and repetition of essential messages; active participation by physicians; and positive feedback on improved practice. The approach is built on marketing strategies used by pharmaceutical companies.

weighed against costs. Yet many studies of educational strategies do not report useful data on the cost-effectiveness of the strategies. Eisenberg (1986) notes that despite the appeal of personalized face-to-face feedback, it may not generate savings that exceed its cost. This is a serious problem if the primary object is cost containment rather than quality assurance or some other purpose. Even when cost containment is not the objective of an education strategy, managers need information on benefits and costs of the alternative strategies available to them.

Educational strategies for patients or consumers tend to emphasize impersonal and relatively inexpensive mass information campaigns or to rely heavily on the physician-patient relationship, although this reliance is rarely reinforced by specific reimbursement for patient education (Green, 1991). At its best, the latter is personal, interactive, ongoing, and decision oriented (if not change oriented). The interactive videos now being developed and tested for prostatism and other conditions promise an attractive supplement to direct physician education of patients (see Chapter 6). Evaluations of the effectiveness and costs of this tool will be received with much interest.

Educational tools for both physicians and consumers are relying increasingly on computers. A recent publication on pharmaceuticals (National Council on Patient Information and Education, 1991) lists an array of products ranging from a self-medication screening program developed at the University of Florida to commercial software that pharmacists can use to generate easy-to-understand educational materials for patients.

Williamson (1991) has emphasized the importance of educating physicians on the needs of their patients for better information and education about the rationale for a course of care and the expected or possible physical and psychological consequences of compliance (including side effects) or noncompliance. He describes one specific hypertension treatment program, built on some of the quality improvement principles described in the next chapter, that includes education for physicians (in particular, specific information about patients' beliefs and behavior), an outcome-oriented plan for improving communication, feedback to practitioners on outcomes, and reevaluation of the program and its statement of the maximum acceptable level of patient noncompliance.

Informal educational processes (such as telephone consultations with respected colleagues, bedside conversations, or lunchtime discussions) should not be ignored. The power of respected leaders to facilitate the diffusion, acceptance, and application of new information and technologies is undoubtedly felt in both deliberately organized and less formal ways (Eisenberg, 1986; Lomas et al., 1991). This applies as well to patients and consumers.

Repeating the point that introduced this section, education is an essential component of most other strategies for effective application of guidelines. This report acknowledges the central role of educational strategies but, consistent with its charge, has attempted only to frame issues and options rather than to explore them in depth. As developers of guidelines improve the documentation that accompanies guidelines, as well as the clinical specificity and the explication of the reasoning that went into their formulation, the task of educators ought to become easier. Likewise, as this happens, those who develop and manage clinical information and decision support systems will find it easier to incorporate guidelines into these systems.

INFORMATION AND DECISION SUPPORT SYSTEMS

In manufacturing and financial services, computer systems oversee and control millions of individual actions. Such systems are ubiquitous and cover all activities associated with the function of an institution—as they do, for example, banking. In the medical care arena, however, even those settings with the most advanced computer systems have not automated the majority of their core clinical and other activities (IOM, 1991b). To the extent that automated systems support patient care, such support generally consists of clinical data rather than guidance about appropriate care; generally, it is hospital based and does not extend to the physician's office and similar settings.

Information and decision support systems are crucial elements in long-term strategies for promoting the application of guidelines, the evaluation of their impact, and the feedback of such evaluation to revise and improve guidelines. The very translation of guidelines into algorithms and computer-based formats can spotlight deficiencies in guidelines (such as lack of specificity) and lead to revisions that will make guidelines more usable (Margolis et al., 1991). Although the following discussion emphasizes computer-based information systems, guidelines should also be available, understandable, and usable in conventional hard-copy forms.

Current Systems

The committee visited several institutions that already have or are implementing effective clinical information and decision support systems. An example is the Regenstrief Medical Record System (RMRS), used by University of Indiana house staff in the Wishard Memorial Hospital and its outpatient clinics (McDonald, 1976; McDonald et al., 1984, 1988; Tierney et al., 1990). The RMRS includes modules designed to record, retrieve, sort, and display medical encounter, treatment, and diagnostic study data as reports and flowsheets. The system also provides real-time clinical reminders and alerts (based on patient-specific data) using protocols for pediatric, medicine, and obstetrics and gynecology clinics.[3] For instance, reminders can alert physicians to preventive care needs or untreated hypothyroidism in patients seen for other ailments or reasons; they can also describe alternative diagnoses and therapies, calculate medication dosages, and estimate Framingham Risk of Cardiovascular Disease probabilities based on patient laboratory values. Regenstrief has developed more than 1,400 rules and has documented their rationale and scientific base (McDonald et al., 1988). In addition, users can create their own protocols.

Some evidence about the impact of such systems is available. For example, at Regenstrief, a large, two-year randomized clinical trial found increases of up to 400 percent in the delivery of preventive care associated with use of the reminder system (McDonald et al., 1984). Other researchers, including those at Latter Day Saints Hospital in Salt Lake City and Massachusetts General Hospital in Boston, report similar results with computer-based reminder and decision support systems (Barnett et al., 1978; Hattwick et al., 1981; Pestotnik et al., 1990; Elliott, 1991; Williamson, 1991).

Existing computer-based information and decision support systems differ in significant ways. These differences involve the degree to which the systems

• come into play automatically or at the discretion of the practitioner or patient—for example, an on-line reminder or surveillance system versus a user-initiated inquiry system;

• are more or less intrusive, a case in point being computer-based systems for ordering laboratory tests that request only the reason for a test versus systems that also require approval of the reason;

• emphasize information or control of behavior—for instance, on-line reminders of appropriate practice versus on-line limits on ordering certain services; and

• link practice guidelines to patient-specific information, a comparison being a general reference system versus an interactive protocol that uses specific information about a particular patient.

As discussed later in this section, change is occurring on two fronts—technical and psychological—which should make computer-based information and decision support systems far more useful and attractive to clinicians. Nonetheless, the following constraints still apply to a considerable

---

[3] Computer-supported reminder systems are not limited to practitioner use, although patient applications are still relatively limited and untested. The simplest systems provide medication storage containers with monitors that beep or otherwise alert patients to medication schedules and record use. A telephone-based reminder system for pharmacists is also available (National Council on Patient Information and Education, 1991).

extent to most of the health care system; overcoming them is one aim of the recommendations in the IOM's 1991 report on the computer-based patient record (IOM, 1991b).

First, practitioners, institutional administrators, and others are wary of the expense of the requisite computer hardware and software. The track record (or at least the perceived record) of computer-related technology is one of failing to meet expectations or of becoming out of date rather quickly, both of which intensify investment concerns (Gardner and Perry, 1989; GAO, 1991a; Gardner, 1991).

Second, computer hardware and software remain threatening or unappealing to many practitioners and patients. Even computer-literate practitioners object to systems that make it onerous to enter data or to retrieve accurate and useful clinical information and guidance on a real-time, interactive basis (Lundsgaarde et al., 1981; Brightbill, 1990; Fliegel, 1990; Gardner, 1990b).

Third, current systems do not generally link all of the many sources of patient data (e.g., the physician office, commercial laboratory, hospital). Even when the source information is computer based, differences in data storage structures, record identifiers, and coding systems may make information exchange difficult across or within patient care settings (see, generally, Brodnik and Johns, 1991, which includes many of the articles cited here). In addition to deficient linkages to support clinical decisionmaking for individual patients, linkages to support outcomes research and guidelines development and revisions are still limited.

Fourth, independent of hardware or software limitations, guidelines themselves are often too incomplete for translation into computer-based decision aids (Margolis et al., 1991). A related problem is that computer-supported use of guidelines may require integration of information on specific patients that is not accessible automatically—for example, handwritten notes.

Promising Developments

Information and decision support systems are advancing on many fronts and in many ways (Gardner, 1990a; Grossman, 1991; IOM, 1991a; McDonald et al., 1991). These advances will make such systems more useful for many purposes, including support for the application of clinical practice guidelines. Several areas of progress can be cited.

First, standard definitions and ground rules for transferring and using information from different computer systems are still limited but are emerging in such forms as Health Level 7 (HL 7) and draft standard 1238 of the American Society for Testing and Materials (ASTM, 1991; Hammond, 1991; McDonald et al., 1991). For practice guidelines, the ARDEN syntax provides a formal way to define guidelines so that they can be tested and executed automatically and shared across different computer systems (Hripcsak et al., 1990).

Second, although most information and decision support systems are now based in hospitals, hospital expansion of ambulatory activities and partnerships with physicians are making computer-based information systems more available to physicians in their offices. Starting at the other end, group practices and health maintenance organizations are beginning to extend their systems to cover hospital care. The Harvard Community Health Plan with its long history of computerization and its link to Brigham and Women's Hospital is an example. These developments make coordination of care easier and collection of data on episodes of care more feasible.

Third, data collection and analysis strategies for laboratory, radiology, and pharmacy departments in patient care settings have become increasingly sophisticated. As information and decision support strategies are used in tandem with other kinds of implementation approaches, they can simultaneously present information and shape and control its uses.

A case in point is a test- or drug-ordering protocol programmed into a computer-based decision support system, which can both display data and options and limit the orders that will be accepted for certain combinations of clinical problems. Today, most systems appear to be far less directive than this, but they are likely to change as systems become more sophisticated and as the emphasis shifts from merely providing information to producing desired changes in behavior and outcomes. The committee expects that clinical information and guidelines will become more integrated in such forms as expert rules, normal limits, contraindications, drug interactions, and other supports for decisionmaking (Eckman et al., 1991).

Fourth, information input and retrieval technologies are becoming less intimidating. Practical voice-recognition systems may be essential to widespread clinician involvement in timely entry of key patient information. Such systems are advancing, although they generally remain unable to handle normal, continuous speech and the large vocabularies required by medicine.

Developments in the arena of information and decision support systems are important because they can support the application and, for that matter, the development of guidelines in at least three important ways. They can provide

- centralized storage, maintenance, and retrieval of guidelines;
- decision aids for practitioners (and, less commonly, patients) that are based on authoritative guidelines; and
- means for collecting clinical information for effectiveness, outcomes, and biomedical research that can, in turn, feed into the development or revision of guidelines.

Access to Information

Perhaps the best developed and most easily improved of these three elements is the central clearinghouse function that permits access to good practice guidelines through remote computer links. The National Library of Medicine (NLM), various commercial vendors, and others are increasing the availability of clinical information through on-line literature search systems, floppy disks, and CD-ROM disks.[4] To date, these systems appear to include guidelines only incidentally, but this state of affairs is changing as guidelines become more visible (Brightbill, 1990; Frisch, 1991).

The Omnibus Budget Reconciliation Act of 1989 requires AHCPR to promote dissemination of guidelines through organizations that represent health care providers or health care consumers, and through peer review organizations, accrediting bodies, and other appropriate entities. Among the first steps that the agency took to fulfill this mandate was to begin work with the NLM for inclusion of guidelines in various NLM bibliographic and information systems. The NLM is arranging for easy access to AHCPR-sponsored (and eventually other) guidelines by

• staffing its recently established Office of Health Services Research Information;
• developing bibliographic headings (Medical Subject Headings, or MeSH) related directly to guidelines;
• creating in its indexing system the label "practice guideline" to identify guidelines as a type of publication;
• highlighting citations for AHCPR guidelines in GRATEFUL MED (an on-line software package for searching medical literature);
• providing on-line access (through its LOANSOME DOC system) to full texts of the "short-form" versions of AHCPR guidelines; and
• allowing on-line requests for mailing of the complete text of AHCPR guidelines and providing instant facsimile transmission of summaries or short versions of guidelines.

Decision Support

Not a new feature but also not commonplace is the programming of guidelines into management and decision support systems (Adams, 1986). Decision analysis software also has a role to play in the application of practice guidelines. These efforts can take several forms including the following:

---

[4] CD-ROM (which stands for computer disk-read only memory) disks are computer storage hardware that runs on personal computers and has a vast storage capacity. Currently available CD-ROMs can store 500 million bytes of information, which could translate into as much as 250,000 pages of data or up to 1,500 floppy disks. CD-ROM systems also allow the user to consult several "books"—major diagnostic texts, compendia on the use of medical therapeutics or pharmaceuticals, and so forth—at once.

• **Reminders and alerts**. For example, a system that integrated information from a patient's medical record with guidelines about appropriate care might be able to state, "Patient had Class III Pap smear four months ago. Repeat smear was due last month but was not done" (Adams, 1986). A system that had on-line entry of clinical activities or patient status could report, for instance, "Patient's throat culture is positive for beta streptococcus. No appropriate antibiotic has been initiated." A more forceful alert might state, "Tracheal tube cuff pressure greater than 27 cm H_2O. Indicates excessive pressure and potential for destruction of tracheal cartilage, arterial bleeding, and sudden death." (This last example is adapted from Elliott's [1991] detailed description of the respiratory care system at the Latter Day Saints Hospital in Salt Lake City, Utah.)

• **Embedded controls**. For example: "Orders for parenteral nutrition are governed by the following protocol (list). Overrides require (procedures listed)."

• **Decision assistance**. An example might be the following: "Patient has mildly elevated creatinine and is already on quinidine, so a lowered dose of digoxin should be considered" (Adams, 1986). Or, "Patient has positive hemocult. Steps in work-up are (screen displays flowchart)."

• **Risk prediction**. For instance: "According to Goldman's computer protocol for patients with chest pain, this patient has state 'K' and therefore is at high risk for myocardial infarction" (drawn from Goldman et al., 1988).

Outcomes and Guidelines Revision

Several IOM committees have emphasized the importance of revising guidelines in the light of new evidence about health care technologies (IOM, 1989a, 1990c,i). To that end, better clinical information about the efficacy and effectiveness of health care services must be acquired, and a number of organizations are engaged in practical initiatives with that aim. Improved computer-based record systems offer an opportunity to collect, aggregate, analyze, and transmit such data in a more timely and more organized way than ever before (IOM, 1991b). Such data might, in the future, be used to trigger review of an existing guideline or to provide some defensible reason for local adaptation of a guideline. On a broader scale, these data, as they are brought more quickly into the scientific literature, will become the foundation for better guidelines.

Integrating Financial and Clinical Management Systems

What were originally financial management systems are increasingly becoming clinical management systems as well, driven by changes in reimbursement systems (in particular, diagnosis-related groups), managed care contracting, and quality-of-care concerns. Two examples of these approaches are the systems at Intermountain Health Systems (Salt Lake City) and the New England Medical Center hospitals (Boston). Both are moving from retrospective, externally oriented systems toward internal concurrent or prospective systems.

Such shifts require that data be integrated from operational systems (e.g., laboratory, radiology, pharmacy, nursing), medical records, and financial systems to determine the costs of patient care "products." Depending on the quality and scope of the basic information, such integration may also allow practitioners and managers to develop budgets, to project how changes in ways of providing care will affect costs and clinical outcomes, and to evaluate departures from projected costs. For example, "if the laboratory is over budget, variances due to excessive test ordering (the responsibility of physicians) or use of more labor than predicted (the responsibility of the lab manager) can be identified" (Grossman, 1991, p. 242). Practice guidelines offer a benchmark for judging the clinical elements so as to identify problems.

The convergence of financial and clinical management systems motivated by the economic and other pressures described earlier will be a powerful force for moving guidelines into multiple environments, for facilitating comparisons of provider performance and guideline impact, and for feeding back useful information to both developers and users of practice guidelines. The recommendations in Chapter 7 are designed to facilitate and test this proposition.

Directions for Information Systems

At this time, no adequate information infrastructure supports the kind of effective, unobtrusive, easy application of guidelines envisioned by continuous quality improvement models, future-oriented utilization management and cost-containment systems, and patient-centered care proposals. Clearly, however, the information technologies of the future will make the application of guidelines much easier, particularly if other conditions support their use.[5]

The work of the NLM and others to establish some capacity for responding to user-initiated inquiries and dissemination needs should be encouraged. In succeeding years, the NLM may be in a position to expand its

---

[5] The scope of the committee's charge did not permit extensive treatment of information systems. For this discussion the committee drew on the recently published report and background materials of the IOM Committee on Improving the Patient Record (IOM, 1991b) as well as on the committee's site visits and the members' collective experience. The IOM report covers the technical issues of computer-based patient records (CPRs) and CPR systems in some detail.

core responsibilities and activities beyond the collaboration with AHCPR to other guideline development organizations.[6]

The committee also favors efforts to foster the translation and movement of guidelines into computerized decision aids of various sorts. However, it believes those efforts should be in conformance with emerging standards in the computer industry that will permit the guidelines (however transformed) to be used on many different types of computer-based equipment and systems (Gabrieli, 1991; IOM, 1991b; McDonald et al., 1991; Megargle, 1991).

Although comprehensive computer-based patient records and systems do not at present exist, parts of them have been implemented in a small number of health care institutions around the country. Likewise, sophisticated computer-assisted applications of particular guidelines are not common but can be found in a number of institutions at the level of individual departments, units, or practitioners.

More and better use of computer-based information and decision support systems for all these purposes depend on several technical and behavioral developments that are already in motion:

• improvements in the logical consistency and completeness of guidelines through use of algorithms and formalized formats;
• technological improvements (e.g., voice-recognition systems to reduce data input chores);
• integration of records of an individual patient's episodes of care into a single system;
• rules of syntax, data base structures, and communication links that support multiple users and settings of care;
• reductions in hardware and software costs;
• changes in attitudes and skills of prospective institutional and individual users including patients as well as practitioners;
• resolution of confidentiality, privacy, and security concerns; and
• demonstrated clinical utility and practicality of the support provided.

Predicting the specific rate of change along these various dimensions is beyond the capacity of this committee. The technical developments (including voice recognition and better networking hardware and software) are more predictable, and closer to hand, than the behavioral changes. The

---

[6] The IOM has recently completed a study to advise the NLM on new and expanded services for health services research and technology assessment (IOM, 1991c). These services may lie primarily in the area of core library activities related to creating and maintaining literature-oriented data bases, supplying basic guidance to regional and organization-based libraries on sources of information, and suggesting likely information search and retrieval strategies. Practice guidelines are seen as lying well within these clinical evaluation fields.

IOM committee studying the computer-based patient record called for concentrated public-private efforts for the remainder of the decade, many of them to be focused on attitudes and behaviors of users of computer-based patient records and systems. By the end of that time, that committee believed, computer-based information systems in health care could be both widespread and ingrained in the clinical life of many practice settings.

SUMMARY

Among the supporting conditions for the effective application of sound practice guidelines are educational programs and information and decision support systems. The first is tied closely to the dissemination of guidelines but goes far beyond that one role to promote understanding of the evidence base, rationale, and expected consequences of guidelines. Guidelines that are clearly written, specific, based on evidence, and well documented can be powerful tools of medical education, although this application is more potential than real at this time. A critical adjunct to education is to incorporate guidelines into routine information and decision support systems. Both education and decision support have a concrete place in quality, cost, and risk management initiatives. How these programs can support and be supported by practice guidelines is examined next.

5

Implementation: Quality, Cost, and Risk Management

Administration is difficult; agitation is easy.
C. Rufus Rorem, 1946

Although those who plan and manage education programs and information systems can encourage the application of practice guidelines, more central to this effort will be those who design and administer programs to assure quality of care, manage health care costs, and protect practitioners and institutions from malpractice liability. The ways in which these programs can support and be supported by guidelines is, so far, poorly charted, although journal articles, conferences, and similar information sources are beginning to focus on the more practical challenges of incorporating guidelines into programs for quality, cost, and risk management. This chapter explores some of those challenges and presents the rationales for investing resources to overcome or manage them.

Perhaps the most appealing rationale for the development and use of clinical practice guidelines is that they can help improve the quality of health care; certainly, it is the most positive and optimistic reason to invest time, resources, and energy in guidelines development. The first section of this chapter thus focuses on programs to assess, assure, and improve the quality of care and on the potential role that guidelines might have in this area. The committee does not, however, take any formal stance on the several approaches to quality assurance, improvement, and management now being promulgated by various groups; neither its charge nor its deliberations were this expansive.

Despite the near universal appeal of the quality-of-care rationale, cost containment appears to be the most urgent and contentious motive behind calls for guidelines development and use. Were it not for this motive, the recent flood of interest in and support for practice guidelines would probably have been a more modest stream. The second section of this chapter examines how cost management programs may employ guidelines, and the next chapter describes the committee's vigorous debate about what developers of guidelines should do to better support these programs.

Relatively few existing guidelines appear to have been prompted primarily by liability concerns. Nevertheless, the broadly perceived medical malpractice "crisis" has inevitably made the role of guidelines an issue in risk management programs and tort law. The last section of this chapter takes up this topic.

QUALITY ASSURANCE AND IMPROVEMENT

Basic Concepts and Propositions

The IOM has defined quality of care as "the degree to which health care services for individuals and populations increase the likelihood of desired health outcomes and are consistent with current professional knowledge" (IOM, 1990i, p. 21). To the extent that guidelines are based on scientific knowledge, estimate expected health outcomes, and delineate current professional judgment, they clearly have a role to play in assessing and assuring the quality of care.

Efforts to ensure high-quality care must prevent or, alternatively, detect and overcome three main problems: (1) overuse of unnecessary care and of inappropriate care, (2) underuse of necessary care, and (3) poor performance (in both the technical and interpersonal senses). Most experts now agree that a comprehensive approach to quality of care must address all three problems, perhaps to different degrees depending on the setting or nature of the care and various local or institutional factors. Good practice guidelines have the potential to contribute in each area.

First, guidelines and review criteria that explicitly and clearly describe appropriate care for particular clinical problems provide a solid base for detecting patterns of overuse or underuse. Second, detailed guidelines may improve the technical provision of care. Certainly, some aspects of technique have to do with physical capacity, skill built on experience and repetition, attention to detail, and similar factors. Good performance, however, depends on a solid understanding of what constitutes appropriate care (e.g., choice of antibiotic) or correct performance of a technical task (e.g., sterile technique). Finally, when guidelines include good estimates of outcomes (risks, benefits, harms), they can contribute to better communication and shared decisionmaking on the part of patients and practitioners. These interpersonal processes lie at the heart of the humanistic "art of care" vision of quality.

Traditional programs of quality assurance (QA) (see Donaldson and Lohr, 1990) derive from a conceptual framework advanced more than a quarter-century ago by Donabedian (1966). This conceptualization (further explicated in Donabedian, 1980, 1982, 1985) emphasizes (1) the structure of care—that is, characteristics of practitioners, institutions, and the health care system including regulatory mechanisms; (2) the process of care, meaning at least patient care activities and, in some formulations, the housekeeping, administrative, and other activities that may affect quality of care; and (3) the outcomes of care, including patient health status and functioning, well-being, and satisfaction.

Clinical practice guidelines, medical review criteria, and standards of quality relate more directly to the processes of care than to outcomes because they describe what constitutes appropriate management of specific clinical problems. Performance measures describe the data needed to evaluate whether actual behavior conforms to guidelines, criteria, and standards. Utilization and quality review programs may employ all these instruments to identify and deter unnecessary and inappropriate services. As more and more guidelines explicitly estimate expected benefits and harms of care (that is, possible outcomes), they may more directly contribute to the specification of sophisticated criteria that relate good quality of care to expected (good) patient outcomes. The use and development of review criteria are discussed further in a later section.

At a systems level of quality assurance strategies, the potential role of guidelines in certification and recertification programs and examinations should be noted. For example, as mentioned in Chapter 4, the American Board of Family Practice has for many years administered a recertification process that involves review of office records against a predetermined list of performance criteria (Langsley, 1991). In Canada, the College of Family Physicians and McMaster University have been involved in an extensive effort to develop and apply chart audits, tests of basic clinical skills, and other methods. These criteria and assessments do not appear to be based explicitly on published practice guidelines, but such guidelines could certainly be factored into the certification and recertification processes. As specialty boards continue their work on methods to judge qualifications accurately, attention to practice guidelines as one base for performance evaluation is an obvious step.

Continuous Quality Improvement

The case studies in Chapter 3 reflect the extent to which the use of guidelines to improve quality of care is a subtext in a managerial and policy debate over the relative contributions of traditional QA strategies and newer quality management approaches. These approaches are variously called total quality management (TQM) or continuous quality improvement (CQI). This discussion, which employs the latter term and abbreviation, relies on a composite model of CQI based on principles described in recent literature[1] and on observations drawn from the health care press, committee site visits, and other discussions. (The IOM committee that studied issues of quality assurance in Medicare [IOM, 1990i] compared traditional QA and CQI models in more depth.)

The growing interest in CQI is reflected in statements by the Joint Commission on Accreditation of Healthcare Organizations that it intends to shift from a QA to a CQI perspective and develop new principles and standards of hospital accreditation to reflect this shift (O'Leary, 1991). In describing the Joint Commission approach, O'Leary (1991) says, "We tend to use CQI . . . because to us the term means a way of life in an organization. Total quality management . . . might imply that there is a single management style that is necessary for all of this change to happen" (p. 74). A recent American Hospital Association survey states that more than 40 percent of reporting hospitals say they are engaged in continuous quality improvement (*Utilization Review Newsletter*, 1991b). The Maryland Hospital Association's ambitious quality indicator project is cast in a continuous quality framework (Maryland Hospital Association, 1990). In addition, the Robert Wood Johnson Foundation supports a program for "Improving the Quality of Hospital Care"; a quarterly newsletter for that program, entitled *Quality Exchange*, is produced at the Johns Hopkins University.[2]

CQI models are generally described in terms of a set of reinforcing principles for implementing change. They aim to make nonpunitive tactics for quality assurance more usable and, it is hoped, more effective than they have been under traditional approaches. Each of these principles has impli-

---

[1] See Deming, 1986; Walton, 1986; Garvin, 1988; Batalden and Buchanan, 1989; Berwick, 1989; Berwick et al., 1990; Gottlieb et al., 1990; Nash, 1990a,b; Jennison, 1991; Williamson, 1991.

[2] Interest in CQI is not confined to the hospital community. For example, the American Medical Record Association (AMRA; now the American Health Information Management Association) has recently compiled a useful bibliography of QA and CQI sources (AMRA, 1991) and distributed *The Memory Jogger*, a pocket-sized guide to basic CQI tools and methods (Brassard, 1988). The CQI movement has also spawned at least two newsletters. One is *QI/TQM*, which describes itself as the health care executive's guide to quality improvement through total quality management (*QI/TQM*, 1991). *Quality Connection* is a quarterly produced by the National Demonstration Project (NDP) on Quality Improvement in Health Care; NDP also sponsors a Quality Management Network and an electronic "Quality Information Support System." In this same vein, the Healthcare Forum, which offers educational programs for health care leaders, has launched the Quality Improvement Network project; its aim is to use quarterly meetings to link hospitals and hospital systems to permit them to share QI models and ideas (QRC, 1991).

cations for the way practice guidelines may be incorporated into the fabric of health care organizations.[3] The principles emphasize the following:

- close relationships between so-called customers and suppliers, that is, the partners in any given health care transaction;
- errors being more often the result of defects in systems (e.g., those for reporting test results or scheduling operating rooms) than the consequence of individual deficiencies ("bad apples");[4]
- planning, control, assessment, and improvement activities grounded in statistical and scientific precepts and techniques;
- reliance on internal (self-) monitoring—as opposed to external (regulatory) inspection—with mistakes viewed as "treasures" that should be used for learning and for resolving problems rather than as an occasion for punishment;
- standardization of processes (decreasing their variability) to reduce the opportunity for error and to link specific care processes to health outcomes;
- feedback to practitioners of statistical information on how their practices may differ from those of their peers or depart from evidence-based standards for practice;
- visible commitment to quality by the top leadership of the organization and involvement by all parts of the organization in processes of quality improvement; and
- a striving for continuous improvement in contrast to simply achieving preset goals.

Within this framework, sound practice guidelines and medical review criteria have several possible uses. First, to the extent that guidelines become more sensitive to patient preferences and participation in decisionmaking, they should improve patients' informed consent, their participation in decisionmaking and, ultimately, their satisfaction with both the processes and outcomes of care. Guidelines could also help identify important patient outcomes to incorporate in patient satisfaction surveys and other instruments designed to improve or assess "customer-supplier" relationships. Second,

---

[3] CQI has tended to assume an organizational context, that is, a hospital or large group practice. Its application to individual and small group practice has been little explored, although many of its principles, if not its techniques, appear relevant and worth considering in these settings (Stocker, 1989).

[4] Jennison (1991) notes that it is also important to study why competent physicians make errors. For example, she cites one hospital that identified "inadequate hypothesis generation" (consideration of possible diagnoses) as a major source of error in managing patients with congestive heart failure; for patients with pneumonia, "mismanagement of therapy" was the major problem (p. 453).

guidelines and review criteria could play a role in identifying possible quality problems arising from underuse, overuse, or incompetent provision of care. They may be particularly useful in instances in which short-term health outcomes (those that are most readily employed) may not be good indicators of long-term results.

Third, to the extent that guidelines identify how compelling is the evidence for certain clinical practices, they will help in determining priorities for improving or standardizing specific patterns of clinical care and in sorting out competing claims for funding for biomedical and outcomes or effectiveness research. Fourth, participation by clinicians in the review, critique, and improvement of practice guidelines can help bring the science of medicine more forcefully into the equivalent "cycles" emphasized by CQI.

Just as guidelines have the potential to contribute to continuous quality improvement, the application of CQI principles and processes can support the effective implementation of practice guidelines. Schoenbaum notes (1990, p. 102) that between the step in an algorithm (guideline) directing a colonoscopy and the actual procedure lie "dozens or hundreds of steps," such as locating, notifying, scheduling, and preparing patients. At all of these points things can and sometimes do go awry in ways that may undermine the successful application of guidelines for appropriate care. A number of CQI techniques are designed to uncover such process flaws and to structure activities to correct them. Moreover, because CQI generally tends to have a "quantitative" emphasis and to be detail oriented, it may encourage those who design practice guidelines and medical review criteria to be more explicit, specific, and comprehensive with respect to the clinical content of guidelines and to better anticipate and confront the practical problems that may face prospective users of guidelines. In addition, the CQI stress on cycles of planning, testing, evaluating, and revising of procedures—the "Plan/Test/Check/Act" cycle—can encourage the processes of guideline assessment and improvement called for in this report and elsewhere.

Although practice guidelines have a potential role in CQI, some aspects of CQI models or strategies may deflect attention from guidelines. To date, CQI efforts have tended to focus more on nonclinical than on clinical issues. Quality problems arising from poor clinical performance and decisionmaking thus have not been highlighted (Causey, 1991). In discussing a series of quality management projects, Berwick and colleagues (1990, p. 24) reported that few of the project teams tackled clinical processes; rather, they focused on problems similar to those found in other industries, problems that were on the "comfortable fringes" of clinical processes. Typical of the problems to which these and other projects gave attention were the length of time needed to get X-rays posted to the medical record department, the late arrival of patient meals, and delays in patient discharge or admission. Williamson (1991) cites a study of TQM prepared for the federal Office of Management and Budget that reports that "nearly 40 of 44 examples [almost 90 percent] of improvement achieved focused specifically on administration process variables as opposed to outcomes, especially health outcomes" (p. 55).

How much this near-total emphasis on administrative rather than clinical processes will change as CQI becomes more institutionalized is unknown. Also unclear is how much the focus should change given the unknown magnitude of clinical versus nonclinical quality programs and the relative susceptibility of each to improvement. The focus on nonclinical issues is, in any case, understandable. CQI is still relatively new, users are looking for easier rather than harder targets of opportunity, and nonclinical problems are likely to be easier to solve from both technical and behavioral perspectives.

Nonetheless, even when clinical outcomes are at issue, practice guidelines and outcome measures do not appear to be widely perceived or explicitly applied as benchmarks for informing or assessing performance. For example, in a recent article examining CQI concepts and applications for physician care, the only reference to practice guidelines occurred in a discussion on the need for chart review and other monitoring activities to supplement CQI (Kritchevsky and Simmons, 1991).

Among the hospitals visited during this study, several were using or trying to develop clinical protocols or pathways that specified the sequence and timing of various interventions for different clinical problems; the object was to standardize practice and reduce errors. (Appendix A presents a pathway for coronary artery bypass surgery.) Most pathways in these hospitals and elsewhere appear to be built on implicit clinical judgments and local statistical data rather than on systematically developed practice guidelines (Coombs, 1991). This reflects the highly operational environment of pathway development and the relatively immediate opportunities for incremental action, monitoring, and adjustment. The focus of most pathways appears to be when and how to undertake a particular intervention (such as cardiac monitoring or respiratory therapy), not whether the intervention is appropriate.

Similarly, in confidential materials reviewed by the committee, several organizations structured their feedback to physicians almost entirely in statistical terms, in part because they feared that substantive guidelines might antagonize physicians, at least initially. An individual physician might be informed how often he or she performed a particular procedure compared with patterns of care for the same procedure by peers—without an explicit accompanying statement of the appropriate indications for the procedure.

Notwithstanding that the principle of variation reduction may be generally sound, specific reductions in practice variation and moves toward consistency are not inevitably shifts toward more appropriate care. Quantitative analyses of variation ideally should consider explicit practice guidelines as one reference point, given that soundly developed guidelines represent the best current understanding of which health interventions will produce desired results (Coombs, 1991). This understanding, in turn, can be evaluated and revised based on a systems study of the link between practice choices and short- and long-term changes in health outcomes.

To some degree, reliance on statistical feedback may reflect the lack of credible, relevant, and specific guidelines for problems targeted by a quality improvement effort. However, other explanations are also likely to apply. One anonymous reviewer of this report observed that many advocates of CQI see practice guidelines as "outdated." This view may reflect an identification of guidelines with the procedures for external review that have been widely criticized by CQI proponents, both on grounds of general principle and on grounds of poor administration. In stressing internal strategies for improvement and rejecting outside review, advocates of CQI may disregard the legitimate interest of other parties in external oversight and systems-level monitoring through retrospective, concurrent, and prospective review programs.

In this context, it is important to recall the observation in the IOM report (1990i) on quality of care in the Medicare program that the superiority of specific CQI techniques, although plausible, has not been demonstrated. Further, and consistent with the sense of the committee, Williamson (1991) reports that "many [CQI] advocates whom I have queried acknowledge that they have had difficulties adopting industrial [quality improvement] methods to clinical outcomes" (p. 55). As a practical matter, people are still trying to grasp what CQI means, how to use it, and how to assess its impact.[5] As one hospital manager said, "We are only at mile two on a never ending journey" (Causey, 1991, p. 3). The stress on guidelines is even more recent than the promotion of CQI and postdates the initiation of CQI projects in many institutions. As credible and relevant practice guidelines become more available and more widely known, they should be perceived as more relevant to those attempting to implement quality improvement models in health care settings.

Medical Review Criteria

Although CQI programs may emphasize professionalism and internal quality improvement rather than regulation and external inspection, both

---

[5] One result is a thriving business for consultants as health care institutions call on them for assistance in understanding and using the CQI model. One observer pungently reflected on the quality of this business: "Some consultants are real gems; some are semi-precious; and some are rocks" (Curt Lindberg, quoted in Burda, 1991a, p. 27).

approaches are needed for a public program such as Medicare and for private health plans that are accountable to employers and others for their performance. How well a continuous improvement mentality can dovetail with outside monitoring, periodic audits, and externally developed review criteria is an important—and unanswered—question. The characteristics of specific medical review criteria and the processes for developing and applying them can make coexistence either easier or more difficult.

General Issues in the Use of Medical Review Criteria

Medical review criteria may be used for quality assessment and improvement purposes and also as part of utilization management programs that aim to reduce spending for unnecessary and inappropriate care. Some will be derived from existing practice guidelines; others may be developed de novo. Like guidelines for clinical practice, some review criteria will be more credible, sophisticated, and useful than others.

Although quality and utilization review require specificity in review criteria, these criteria will not necessarily incorporate every recommendation or specification contained in a set of guidelines. For example, in the judgment of a review organization, some elements of a set of guidelines to assist clinical decisionmaking may not provide sufficient additional information to justify the cost of using them in the review process.

Review programs may add to as well as subtract from particular practice guidelines. As a case in point, review programs directed at patterns of care may employ quantitative thresholds that do not appear in guidelines to assist individual patient or practitioner decisionmaking. Thus, such programs may specify institutional rates of infection or percentages of surgery with normal tissue removed that will trigger remedial actions or further investigation.

Processes for creating review criteria from scratch or for transforming guidelines into review criteria and related tools have been little documented and appear to vary considerably. Many review criteria are not based on clinical practice guidelines at all but originate in "global" judgments about the "proper" frequency of certain tests or the acceptable interval between office visits. Such judgments may involve some kind of systematic process of expert judgment, or they may involve only an organization's medical director or consultant. Organizations that consider their review criteria proprietary may reveal little of the processes they use to create them.

The lack of external scrutiny of review criteria is a major criticism of many public and private utilization management programs (IOM, 1989a). Practitioners complain that they cannot find out in advance what are the criteria for review decisions; this particular criticism has been leveled frequently at the actions of Medicare carriers and fiscal intermediaries (but not at Medicare peer review organizations, or PROs). Clinicians also complain that criteria differ from organization to organization and sometimes conflict, even when they are said to be based on the same starting point.[6] Nonpublic criteria also preclude the kinds of education efforts described in the preceding chapter. Review organizations, in turn, express concern about physicians who may try to "game the system" if they know the review criteria in advance.

Selected Illustrative Activities Related to Medical Review Criteria

Public Sector Medicare peer review organizations have for the past few years been expected to carry out a variety of utilization review activities, chiefly preprocedure and preadmission review as well as some retrospective review (IOM, 1990i, see especially vol. 2). The PROs, which are regulated and directed in great detail in many respects, have been explicitly granted considerable freedom either to use national criteria or to develop their own criteria for these tasks, based on local patterns of practice.

PROs have submitted their criteria to the Health Care Financing Administration (HCFA) for approval, but variability among PROs and between PRO criteria and national guidelines has nevertheless been considerable (Project Hope, 1987; IOM, 1990i). PRO review criteria have also been criticized for lack of precision and specificity and poor documentation. A recent study of PRO preprocedure review criteria found considerable variability in criteria for carotid endarterectomy and cataract removal but less for cardiac pacemaker implants (Kellie and Kelly, 1991). In an effort to move toward greater consistency (and efficiency), the American Medical Peer Review Association in early 1991 drafted a two-volume set of review criteria for some 3,000 surgical procedures.[7] Further, HCFA-funded pilot projects to develop methods and criteria for evaluating office-based care are being undertaken with a level of conscientiousness that reflects the sensitiv-

---

[6] Criteria for reviewing the appropriateness of hospital admissions and continued hospital stays are often based on the AEP or Appropriateness Evaluation Protocol (Gertman and Restuccia, 1981) or the ISD-A criteria set (Intensity of services, Severity of illness, Discharge and Appropriateness screens; InterQual, 1987). These systems ostensibly provide the same or similar guidance about appropriateness of inpatient care, but depending on the interpretations of information made by those who apply the criteria, they may yield quite different findings.

[7] The use of this document in actual PRO activities may prove moot if PROs do not continue to conduct preprocedure reviews. The so-called Fourth Scope of Work issued by HCFA for the PRO program eliminated all preprocedure review (as of October 1991). The PRO community objected greatly to this change in their usual required activities, believing that preprocedure review had been a successful aspect of their work. PROs are permitted to propose to continue such activities as part of special review objectives.

ity of the quality assurance community to charges of poorly developed or "black box" criteria (Darby, 1991a).

Consistent with its charge to arrange for the development of medical review criteria as well as practice guidelines, AHCPR in August 1991 issued a request for proposals (RFP) with three major aims: (1) to derive review criteria from AHCPR guidelines on benign prostatic hypertrophy (BPH), urinary incontinence, and postoperative pain management; (2) to apply these criteria to samples of hospital or nursing home records that have already been reviewed by the PROs to determine how using these criteria will affect current PRO processes to identify quality and utilization problems; and (3) to evaluate practitioner education programs related to the parent BPH guideline document and its associated review criteria. The work will begin in late 1991 under the direction of the American Medical Review Research Center with the assistance of four PROs (Alabama, Massachusetts, Michigan, and Pennsylvania) and a large group of consultants; it is scheduled to be completed by September 1993. It is expected that the three (original) guideline panels will evaluate the review criteria developed in this project. At the time this report was being prepared, a similar "non-PRO" RFP was expected as well.

In addition to these efforts, the agency will create a new expert panel to develop criteria for evaluating medical review criteria. The panel will consist of representatives of Medicare PROs, health maintenance organizations, private insurers, and others in the private sector, as well as HCFA staff.

Private Sector   Value Health Sciences (VHS), a for-profit utilization management company, creates its preprocedure and other prior-authorization review criteria in a formal manner. Originally it based its Medical Review System (MRS) criteria on appropriateness indications developed by a team of researchers at the RAND Corporation and the University of California at Los Angeles. VHS incorporated those very complex indications through a specific set of steps and supporting tools into detailed computer algorithms. The RAND work is in the public domain; the VHS work is not. Other companies are developing somewhat similar strategies linked to the RAND methodology (Winslow, 1990).

The VHS MRS technology has the following components: (1) selection of procedures according to several criteria including risks to patients, financial impact of the procedure, and extent of agreement about appropriateness within the medical community; (2) review of the medical literature with respect to circumstances in which the procedure has been shown to be effective or ineffective; (3) development of a "framework" of clinical criteria of appropriateness for major procedures, using a "catalogue" of indications (detailed descriptions of specific classes of patients who are potential candidates for the procedure); (4) review and refinement of the framework by expert practicing physicians who rate the appropriateness of each indication and define decision rules; and (5) development of "smart questioning logic" and other software that will collect the key clinical data required to apply the criteria as well as a set of detailed guidelines for each question in the logic to ensure that the products are used consistently. VHS has also created a training program to help nurses, administrators, and physicians understand both the clinical standards of care embedded in the criteria and algorithms and use of the MRS itself. VHS updates the criteria regularly.

Directions for Quality Assurance Strategies

The committee believes that well-developed, scientifically based practice guidelines have an important role to play in assessing and assuring the quality of health care services provided in this country. Clear, specific guidelines and associated review criteria should help deter or remedy problems of overuse of care, underuse of care, and poor technical and interpersonal provision of care. Guidelines accepted by those responsible for providing care, those responsible for financing it, and those responsible for monitoring care in the public interest are one means of bridging the chasm between internal and external quality assurance strategies.

With respect to models of quality assurance as discussed earlier, the committee urges that their focus on systems problems, on improvement of average performance, and on variation reduction be more systematically and explicitly joined with an effort to apply and improve sound guidelines for clinical practice. Specifically, the committee urges the following:

• Guidelines, medical review criteria, and other evaluative tools should be used both to improve average performance and—as is still important—identify substandard performance.

• Analyses of how individual practice patterns differ from average patterns should go beyond statistical analysis to consider relevant practice guidelines as benchmarks for performance.

• Both the statistical information from such analyses and the pertinent guidelines should be part of educational feedback on practice patterns.

• Evaluations of performance and outcome data should seek to determine the sources of poor outcomes and deviations from guidelines so that systems problems can be corrected, information efforts strengthened, and, if necessary, impaired practitioners dealt with through counseling, limiting of privileges, or other appropriate mechanisms.

• Evaluations of performance and outcomes data should also be used to determine whether practice guidelines ought to be updated or revised.

• Developers of guidelines and health care institutions should convene educational conferences to acquaint practitioners with specific guidelines and provide an opportunity for them to discuss and plan setting-specific applications.

• Institutional activities to develop guidelines or adapt national practice guidelines should aspire to the attributes for guidelines described in Chapter 1 of this report.

The committee suggests that the popularization of continuous quality improvement in the health arena may have underemphasized a principle that was clearly articulated by Deming and others in their original discussions of CQI in the industrial sector. This principle is that an organization must integrate the science of its field into its day-to-day workings. When applied to health care, the principle brings the role of science-based guidelines more to the fore. In other words, each of the activities listed earlier is a vehicle for bringing science-based guidelines into efforts at quality management and improvement.

In addition, the committee recognized the controversy that has developed over the use and content of medical review criteria, and consequently identified several desirable attributes of such criteria. These eight attributes are analogous to those described in Chapter 1 for clinical practice guidelines. They are listed in Table 5-1. Both sets of attributes build on the IOM report on quality assessment and assurance for the Medicare program, which identified 23 desirable attributes of what it termed appropriateness indicators, case-finding screens, and evaluation and management criteria.

Generally, the committee would prefer carefully devised "national" review criteria to those developed locally, for reasons that are discussed more thoroughly in Chapter 7's examination of local adaptation of practice guidelines. In addition, like guidelines, review criteria should be accompanied by documentation of the procedures followed, the participants involved, and the evidence or guidelines used as a basis for designing them. By providing such information, review organizations can respond to some of the more serious criticisms of their credibility.

COST MANAGEMENT

Virtually everyone involved in health care stands to benefit from guidelines that offer decisionmakers careful estimates of the costs of alternative courses of care in relation to their benefits. Health care institutions may refer to such guidelines in making investment and other decisions. For example, although recent reports about the costs and benefits of alternative thrombolytic drugs are not formal guidelines, they may influence purchasing decisions by hospitals as well as patient management decisions by individual practitioners (O'Donnell, 1991). Similarly, hospitals may look to similar reports about anti-infective agents to control nosocomial infections

TABLE 5-1   Desirable Attributes of Medical Review Criteria

Attribute	Explanation
SENSITIVITY	Review criteria are sensitive when it is highly likely that a case will be identified as deficient given that it really is deficient. (This assumes that a guideline or other source provides a "gold standard.")
SPECIFICITY	Review criteria are specific if it is highly likely that they will identify truly good care as such.
PATIENT RESPONSIVENESS	Review criteria specifically identify a role for patient preferences or the process for using them allows for some consideration of patient preferences.
READABILITY	Review criteria are presented in language and formats that can be read and understood by nonphysician reviewers, practitioners, and patients/consumers.
MINIMUM OBTRUSIVENESS	Review criteria and the process for applying them minimize inappropriate direct interaction with and burdens on the treating practitioner or patient.
FEASIBILITY	The information required for review can be obtained easily from direct communication with providers, patients, records, and other sources, and the decision criteria are easy to apply. Review criteria are accompanied by explicit instructions for their application and scoring.
COMPUTER COMPATIBILITY	Review criteria are straightforward enough that they can be transformed readily into the computer-based protocols and similar formats that can make the review process more efficient for all involved parties.
APPEALS CRITERIA	Criteria provide explicit guidance about the considerations to be taken into account when adverse review decisions are appealed by professionals or patients.

as a means of selecting a cost-effective agent (Weinstein et al., 1986). New research findings in turn may challenge these results—a fact of life for clinicians and those trying to advise them.

Public and private payers are clearly interested in guidelines as potential instruments to control costs. That kind of attention is a major source of anxiety for professional groups that are involved in developing guidelines and for individual professionals who are exposed to payer efforts to influence practice in conformity with guidelines.

Others involved in guidelines development and related technology assessment efforts see payer interest as a major source of support. One analysis of the potential gains to be made by eliminating unexplained variation in 25 common medical interventions argues that the savings produced by convincingly executed technology assessments of these services would greatly outweigh the cost of the assessments (Phelps and Parente, 1990). Whether reality can be so ordered that it comes close to matching this potential is untested. The committee reiterates its earlier caution against overly optimistic expectations that guidelines, taken collectively, will produce net reductions in the rate of increase in health care spending.

Payers can use guidelines in various ways: (1) to help determine health insurance coverage and avoid payment for unnecessary or inappropriate care, (2) to aid in selecting or credentialing practitioners for participation in various health plans or institutions, and (3) to tailor other economic incentives to affect practitioner or patient behavior. Such approaches usually do not depend on a specific organized practice setting; that is, they can affect practitioners and patients in solo or group practice settings as well as those in larger organizational or institutional settings. Some approaches may be more or less confined to third-party payers whereas others may be shared by health care institutions, quality review programs, and others.

The following sections discuss how these cost-management strategies may support and be supported by practice guidelines and review criteria. One section discusses legal liability issues for third-party payers and others, particularly as these issues relate to decisions about payment.

Coverage Policy and Administration

As described in the second case study in Chapter 3, health benefit plans are a clear "market" for guidelines and review criteria. These plans apply guidelines in various ways to limit their liability for particular expenses and to influence practitioner or patient behavior (IOM, 1989a). When existing guidelines do not meet their needs, health plans may undertake their own development initiatives.

In this context, health benefit plans include traditional indemnity insurance and Blue Cross/Blue Shield programs, self-insured employer plans, preferred provider organizations (PPOs), and health maintenance organizations (HMOs), as well as the various organizations that may provide these plans with such services as claims administration and utilization management. Although public plans such as Medicare and Medicaid may operate under special legal and other constraints, much of this commentary applies to these plans as well.

Types of Coverage Decisions

In considering how health plan features may affect the application of guidelines by practitioners and patients, several distinctions are useful. First, coverage policy as explicitly delineated in health insurance contracts often is not specific to particular clinical problems; rather, policies typically describe broad ranges of covered services—for example, hospital care, physician services, or prescription drugs.

Second, health plan contracts may state that coverage is limited to care that is medically necessary or appropriate and not experimental. This kind of policy requires criteria that allow payers to distinguish instances in which particular services are not necessary or appropriate for patients with specific clinical problems. Although these criteria may also be used for educational purposes and in contracts that explicitly exclude the use of particular procedures for specific conditions, they typically come into play in case-by-case examinations of care that has been proposed or already provided.[8] Without a general contractual provision limiting care to that which is medically necessary, denials of payment based on prospective, concurrent, or retrospective utilization review may not be upheld. In fact, because provisions in insurance contracts must, in common law, be interpreted in favor of the insured in borderline or ambiguous situations, failure of a contract to authorize prospective, concurrent, or retrospective review may lead to a similar finding.[9]

Third, when contracts exclude coverage for a specific type of procedure or other service, the intent may be simply to contain costs by precluding or limiting payment rather than precluding or discouraging behavior. Thus, traditional insurance plans have often excluded immunizations from covered physician care; the intent is to limit insurance payments for routine, inexpensive, predictable, and thus budgetable services rather than specifi-

---

[8] One recent judicial ruling, if widely followed, could significantly increase the burdens on insurers seeking to deny coverage for new treatments. A U.S. District Court held that an insurer had to obtain data to show whether a procedure would work rather than wait "until somebody chooses to present statistical proof that would satisfy all experts that a treatment will work" (*Pirozzi* v. *Blue Cross and Blue Shield of Virginia* 741 F. Supp 586 [E.D.Va. 1990]). The procedure in question involved near lethal doses of chemotherapy combined with a bone marrow transplant for a patient with breast cancer.

[9] In one of the better-known cases on the liability of utilization review organizations, *Wilson* v. *Blue Cross of California* (222 Cal. App. 3d 660 [1990]), a major issue is the plan's apparent lack of a contractual basis for conducting a prospective review of medical necessity. The case is more commonly cited for the appeals court decision saying that physician failure to appeal a negative review decision is not a sufficient basis for precluding a review program's liability for harm to a patient. An earlier case, *Wickline* v. *California* (228 Cal. Rptr. 661 [Cal. App. 1986]) was widely viewed as suggesting such protection might exist.

cally to discourage patients from obtaining them.[10] Particular services may be excluded, however, because of concerns that they have a high potential for inappropriate or unnecessary use.

In sum, health plan coverage is a general term. Health plan contracts may describe coverage in terms of (1) very broad categories of included services, such as hospital or physician care, or excluded services, such as dental care; (2) specifically named treatments or types of care that are covered or excluded, such as particular transplants; or (3) care that is medically necessary or appropriate without explicit contractual reference to specific services and conditions. Guidelines are most relevant to decisions involving the last two categories.

Medical Review Criteria and Managing Benefit Costs

The general issues in medical review discussed earlier are also relevant to the use of medical review criteria in programs to limit payment for medically unnecessary or inappropriate care. For both quality assessment and cost containment purposes, review programs have relied primarily on retrospective utilization review (i.e., review after care has been provided) and secondarily on concurrent review of inpatient care (Fitzpatrick, 1965; Young, 1965; Gosfield, 1975, 1989; IOM, 1989a).

Retrospective utilization review by third-party payers may comprise either the review of individual claims for payment (and sometimes related patient medical records) or the profiling of provider practice patterns. In some cases, payment may be denied for services that are judged to be unnecessary; in other cases, efforts may be made to inform physicians about practices that are viewed by the payer as questionable. (Retrospective utilization review programs mounted by hospitals and other organizations for their own purposes work somewhat differently, in part because the results of such reviews are unlikely to affect reimbursement and are more likely to feed into educational or management activities.)

Many health plans have shifted their emphasis to prior review programs. One rationale for this shift is that such programs could have a sentinel effect, deterring practitioners from proposing or performing certain unnecessary services in the first place and thus shielding patients from needless medical risk and inconvenience. Another rationale is that prior review programs are less negative or punitive than denying payment for care that has already been delivered. Yet any familiarity with the popular medical press, with legislative hearings, and with medical society meetings will suggest that practitioners resent the intervention and second-guessing

---

[10] To encourage these services and to compete with HMOs, many of these plans are now covering selected preventive services.

of such programs as much (or more) than they ever resented retrospective payment denials. Many of the criteria used for prior review are adapted from criteria used for retrospective review—in theory, with due regard for the greater uncertainty about a patient's condition that exists before a hospital admission or other action.

Whether utilization review programs control costs has not been clearly demonstrated (IOM, 1989a). The case is more convincing for prior review of inpatient admissions; when administrative costs and costs for outpatient or other alternative (or delayed) care are considered, the results are mixed.

In any case, the availability of sound guidelines for clinical practice and their competent translation into criteria, software, and other elements of a review program are clearly critical for the effective, responsible use of utilization review programs. Conversely, the use of good guidelines and review criteria in well-administered review programs can be an important vehicle for rationalizing care and, perhaps, controlling costs.

Review criteria and programs have been criticized on many grounds, both substantive and procedural. This report has noted the "hassle factor" at several points and the nonpublic nature of the criteria used by many programs. Many of the criticisms of review criteria parallel criticisms of guidelines: review criteria have been described as subjective, arbitrary, vague, inconsistent with scientific evidence, insensitive to patient preferences, and unevaluated with respect to health outcomes.

To the extent that review criteria reflect the eight attributes discussed earlier in this chapter, organizations using these criteria should generate less hostility and more acceptance (assuming open and sensitive application techniques). Similarly, to the extent that the guidelines development efforts of public and private organizations are shaped by the attributes identified in Chapter 1, the committee expects that their products will generally be welcomed and used by review organizations and payers; that, in turn, should make the criteria more credible.

Concerns about Tort Liability

Although developers of guidelines should expect to be treated as legally accountable for exercising due care in formulating their recommendations and in updating them in the light of new knowledge (Brennan, 1991b; Hall, 1991), this committee at this time knows of no cases in which they have been sued or held liable for harm to patients resulting from negligent standard setting (AMA, 1990b; Miller, 1991). Even insurers, who have faced and lost many cases related to their cost-containment programs, have been involved in few cases that involve allegations of medical harm. Rather, most cases focus on financial harm, that is, denials of payment for care.

The primary issues are whether the denials were supported by contract language and were administered competently and in good faith.[11]

However, as insurers and review organizations have moved more aggressively to apply guidelines, medical review criteria, and similar tools, they have been the subject of some highly publicized litigation alleging that review determinations have caused medical harm. Unfortunately, this litigation has, to date, produced more questions than answers about when reviewers—to say nothing of developers of guidelines—might be held negligent for medical harm to a patient (Helvestine, 1989; Gosfield, 1991a,b; Miller, 1991).

For a developer or third-party user of a guideline to be held liable for medical harm to a patient, four questions must be answered positively (as in all negligence cases; Miller, 1991). Do the guidelines developers or review programs applying guidelines have a duty of care to patients? Has that duty been breached? Was there injury? Was the breach of duty a proximate cause of the injury?

The answer to the first question about the duty of care appears fairly clear in the case of review programs, despite the paucity of specific cases. For example, in *Wickline* v. *California* (228 Cal. Rptr. 661 [1986]), the court held that "third party payers . . . can be held legally accountable when medically inappropriate decisions result from defects in the design or implementation of cost containment mechanisms" (p. 670). The third party in this particular case was the state Medicaid program, whose application of length-of-stay criteria during concurrent review was alleged to have resulted in patient harm (specifically, an avoidable amputation) that resulted from the patient's premature discharge from the hospital.

The Wickline case, however, never directly addressed the question of whether the Medicaid review program breached a duty of care—in particu-

---

[11] In this regard, some recent cases should be noted involving the Employee Retirement and Income Security Act of 1976, which generally has been interpreted as exempting employers' self-insured health plans from state regulation and tort claims (Costich, 1990-1991). In some cases, courts have rejected some denials of benefits by such plans as being "arbitrary and capricious"; this standard substantially defers to the judgments of plan administrators. In other cases, courts have more fundamentally challenged the judgments of plan administrators, declaring certain determinations as inconsistent with expert medical judgment on the basis of de novo judicial review of the evidence. The cases have involved what the health plans have deemed noncovered "experimental" or "investigational" services including some types of autologous bone marrow transplants, radial keratotomy, and "coma arousal" programs: See, for example, *Pirozzi* v. *Blue Cross-Blue Shield of Virginia* (741 F. Supp. 586 [1990]) and *Rollo* v. *Blue Cross-Blue Shield of New Jersey* (D.N.J., March 22, 1990). Although the court in the Pirozzi case indicated that health plan decisions based on medical necessity rather than on the experimental nature of a service were due more deference, it is not clear that health plans should count on other courts following this principle.

lar, whether its review criteria were defective. The court held that the injured patient's physician was "acting within the standards of the medical profession" (p. 667) in discharging the patient even though he disagreed with the Medicaid length-of-stay criteria. Because the early discharge did not violate the standard of care and was not a proximate cause of injury, the court did not need to consider the role of the Medicaid directive itself.

For review organizations, the question of proximate cause seems to hinge largely on the degree to which physicians are held responsible for care prompted by review determinations and for failure to appeal a medically inappropriate determination. The Wickline case seemed to suggest that, even if a review determination was faulty, the action of the reviewers would not be viewed as a proximate cause of harm if the patient's physician acquiesced to the review determination without protest. It stated that "the physician who complies without protest . . . when his medical judgment dictates otherwise, cannot avoid his ultimate responsibility for his patient's care" (p. 671).

In contrast, in an as yet unresolved case, *Wilson* v. *Blue Cross of California* (222 Cal. App. 3d 660 [1990]), an appeals court held that a physician's failure to protest did not automatically protect a private review organization from tort liability (even though a state government might set different rules for public programs); it sent the case back to the trial court for further proceedings. It is unclear whether this case, once it has been fully litigated, will provide more specific precedents on such matters as negligent application of standards for appropriate care because other facts of the case appear likely to determine the outcome.[12] The issue of negligent setting or selection of standards by the review organization apparently has not been raised.

Overall, prudence dictates that those developing guidelines or review criteria and those applying them in medical review programs should expect to be held legally accountable for their actions and should manage their affairs accordingly. In the words of the IOM report on utilization manage-

---

[12] The Wilson case, which is emotionally charged because the patient in question committed suicide, is factually complicated. The review organization (Western Medical) that had advised that further hospitalization for the patient was unnecessary was an agent of the California Blue Cross plan. The California plan, in turn, was acting for Blue Cross/Blue Shield of Alabama, by which the injured party was insured. The plaintiffs argue that the Alabama plan's contract with the patient had no provision for utilization review and, in fact, explicitly defers to the attending physician to determine when hospital care is necessary. Such contract provisions provide the basis for charges that the defendants acted in bad faith—regardless of the soundness of the review procedures or criteria employed. The reasonableness of those review procedures and criteria has also been challenged, but this issue will not necessarily be addressed if the bad faith arguments are successful. The physician in this case was not initially sued for malpractice for having discharged the patient without protest; he has since been brought into the case as a cross-defendant by the original defendants (Peter Aronson, attorney for the plaintiffs, personal communication, December 10, 1991).

ment (1989a), they should seek the general—but not infallible—protections against liability offered by "good management, good judgment, good faith, and good documentation."

Review programs almost certainly have more to worry about than independent developers of guidelines such as medical specialty societies. Moreover, the potential for liability related to the application of guidelines "can logically be extended to cover any . . . entity—such as a hospital or malpractice insurer—offering benefits or imposing sanctions for professional behavior related to specific guidelines" (Miller, 1991, p. 32). For example, one might question with respect to an HMO whether its financial inducements for parsimonious care were so strong that "they could be anticipated to corrupt clinical judgment" (p. 31). Those using the selective contracting and credentialing techniques described below should also be aware of the potential liability for defects in their application of guidelines and review criteria.

Credentialing, Selective Contracting, and Related Strategies

In theory, guidelines may inform decisions made by health care institutions, HMOs, and other organizations about the selection and retention of practitioners. Such decisions may involve the initial credentialing of physicians and ongoing delineation of clinical privileges in hospitals and other institutions. They may also involve hiring and contracting decisions in a variety of contexts. Most selection or credentialing decisions are based on educational qualifications, licensure, board eligibility or certification, previous positions, willingness to abide by organizational policies, and similar factors. However, quality objectives, liability concerns, and cost-management objectives are providing the impetus to develop and apply more direct measures of medical competence and performance (Gosfield, 1991b). The specifics of this process, including the role of practice guidelines, are still being defined (Langsley, 1991).

Health benefit plans and health care institutions that somehow select or "credential" practitioners have several opportunities to encourage the application of practice guidelines.[13] For example, they can make employment, participation, or privileges contingent on a practitioner's prior agreement to practice in accord with the organization's clinical policies. Among the sites visited by the study committee was a group of primary care clinics that employed physicians with the understanding that they would practice in

---

[13] A variant on this theme is for the employer, rather than a health care institution, HMO, or insurer, to hire or contract with practitioners directly to provide routine health care services to employees. A practice with a long history in certain companies that operate in geographically isolated areas, its revival as a concept apparently reflects its cost-containment appeal.

conformity with the clinic's primary care manual and that their practice would be evaluated annually. The group's primary care manual is a collection of both what this committee considers systematically developed guidelines and protocols and policies that reflect the system's patient population, resources, and objectives.

Guidelines can be worked into credentialing and other decisions in several ways. Depending on the access of a health benefit plan to relevant data sources, a plan can examine or profile the practice patterns of candidates for new or continued employment, contracts, or privileges to determine whether they already practice in accordance with selected guidelines. This review of practice may be based on claims data, medical records, and on-site observation (Stocker, 1989). Currently, however, nonclinical factors, such as geography and the willingness of providers to agree to health plan terms, may play the major role in selection and deselection decisions. The committee knows of no good evidence on the subject, but it suspects that profiling based explicitly on clinical practice guidelines is less common than simpler profiling based on utilization rates or levels.[14]

To the extent that credentialing, selective contracting, and similar strategies work well and are supported by ongoing health plan structures and processes, they presumably should bring into health plans and institutions those practitioners who are already committed to the desired practice patterns and then help to maintain that commitment. To maintain or redefine desired performance, other strategies are necessary. These may be both negative (e.g., financial penalties or even dismissal from the plan for unacceptable performance) and positive (e.g., education and feedback consistent with quality improvement models). Guidelines may contribute to the definition of what constitutes acceptable clinical performance for purposes of education, feedback, or evaluation.

Interestingly, one major initiative that is very strongly linked to the concept of selective contracting or purchasing, InterStudy's Outcomes Management System, makes little explicit reference to practice guidelines (InterStudy, 1991). This system is built on four main elements: (1) protocols and instruments for collecting data on patient satisfaction, functional status, demographic and other characteristics of patients, insurance status, and treatment setting; (2) condition-specific measures of changes in patient status over a course of treatment; (3) construction of a national data base; and (4) practitioners and analysts working in participating organizations to analyze information and promote change.[15] With InterStudy acting as coordinator,

---

[14] What has been called economic credentialing may involve primarily comparisons of costs and revenues generated by a practitioner.

[15] The system has 16 data collection protocols, 3 of which were provided to the committee. Only the protocol on diabetes made direct reference to practice guidelines; the protocols on cataracts and prostatism did not (Hoogwerf, 1989; Javitt and Ware, 1990; Fowler, 1991).

two consortia, one involving six large group practices and another (in the planning stage) involving 24 employers, are engaged in a major effort to test this system.

One appealing feature of selective contracting is that it can reach beyond the hospital and large group practice to office-based practitioners in small group practices, at least when it is used by independent practice associations (IPAs), PPOs, and similar groups. Thus, it can encourage conformity with good guidelines in settings less readily reached by other strategies. However, one question about the use of guidelines in closed panel systems with incentives for physicians to control costs is what information should be provided to consumers about the incentives, guidelines, or other components of these plans. This question is explored in the next chapter.

Other Economic Incentives

Many health plans and public programs use explicit financial incentives to influence practitioner or patient behavior without explicitly attempting to encourage specific appropriate care and discourage specific inappropriate care (Brook, 1991). For example, in and of itself, typical patient cost-sharing in the form of deductibles and coinsurance applies equally to appropriate and inappropriate care. Likewise, capitated and per-case methods for paying health care practitioners and providers do not, in themselves, explicitly differentiate between appropriate and inappropriate care. When, however, such provider payment methods are used in conjunction with monitoring, educational, and other programs to detect poor quality care and to promote specific types of appropriate care, they may play an important strategic role in encouraging the application of sound guidelines.

Although explicit financial incentives have been rejected by many as philosophically objectionable or simply too controversial, some employers and insurers have designed positive or negative financial incentives to change specific consumer or patient behaviors that are inconsistent with recommended health practices and that are thought to lead to higher health care costs (New York Business Group on Health, 1990; Becker, 1991; Sipress, 1991; Terry, 1991). For example, some payers employ such incentives as insurance premium rebates (positive) or higher insurance premiums (negative) for individuals based on the results of blood, urine, and other tests related to recommended cholesterol and blood sugar levels, blood pressure, weight, and smoking. Some health plans cover or provide counseling for individuals who "fail" the tests; others do not. An unknown number of employers go further and refuse to hire individuals who are thought to be at higher risk of illness or injury because of their behavior or genetic inheritance.

Taking a different but also controversial approach, some theorists have proposed that consumers could be discouraged from demanding marginally beneficial care if they were offered choices among health plans that offered more or less generous levels of care as defined by different practice guidelines (Havighurst, 1990a, 1991a; Blumstein, 1991). To be covered for care for which the expected benefit is slight or questionable, consumers would buy a more expensive plan governed by more generous guidelines; if a less generous plan were chosen, consumers could, in principle, pay for such care on their own. Potentially, the guidelines could be incorporated into the health plan contract itself and referenced by specific name or they could be developed according to a process defined in the contract.

This contract-based strategy would offer direct economic incentives to the consumer in the first instance, with provider behavior affected as a consequence.[16] Whether policymakers would agree that patients and consumers are able to make informed choices about these important matters and that they should be held to their choices is an open question that demands thorough debate. Research and experience suggest that people frequently find some basic provisions of existing plans difficult to comprehend (McCall et al., 1986; National Association of Private Psychiatric Hospitals, 1991). Even if people understand their choices, is it fair to expect healthy people to make good choices about health insurance that would apply in the future, should they or their family members become ill? Aaron (1991) notes that "health insurance and health care pose special problems [for economic analysis because] health insurance typically is purchased by healthy people, while most health care is consumed by sick people. Society normally has little interest when people gamble and lose. But when the gamble concerns events that change basic preferences and that affect the life and health of oneself and one's family, it is not clear why past consumer decisions deserve priority over new preferences" (p. 17).

The more drastic the consequences of the choices people make about health care, the more compelling are these kinds of questions and arguments. Similar issues arise, for example, with respect to decisions involving living wills and advance directives about the use of life support in cases of terminal illness or injury. Judgments on such matters require a mix of empirical evidence (which may not be available), ethical judgments, and practical wisdom.

---

[16] As noted earlier, such contracts could very well conflict with the tendency in tort law toward a uniform standard of care (Morreim, 1989). Havighurst (Havighurst and Metzloff, 1991) suggests that malpractice determinations for contract-based care be taken out of the courts and dealt with under an arbitration system that would base its judgments on the standard of care specified in the contract.

Directions for Cost Management

On both philosophical and strategic grounds, this committee believes that thoughtfully designed and applied programs to encourage cost-effective use of health care have an important role to play in supporting the wider application of guidelines for clinical practice. Such programs need guidelines and related materials that provide information on the cost-effectiveness of alternative ways of managing particular clinical problems. They also need to be supplemented by explicit programs that employ guidelines and medical review criteria to monitor the quality and appropriateness of care.

Those who develop review criteria should be guided by the attributes for such criteria that were discussed in the section on quality assurance and improvement. Review organizations that allow these attributes to govern their work on criteria will make their review activities as manageable and as unintrusive as possible for both patients and practitioners. They will also make their review criteria available to practitioners and others. Furthermore, these organizations will provide an explicit process for appealing negative decisions that is free from unreasonable complexity, delay, or other barriers. If a review organization identifies quality-of-care problems, it should have procedures for, at a minimum, discussing these problems with the practitioner or provider involved and, perhaps (with due regard for legal risks), raising the matter with the relevant PRO.

It is the committee's hope that economic incentives and quality review mechanisms will, in the future, reduce the need for so-called micromanagement of professional and institutional behavior. Utilization review still may have a role in monitoring practice and targeting problems, but many payers will readily admit that they would prefer to rely more on effective self-regulation by practitioners and providers. Consistent with the principles of quality improvement, they can stress education and feedback to physicians aimed at improving practice rather than punishing missteps.

RISK MANAGEMENT, MEDICAL LIABILITY, AND PRACTICE GUIDELINES

Given the context in which clinical practice guidelines are being promoted, concerns about medical liability loom large. Any strategy to encourage the application of sound guidelines ought to consider the opportunities and obstacles presented by risk management programs and medical liability reforms. Such a strategy must also recognize the complexities introduced by quality assurance and CQI principles and by the existence of multiple and potentially conflicting guidelines (see Chapter 7).

Risk Management

Risk management programs attempt to evaluate and decrease liability risks related to clinical care, housekeeping functions, management decisions, and other sources. Liability claims may arise from adverse events experienced by patients, visitors, staff, and others—even by prospective patients turned away from care. Across health care institutions, risk management programs and quality assurance programs are generally distinct organizational functions with varying degrees of interaction (Donaldson and Lohr, 1990). The wider availability and application of clinical practice guidelines should provide a stimulus for closer coordination.

For risk management programs, clinical practice guidelines offer several potential benefits, as shown in Figure 5-1. First, the wider application of good guidelines should improve clinical performance and thereby reduce

---

HYPOTHESIS AND HOPE: Good Practice Guidelines, When Widely Disseminated and Integrated into Good Quality Assurance and Improvement Programs, Will Help

(1) IMPROVE MEDICAL PRACTICE AND QUALITY OF CARE
    (a) BETTER TECHNICAL CARE (less iatrogenesis, negligence)
        ↓ medical costs, ↓ legal costs
    (b) LESS OVERUSE (INCLUDING DEFENSIVE MEDICINE)
        ↓ medical costs, ↓ exposure to iatrogenesis
    (c) LESS UNDERUSE
        ↑ medical costs (short-term at least), ? legal costs*
    (d) BETTER ART OF CARE, PATIENT SATISFACTION
        ↓ legal costs, ? medical costs (net)

(2) STRENGTHEN ACCURATE EVALUATION OF CARE BY PEERS, PATIENTS, AND OTHERS
    (a) MORE NEGLIGENT CARE IDENTIFIED
    (b) LESS NONNEGLIGENT CARE MISLABELED

(3) IMPROVE QUALITY OF LITIGATION AND COMPENSATION FOR NEGLIGENCE
    (a) EARLIER RESOLUTION OF WORTHY CASES
        ↓ legal costs, ? medical costs
    (b) REDUCED PURSUIT OF UNWORTHY CASES
        ↓ legal costs, ↓ medical costs
    (c) FAIRER LIABILITY DETERMINATIONS
        ? legal costs, ? medical costs

*Question marks indicate that the net impact (increase or decrease) cannot be readily predicted.

FIGURE 5-1 Guidelines and Malpractice Incidence and Costs.

the number of adverse events. These outcomes have been one objective of guidelines for anesthesiology and emergency room care. An important corollary aim has been to have malpractice insurers recognize adherence to such guidelines as an indicator of lower risk and a basis for lower premiums (Eichorn et al., 1986; Holzer, 1990).

Second, practitioners and health care institutions should find well-developed, condition-specific or treatment-specific guidelines useful in communicating to patients the risks and benefits of treatment alternatives, thus helping patients to make informed choices among alternative courses of care. From a risk management perspective, among the objectives of such communication should be the reduction of litigation inspired by poor communication and of disappointment resulting from unrealistic patient expectations of perfect or guaranteed outcomes.

Third, guidelines that define appropriate care for specific clinical conditions can help in determining whether identified adverse events are the result of poor care rather than the unfortunate consequence of medical uncertainty. An adverse drug reaction following first-time administration of a drug to a patient with no ascertainable contraindications would fall in the latter category; a second use of the drug followed by another adverse reaction would, absent qualifying circumstances, likely be judged negligent (Brennan, 1991b). Sound guidelines should provide a strong basis for distinguishing negligent from nonnegligent care, which, in turn, should help deter unjustified malpractice claims, resolve justified claims earlier, and improve decisions for cases that go to trial.

Fourth, if practitioners have confidence in particular clinical practice guidelines and expect that documented conformance with these guidelines will do much to protect them against unwarranted claims (and findings) of malpractice, the anxieties that give rise to defensive medicine should diminish and the willingness to apply guidelines should increase. Given that defensive medicine occurs when practitioners provide or order services that are unnecessary except as potential malpractice protection, a reduction in defensive medicine should both improve quality of care and help contain health care costs.[17]

---

[17] The extent and consequences of defensive medicine have been the subject of much debate and are difficult to document empirically. A 1990 congressional report on medical malpractice cited two estimates of the costs of defensive medicine (U.S. House of Representatives, Committee on Ways and Means, 1990). First, it cited the American Medical Association's estimate that defensive medicine accounted for $11.7 billion (about 75 percent) of the total $15.4 billion cost for the medical liability system in 1985. Second, it reported HCFA's estimate that defensive medicine cost the Medicare program $2.5 billion in 1987. Such cost estimates are notoriously slippery (Mills and Lindgren, 1991) because they are based on physician self-reports, they ignore certain costs, and they do not reflect offsetting savings from avoided adverse events. A full discussion of the economics of malpractice must also acknowledge evidence that much negligence is never identified or compensated (Harvard Medical Practice Study, 1990; Brennan et al., 1991; Localio et al., 1991).

Medical Malpractice

The second, third, and fourth points above bring clinical practice guidelines directly into debates about medical liability, standards of care, and malpractice reform. Most proposals for malpractice reform concentrate on such issues as limits on punitive damages and use of alternative dispute resolution mechanisms; many, if not most, make no mention of practice guidelines (GAO, 1987; Macchiaroli, 1990; U.S. House of Representatives, Committee on Ways and Means, 1990; Miller, 1991). Nonetheless, the increasing interest in guidelines has prompted several analyses of their potential for improving decisionmaking in cases of alleged malpractice. Although opinions about this potential are mixed, the precept that "good medicine is good law" is widely accepted (Miller, 1991, p. 1).

The legal theory of liability provides a deterrent to wrong behavior as well as a form of redress for such behavior when it occurs. To influence behavior, the liability strategy relies on economic penalties and fear. In this context, the role for guidelines is not to motivate but rather to assist decisionmaking—prospectively in the case of clinicians and retrospectively in the case of those evaluating claims of malpractice.

The potential impact of guidelines on the incidence and resolution of cases of medical negligence depends on many factors that have already been discussed and questioned here. These factors include the soundness of guidelines (e.g., their validity, reliability, precision), the degree to which practitioners accept and effectively employ them, and the extent to which guidelines exist for particular types of care—in this case, care that is likely to incur negligence and give rise to legal claims of negligence. On this last point, one recent article estimated that existing guidelines could provide relevant evidence for 20 percent of the medical injuries identified in a major study of adverse medical events and related litigation (Garnick et al., 1991). Since the availability of practice guidelines is growing, this percentage should also grow somewhat—even if malpractice concerns are not the key factor motivating the development of most guidelines.

In addition, for guidelines to influence legal decisionmaking, courts have to accept guidelines as important evidence of the standard of care. Some argue that the potential of guidelines to reduce defensive medicine, improve decisions in liability cases, and discourage unwarranted claims cannot be adequately realized unless courts accord clinical practice guidelines more weight than they currently do in determining the standard of care to be applied in assessing claims of malpractice (Hall, 1989; Brennan, 1991b; McCormick, 1991). This committee agrees generally with that proposition. The rest of this section presents definitions and describes options for granting guidelines more weight in malpractice decisionmaking. The next section presents the committee's assessment.

Malpractice Defined

Medical malpractice is conventionally described as a deviation from the accepted medical standard of care that causes injury to a patient for whom a clinician has a duty of care (Kinney and Wilder, 1989; AMA, 1990b; U.S. House of Representatives, Committee on Ways and Means, 1990; Miller, 1991). The definition of the accepted standard of care may be supplied by case law (i.e., judicial precedent) or by state statute or regulation (Brennan, 1991b; Miller, 1991).

In case law, the accepted medical standard of care traditionally has been described as that degree of care exercised by physicians of good standing in the same or in a similar locality as the defendant physician—in essence, medical custom. More recently, case and statutory law have moved away from geographically delimited standards of care (in legal terms, the "strict locality rule" and the "similar locality rule") to national standards of care, particularly for specialists (Bovbjerg, 1989; Hall, 1989; Kinney and Wilder, 1989).[18] Geographical factors, however, may still be considered—for example, if they affect the availability of medical facilities and resources.[19] In addition, traditional case law allows for some divergence from common practice when that divergence is backed by a "respectable minority" of professionals. What a "respectable minority" is and will be in the future is far from clear (Hall, 1991; Miller, 1991). For example, if guidelines conflict, how will courts determine whether the respective sponsors are respectable?

For other areas of tort law, the standard of care for evaluating someone's conduct is quite different from that applied in medical malpractice cases (Kinney and Wilder, 1989). It is usually defined as what a reasonable person would have done under similar circumstances. Industry customs may be cited to help juries and courts assess what is reasonable, but evidence of customary practice carries far less weight than it has in medical malpractice.[20]

---

[18]Traditionally, the "strict locality" rule has referred to customary practice of physicians in the same geographic area as the defendant. The "similar locality" rule has been less delimiting; for example, it allows practice in rural areas generally to be cited as the basis of comparison for the practices of a particular rural physician.

[19]At this time, the consideration of available resources is fairly limited and does not extend to any broad balancing of patient needs against any social interest in limiting resources for services of uncertain or limited benefit (Hirshfield, 1990a,b). Whether this will and should change and how practice guidelines will figure in any change are issues in the general discussion of the role guidelines should have in determining medical liability (Hall, 1989; Morreim, 1989).

[20]As Kinney and Wilder point out (1989, pp. 439-440), the rationale for not automatically deferring to custom was described by Justice Oliver Wendell Holmes: "What usually is done may be evidence of what ought to be done . . . [However] what ought to be done is fixed by a standard of reasonable prudence, whether it is usually complied with or not."

The legal standard of medical care is, for the most part, established by expert physician testimony based on the expert's judgment. Because both plaintiffs and defendants usually present their own experts, this practice is informally described in legal circles as a "duel of experts" or "swearing contest." Subject to some limitations, experts may also cite published standards or textbooks (in legal jargon, "learned treatises"). Some states have given the courts explicit discretion to admit such standards without accompanying expert testimony, apparently to make it easier for plaintiffs to use their sources without running afoul of prohibitions against "hearsay" evidence (Kinney and Wilder, 1989; Brennan, 1991b). It is in the guise of learned treatises that clinical practice guidelines can be cited as evidence.

In theory, in medical malpractice, judges and juries evaluate only the persuasiveness of the expert's testimony; they are not supposed to evaluate directly the reasonableness of physician conduct.[21] Hall (1991), however, argues that conflicting expert testimony and the lack of definitive scientific standards in most cases give juries ample opportunity to apply their own judgments about what is reasonable. The hope is that the development and adoption of soundly based practice guidelines will permit a better fit between theory and fact.

According Guidelines Greater Weight in Determining the Standard of Care

Although the definition of standard of care in medical liability law has been changing—moving away from local toward national standards and permitting published standards to be cited as evidence—change based on case law tends to be neither quick nor predictable. Some statutory or administrative mechanism may well be needed to give guidelines based on sound, documented scientific evidence and analytic processes greater weight in litigation than they now have. In particular, such a mechanism may be needed to provide immunity from malpractice liability for performance in accord with practice guidelines. Immunity means that a conforming clinician, if sued, would not be held liable absent some other basis of liability.

Assuming the existence of good guidelines that can be used in everyday medical practice and as a basis for evaluating performance, what else may be necessary to accord guidelines greater weight in determining the legal standards of care? Table 5-2 lists some options and considerations for

---

[21] In one exception, *Helling* v. *Carey* (83 Wash. 2d 514, 519 P.2d [1974]), the Washington State supreme court held that a jury could find a defendant liable for not testing a 27-year-old woman for glaucoma—even though experts for both plaintiff and defendant stated that it was not customary to start routine testing until age 40. This case has not, to date, been taken as a precedent for similar decisions by other courts.

action. They relate to (1) how guidelines might be granted special recognition, (2) what authoritative status guidelines might have, (3) what parties could use the guidelines in the prosecution or defense of a malpractice suit, and (4) what weight might be granted guidelines.

Proposals for legislation that would confer malpractice protection on clinicians who practice in conformance with guidelines have a precedent dating back to the 1972 law (Public Law 92-703) that created professional standards review organizations (PSROs); the relevant provision continues to apply to the successor peer review organizations (Gosfield, 1975). That provision declares that if a doctor has exercised due care, he or she cannot be held liable for actions that conform to norms developed by PSROs. It appears, however, that this "immunity" provision has never been used as a defense against a malpractice claim (Gosfield, 1989). Perhaps the due care

TABLE 5-2 Options For Recognition of Guidelines in Medical Malpractice Law

---

SOURCE OF RECOGNITION
1. Legislation
    a. Federal
    b. State
2. Rules of evidence developed within or by the judiciary and promulgated through administrative rulemaking
    a. Federal
    b. State
3. Judicial precedent (case law)

AUTHORITATIVE STATUS
1. Guidelines developed by a specific entity are authoritative.
2. Guidelines developed according to specified criteria are authoritative.
3. Judges have case-by-case discretion to determine whether a guideline is authoritative.
4. Juries can decide as a matter of fact whether a guideline is authoritative.

RIGHT TO USE
1. Only the defendant(s) can cite and use guidelines as a "shield" to claim immunity from liability for care delivered in accordance with guidelines.
2. Only the plaintiff(s) can cite and use guidelines as a "sword" to claim malpractice for defendant failure to deliver care in accordance with guidelines.
3. Both defendant(s) and plaintiff(s) can cite guidelines.

WEIGHT
1. A guideline provides per se or conclusive definition of an applicable standard of care.
2. A guideline raises a rebuttable presumption; proof to counter this presumption can be offered.
3. A guideline can be considered as some evidence of an applicable standard.

SOURCE: This table was suggested by Arnold J. Rosoff in a discussion of legal implications of practice guidelines.

reference raises the specter of continued argument about whether the standard of care was met, thus making the immunity promise appear dubious. More important may be the general low representation of Medicare patients among litigants and the lack of knowledge among attorneys of this provision of the Social Security Act and its amendments.

More explicit and more controversial than the PRO immunity provision is the approach taken by the state of Maine. The state legislature has initiated a 5-year demonstration project to produce "standards of practice designed to avoid malpractice claims and increase the defensibility of the malpractice claims that are pursued" (Edwards, 1991, p. 3).[22] Unlike the federal legislation that created AHCPR, the Maine statute does not explicitly require that the guidelines that are developed be based on the best available scientific data.

The process was designed by the Maine Medical Association and is defined by statute. The state's Bureau of Insurance and Board of Registration in Medicine oversee the project, which started with three medical specialty advisory committees composed of physicians and public members serving 3-year terms. The advisory committees have, as directed by statute, focused on anesthesia, obstetrics and gynecology, and emergency medicine; radiologists recently asked to be included, and legislation to that effect is pending. Smith (1990), in explaining the legislature's action, states that the first two clinical areas were selected because of the "well-established standards that have already been promulgated nationally" (p. 2).

Once guidelines and protocols are developed, the Board of Registration will adopt them as rules under the state's Administrative Procedure Act. If 50 percent of the physicians in the state agree to practice according to the guidelines, then physicians can cite the guidelines in their defense in malpractice cases. Plaintiffs cannot use the guidelines unless they are first cited by the defense or unless the provisions they cite are identical to those in some other independently developed set of guidelines. At this point, it seems that most of the Maine guidelines will incorporate guidelines already issued by other organizations; one exception may be provisions regarding preoperative tests for patients facing relatively uncomplicated surgery (G. Smith, Maine Medical Association, personal communication, June 10, 1991).

Questions have been raised about the constitutionality of the "defendant use only" aspect of the Maine project. Indeed, one malpractice insurer, nervous over the questions raised about the law, has backed away from the effort. Nonetheless, the legislature does not appear inclined to change this aspect of the law, which was a significant element in the careful, lengthy

---

[22] Voters in California may soon vote on a proposal similar to the Maine model (McCormick, 1991).

process of negotiation among involved parties that led to the demonstration project (State Representative C. Rydell, Maine House of Delegates, personal communication, August 5, 1991).

In 1986, the legislature of Massachusetts took a different approach. It created a risk management unit in the state's medical licensing and discipline agency and required physicians to participate in a quality assurance program as a condition of licensure. Guidelines feature prominently in the quality assurance program, and the statute includes certain requirements for their content and for the development process. Physicians who participate in the program are entitled to reductions in malpractice insurance premiums from the state's liability insurers. Two specialties, anesthesiology and emergency medicine, have developed guidelines that initially qualified participating physicians for a 20 percent discount in liability premiums (McGinn, 1988).

Whether the experience of Massachusetts can be generalized to other types of guidelines is not clear. For example, the anesthesiology guidelines have several characteristics that are not common to most guidelines. Specifically, they were developed as a direct response to problems recognized as sources of liability; they are precise, particularly in their key recommendations for the use of pulse oximeters; and professional support for them was virtually unanimous. (It should be noted, however, that these guidelines do not cite or analyze any scientific evidence of effectiveness.)

Statutes that would allow judicial and jury discretion in determining the admissibility of guidelines or that provide for their consideration as merely some evidence of the applicable standard of care accord little more stature to guidelines than is granted under existing case law. Hall (1991), however, suggests that statutes specifically allow judges to consider, without the jury present, the stature of guidelines offered by defendants. Thus, without being bound by the technical rules of evidence, judges could determine the weight to give guidelines and could, in the case of "authoritative and indisputably applicable" guidelines, direct a verdict for the defense (p. 135). Authority would be assessed according to "the respectability of the issuing organization and its process of promulgation, [separate] from the inherent appropriateness of the standard itself" (p. 140).

At the federal level, several legislative proposals link guidelines to medical liability reform (McCormick, 1991). The most far-reaching would enmesh guidelines in the competition strategy for health care reform (described earlier), using contract law and federal tax policy as leverage (Havighurst, 1990a, 1991a; Blumstein, 1991). This approach would encourage consumers to choose among health plans that could offer different standards of care. Health plans could incorporate (or cite) particular practice guidelines in their contracts, or the contracts could provide for the application of guidelines developed according to specific procedural and substantive criteria.[23] How courts would reconcile this approach with the mostly unitary standard of care that has been developing through medical liability case law is far from clear (Blumstein, 1991; Schulman, 1991). This uncertainty has prompted a proposal that would essentially require, first, that health plans and their participants use an arbitration procedure for dealing with malpractice and, second, that the arbitration process apply the standard of care defined in the health plan contract (Havighurst and Metzloff, 1991).

Directions for Risk Management and Liability Standards

Once again, the committee stresses the desirable attributes of guidelines that were identified in Chapter 1. Regardless of specific statutory developments, guidelines that are based on scientific evidence and judgment and that are clear, specific, and developed by a reputable organization and process should carry greater weight in malpractice decisionmaking than vague, nonspecific, and undocumented guidelines; they should certainly be accorded more weight than isolated expert testimony (Miller, 1991; Hirshfield, 1990b). To the extent that guidelines document the strength of the evidence, the importance of the risks and benefits, and how compelling is the case for a particular intervention, they should help courts distinguish required care from optional or unindicated care.

The committee vigorously debated whether to recommend that federal or state legislation grant immunity to practitioners acting in conformance with practice guidelines. Although some members argued quite forcefully that such a recommendation was warranted now, the committee on balance concluded that it would be premature.

---

[23] Havighurst (1991b, pp. 25-26) has proposed the following contract language for HMOs concerned about malpractice liability: "The Plan warrants that each of its physicians possesses at least the skill and knowledge of a reasonably competent medical practitioner in his or her specialty and undertakes to you that its physicians will exercise that skill and knowledge in a reasonable and prudent manner in your case. In so doing, a Plan physician may sometimes depart from practices customary among other physicians. Such departures shall not be deemed to breach the foregoing undertaking, however, unless they are expressly found to have been unreasonable and imprudent; evidence to support such a finding shall include the testimony of experts knowledgeable about practices customary among physicians in other organized health plans in which physicians are not compensated on a fee-for-service basis. In instances where the Plan has consulted with the Members' Advisory Panel concerning a particular practice or method of diagnosis or treatment and obtained the Panel's approval of a particular clinical policy, adherence by the Plan's physicians to the policy shall not be deemed unreasonable and imprudent unless such approval was obtained by misrepresentation or unless changes in medical knowledge between the time such approval was obtained and the time you were treated indicated that continued adherence to such policy was unreasonable and imprudent. You agree that the undertaking in this paragraph fully defines the duties of the Plan and its physicians to you."

Legislation that provides for immunity, the committee believes, ought to specify either operational criteria for the organizations developing guidelines or particular criteria for the guidelines themselves. Criticism of the variability and weaknesses of guidelines developed by PROs made the committee reluctant to accept organizational imprimatur alone as a sufficient basis for a grant of immunity. More broadly, existing publicly and privately developed guidelines and related organizational processes for developing guidelines vary widely in quality; some are clearly inferior. As discussed in Chapter 8 (and Appendix B), an entity to assess the soundness of guidelines might provide the foundation on which legislation could rest. Such a body could help users of guidelines, including attorneys and courts, to evaluate the merits of different guidelines, and hence the merits of lawsuits that employ guidelines as evidence.

Although the committee understands that allowing only the defense to cite authoritative guidelines in court might reassure physicians and speed acceptance of guidelines, such a restriction is unfair and probably constitutionally suspect (McCormick, 1991). Equally important from the committee's perspective, such restrictiveness is inconsistent with the basic concept of science-based guidelines for appropriate care. Both the evidence and any further credibility offered by a sound process of guideline development should be available to defendants and plaintiffs alike.

The lack of a legislative imprimatur does not mean that guidelines cannot and will not be increasingly used to define the standard of care (Hall, 1991). For example, judges are in a position to consider the reputability of organizations that develop guidelines. As the development and assessment of guidelines become more firmly grounded and more recognized in practice, judges and juries should eventually give them greater weight than isolated expert witnesses, less firmly grounded testimony, or older medical treatises.

The committee urges AHCPR to continue to support scientifically meritorious research on medical liability that could simultaneously examine topics related to guideline development. One question the agency might consider is whether clinical practice guidelines for services of unclear or very marginal benefit could be phrased and explained in ways that would reduce the likelihood of defensive medicine. For example, are judges or juries (or, for that matter, patients, lawyers, or practitioners) likely to make different decisions depending on whether guidelines (a) explicitly state that, given the scientific evidence, a practitioner can prudently forego a specific service under specific circumstances, (b) explicitly state that a practitioner may want to provide the service although evidence does not support a specific recommendation, or (c) are silent on the issue? Chapter 6 suggests how guideline developers might construct recommendations that would be more useful to those who must make decisions in the face of weak or nonexistent evidence.

The committee noted one serious potential problem that medical liability law raises for the CQI model of quality assurance. Current liability procedures and standards could jeopardize implementation of the CQI vision of mistakes as "treasures" to be uncovered, analyzed, and used for learning. In an ideal world, if such mistakes resulted in harm to patients or others, institutions and practitioners would admit liability and compensate the injured party. This practice operates now to some degree, but the financial, reputational, and other potential harms of this aspect of the CQI strategy must be recognized as a powerful disincentive to such behavior.

SUMMARY

Guidelines do not implement themselves. Patients and practitioners make the key clinical choices that determine whether care will or will not be consistent with guidelines. Good guidelines aim to strengthen the scientific basis and consistency of these choices and ensure that patients and practitioners are well informed about the risks and benefits of alternative courses of care. For such guidelines to be more widely and successfully applied, however, patients and practitioners need an extremely broad range of supportive conditions and organizations.

The last two chapters have examined several critical areas of support: educational activities, information and decision assistance systems, quality assurance and improvement programs, cost control strategies, and risk management. In considering these supportive programs, this chapter and the next underscore a theme of this report: successful implementation of guidelines begins with the process of developing guidelines. The more developers of guidelines can anticipate what will make guidelines practical and credible, the more likely it will be that guidelines will be used in the kinds of activities described here.

At several points, the discussion has suggested that cost control, quality assurance, equity, and other strategies may conflict and pose problems for organizations and policymakers seeking coherent programs. The next chapter considers interrelated questions of cost-effectiveness, minimum standards of care, and requirements for informed patient consent.

6

The Inescapable Complexity of Decisionmaking: Ethics, Costs, and Informed Choices

Be Prepared for Sudden Aggravation.

Construction sign,
Maryland Department of Transportation

The strategies discussed in Chapters 4 and 5 can encourage more consistent clinical practice, reduce the occurrence and costs of inappropriate care, and increase the provision of appropriate care. They can thus help improve the value received for expenditures on health care. In themselves, however, these strategies do not necessarily lead to commonly held conclusions about how to distribute, organize, or pay for health care. Decisions in these arenas are thoroughly entangled with debates about reforms in health care financing and delivery.

During its deliberations, the committee became most engaged in debate over health care reform when it considered how guidelines for clinical practice might be used as tools to constrain costs. The committee's consideration of this issue did not—and was not intended to—lead to proposals for financing and delivery system reform. Such proposals would have exceeded the committee's charge. However, the final chapter of this report concludes with a few comments on the relationship between guidelines and some proposed directions for reform.

The first section of this chapter highlights some central ethical questions related to the development and use of practice guidelines in making everyday medical decisions and in adopting social policies that may benefit some people at the expense of others. The discussion then turns to health care costs and the responsibilities of guidelines developers to consider these costs in their recommendations. The last sections of the chapter consider the issue of informed consent and the concept of basic or minimum care. Many controversial issues are raised in this chapter. The intent is to present background information, examples, and different sides of debates on these issues clearly and fairly so that the reader can consider them and perhaps say "I disagree."

The discussion here takes as a starting point the propositions offered in Chapter 1 about how developers of guidelines can improve the knowledge base for making day-to-day clinical decisions and for formulating policies to affect the cost, quality, and availability of health care. To reiterate, every set of guidelines should be accompanied by statements about the strength of the evidence behind the guidelines and by projections of the relevant health and cost outcomes. In building the case for or against particular courses of care, scientific evidence takes precedence over expert subjective judgments. Guidelines should be accompanied by documents that disclose the procedures followed in the development process, the participants involved, the evidence used, the rationales and bases for decisions, and the analytic methods.

More often than not, developers of guidelines will find that particular clinical interventions will not be backed by a clear-cut scientific case. Another, perhaps more difficult challenge will be to distinguish facts from values; self-interest and other biases may be hard to discern even for parties making every effort to be objective. These problems, which are hardly unique to practice guidelines, should be acknowledged candidly and tackled with special sensitivity to their ethical implications.

As guideline developers move in the directions outlined here, they will describe how compelling is the case for the use of specific services in specific circumstances. They will thereby inform but not necessarily dictate answers to ethical or policy questions such as where to draw lines between care that is covered by insurance plans and care that is not.

AN ETHICAL CONTEXT

Members of the IOM committee brought to the study several ethical concerns about the development, use, and evaluation of clinical practice guidelines. These concerns were echoed and amplified in the study's site visits, public hearing, focus groups, and other activities and in a paper (Povar, 1991) commissioned by the committee to help it explore the ethical sensitivities and complexities associated with practice guidelines. A pervasive theme was the real and potential conflicts between individual and collective views about ethical obligations and standards in health care.

Ethical Obligations of Individuals

In discussions about health care, most ethical analysis focuses on the practitioner's ethical obligations to individual patients. These obligations are generally viewed as doing good, avoiding harm, respecting patient autonomy, and treating patients equitably (Beauchamp and Childress, 1983; President's Commission for the Study of Ethical Problems in Medicine and Biomedical and Behavioral Research [hereafter, President's Commission], 1983; Jonsen and Toulmin, 1988; McCullough, 1988; Brennan, 1991a; Povar, 1991).[1] (Professional obligations in the form of honesty, competence, and avoidance of conflict of interest are assumed here.)

Physicians and other practitioners may face conflicts among ethical obligations. A professional's obligations to do good and avoid harm may conflict with the obligation to respect patient autonomy. For instance, competent patients may make choices that appear irrational to physicians but that conform with the patients' own values and priorities (Brock and Wartman, 1990). A case in point is the patient with end-stage renal disease who prefers greater control and freedom in his or her life and so declines to follow difficult dietary, drug, dialysis, and other regimens despite the understood medical risk (IOM, 1991d). When the physician doubts that the various risks and benefits are or can be understood by the patient, he or she may feel even more troubled by conflicting ethical duties.

During the past two decades, patient autonomy has been increasingly emphasized and the paternalistic substitution of professional for patient judgment correspondingly criticized (President's Commission, 1983; Kapp, 1989; Povar, 1991). Single-minded emphasis on autonomy, however, has also been challenged—for three reasons. First, it seems to imply that physicians need only be technicians without being committed to their patients' best interests. Second, it appears to suggest that patients do not need the counsel, judgment, and assistance of physicians and other professionals (McCullough, 1988). Third, it assumes too strongly that patients can always understand the information and the options being presented well enough to make informed decisions. This third issue is not restricted to debates about pa-

---

[1] In the bioethics lexicon, these are often referred to as duties of the following sorts:

- *beneficence*, to promote good care (or, as it is sometimes expressed, to do to others their good);
- *nonmaleficence*, to prevent or avoid harm;
- *autonomy*, the general duty to respect persons or, in its applications in health care, the duty to respect the right of self-determination regarding choices about one's life, mind, and body;
- *justice*, to avoid discrimination on the basis of irrelevant characteristics (sometimes expressed as treating individuals [or equals] equally in morally relevant situations) or, more specifically and commonly, *distributive justice*, the duty to distribute health care resources in ways that are defensible, fair, not arbitrary, and not capricious (in other words, equitable).

Sometimes people also include "fidelity" among these principles, that is, the responsibility of the health care professional to place his or her patients first. This is sometimes described as the "fiduciary" nature of the patient-physician relationship.

tient autonomy and paternalism; it surfaces more directly in discussions of informed consent and in proposals for health care reform based on consumer choice among competing health plans. A different issue is what patient autonomy implies with respect to an individual's assuming financial or other responsibility for the consequences of noncompliance with recommended health practices.

Ideally, practice guidelines should strengthen the dialogue between patient and physician. They should serve the objective of patient autonomy by being as clear as possible about the evidence and rationale for guideline recommendations, the outcomes expected for alternative courses of care, and the ways patients may view these outcomes.[2] For example, guidelines that carefully present evidence about how test results will or will not affect patient management or patient outcomes can help physicians distinguish between a mere "quest for diagnostic certainty" (Kassirer, 1989) and a quest for information that makes a difference in decisionmaking and potential outcomes. In general, guidelines for clinicians and materials developed specifically for patients should be designed to help physicians and patients discuss recommendations more fully in terms relevant to patients; they would thereby demonstrate—rather than merely imply—the "connection between [the physician's] clinical judgment and the best interests of patients" (McCullough, 1988, p. 461).

Ethical Obligations of Collective Social Systems

At the organizational or societal level, ethical analysis becomes particularly complex as it confronts what it means to do good, avoid harm, respect autonomy, and act fairly. Doing good or avoiding harm for a specific individual may sometimes conflict with doing good or avoiding harm for patients (or potential patients) collectively.

For example, when society requires immunizations, reporting of communicable diseases, and similar measures, collective interests in disease prevention generally override personal interests in privacy and autonomy. Less straightforward and less widely accepted are principles regarding services for terminally ill individuals, especially patients with formal "Do Not Resuscitate" orders (Lo, 1991). The individual's (or family's) interest in self-determination may, on the one hand, conflict with traditional professional and social interests in preserving life; on the other hand, the patient's interest may confront institutional interests in limiting resources for care that is seen as nonbeneficial. Other conflicts are possible as well. In the hospice and nursing home case presented in Chapter 3, the regulations re-

---

[2] A recent issue of *Health Management Quarterly* is devoted entirely to the topic of guidelines. In it, Silberman (1991) and Mulley (1991) make these points eloquently.

garding patient restraints were intended to protect individual patient dignity; the institution, however, must also consider the safety of other patients and staff.

Much of the debate over divergent interests revolves around issues of cost-effectiveness and rationing or allocation of limited resources among alternative uses (Weinstein and Stason, 1977; President's Commission, 1983; Pellegrino, 1986; Callahan, 1987).[3] Such debate often highlights trade-offs between providing very expensive services (such as transplants) to a few individuals and providing less expensive services (such as prenatal care) to many more individuals (Redelmeier and Tversky, 1990; Egan, 1991; Fox and Leichter, 1991). The rationing debate, however, should not focus on expensive versus inexpensive health care services per se. The issue is not the expense per unit of *service* but, rather, the expense per unit of *benefit* (for example, years of life or freedom from pain). High-volume services with low unit costs are less dramatic but not necessarily less important than very expensive, low-volume services.

Systems must inevitably make trade-offs among alternative ways of using available resources to benefit large groups (their members).[4] Guidelines, in the form of standards of minimum, necessary, or basic services to be covered by public or private health benefit plans, have been suggested as one vehicle for determining these social allocations (Hadorn, 1991a,b,c). A system that has attempted to use guidelines to inform decisions about resource allocation is the Group Health Cooperative of Puget Sound (GHCPS). GHCPS has developed risk-based guidelines for various preventive services. Its process for developing these guidelines considers the literature on the services, other guidelines, and the organizational objectives and capabilities of GHCPS. A major objective has been to increase the proportion of high-risk individuals who undergo recommended screening. The GHCPS

---

[3] Brown (1991, p. 30) has identified at least three ways in which the term *rationing* is used. First, rationing may be seen as "any set of arrangements that allocate benefits and costs within society. Markets ration. So, inevitably, do public budgets . . . the U.S. health care system is (in)famous for rationing by price." Second, rationing may mean "strategies that make existing or proposed allocation schemes more 'rational' when judged against some principle, often equity." Third, rationing can also mean "the deliberate, systematic withholding of beneficial goods or services from some elements of the population on the grounds that society cannot afford to extend them . . . [the] main justification [being] to respond to perceived crises by making the best of a bad situation." Brown identifies this last meaning as the most common in current debates and suggests that the Oregon Medicaid reform initiative encompasses both of the last two meanings.

[4] To focus on allocations at the systems level is not to deny that individual practitioners must ration the time and attention they devote to their own patients based on relative need (among other factors). By and large, such rationing involves trade-offs across individuals, *not* trade-offs on behalf of a social policy objective between a given individual and a statistically identified group.

screening mammography guidelines, adopted in April 1988, recommend yearly screening for women aged 40 to 49 with previous breast cancer or abnormal breast tissue or with two or more first-degree relatives with breast cancer; biennial screening for women with one first-degree relative with breast cancer; triennial screening for women with at least one minor factor; and no screening for other women in this age group except on physician referral. (This guideline was reproduced in IOM, 1990c.)

GHCPS moved from guidelines development to guidelines implementation when it sent 67,000 female members over the age of 40 a risk assessment questionnaire and invited women to come for screening as indicated by their level of risk (Thompson et al., 1988). A computerized information system recorded the responses and incorporated them in the patient's medical record; the system now provides monthly reports to physicians on the status of the women in their practices. The case-finding rate in this program is considerably higher than the rate reported in non-risk-based programs.

Screening guidelines are to some degree atypical examples of existing practice guidelines. They are commonly accompanied by information about costs, and recommendations often reflect explicit or implicit judgments of cost-effectiveness. That is, social as well as individual benefit is considered, albeit in the context of choices among health services rather than between health and nonhealth services.

Another IOM committee (1990i) has argued that quality care should be evaluated on the same scale for rich and poor systems, rural and urban settings, academic and nonacademic institutions. That panel recognized that resources will affect decisions and actions. It went on to argue, therefore, that quality assurance and improvement programs should be able to identify (1) how and to what degree resource constraints do in fact affect the structures, processes, and outcomes of health care; and (2) which agent(s) are responsible for such constraints (Lohr and Harris-Wehling, 1991). Thus, although judgments about quality are distinct from judgments about appropriate uses of resources, processes of quality assessment and improvement cannot ignore how the latter affects the former.

GUIDELINES, COSTS, AND DECISIONS

The issues raised above involve two somewhat different meanings of *value.* The first meaning conveys the *normative* aspect of the word: what should be the responsibilities of individuals and governments, and how should limited resources be distributed? The second meaning has a more *empirical* slant: given agreement on basic definitions and assumptions, what is the net benefit and cost-effectiveness of a particular intervention? Information about *value* in the second sense contributes to, but does not dictate, decisions about the pursuit of *values* in the first sense.

Why Present Information About Costs?

This report recommends that every set of clinical practice guidelines include information on the cost implications of alternative preventive, diagnostic, and management strategies for the clinical situation in question. The rationale is that this information can help potential users, who must take financial and other resources into account, to better evaluate the potential consequences of different practices. The reality is that this recommendation poses major methodological and practical challenges (Weinstein and Stason, 1977; IOM, 1985; Russell, 1986; Detsky and Naglie, 1990; Eddy, 1990l, 1991c,d).[5]

With respect to the rationale for cost estimates, their purpose is to inform decisionmaking by relating the expected costs of care to the outcomes expected from that care—that is, by projecting the cost-effectiveness or value of the services in question. To be relevant to decisionmaking— that is, to the making of choices among alternatives—cost estimates should cover not just a single option for care but also the major (that is, reasonable) alternative or alternatives. The alternative(s) could be watchful waiting, doing nothing, or a different kind of intervention (e.g., a different drug or medical rather than surgical treatment).

In making cost projections, the estimates should go beyond the immediate costs of managing a clinical problem or completing a procedure to encompass the costs related to follow-up care, supportive services, and other steps *necessary for the service to make a difference* to life expectancy, functional status, or some other result that matters to the patient. For example, the so-called downstream costs of treatment for individuals whose cancers are discovered by screening must be included in the cost of a screening policy, because treatment is essential to make a difference to health. Likewise, cost estimates should include the costs of further testing to pursue false-positive results. The costs associated with *not* providing the screening or other intervention in question need to be estimated so that net costs or savings can be identified. Where estimates are subject to substantial uncertainty, analysts can use different estimates to indicate how sensitive the projections are to different assumptions. (For a discussion of the practical decisions and tradeoffs involved in making projections, see Rettig, 1991a.)

Cost estimates are most helpful if they show separately the cost of each major component of care. For example, estimates for a screening program might show the cost of initial screening, the cost of follow-up for patients

---

[5] One committee member argued forcefully that this recommendation was far too strong, that following the steps recommended here would substantially exceed the capacities of virtually all developers of guidelines, and that efforts to do so would set guidelines development back significantly.

with positive results in the initial screening, and the cost of treatment necessary to affect health outcomes in a clinically meaningful way. Detail such as this helps those who may use the guidelines to understand better the resource implications of different choices. It also focuses attention on areas in which future improvements in the process can make the most difference to costs.

Clearly, cost-effectiveness analysis and estimation must involve both clinicians and experts in cost-effectiveness analysis. Preferably, some individuals who have both kinds of expertise can be involved. As more clinicians are trained in techniques needed for guidelines development, this cad-. re of individuals should grow.

The committee discussed extensively what might be expected of cost-effectiveness analysts in the process of guidelines development. Some committee members took the position that analysts should be involved from the early stages of guidelines development. Such experts might, for example, point out that the panel should provide analysts with assumptions about how a patient will be treated once a problem is discovered through screening. This approach suggests that guideline development work should be done "all at once," by the same group of people. What is closer to reality is a "partitioned" approach that deals with cost-effectiveness analyses and judgments in stages. The drawbacks here are that partitioning increases communication costs (between panel members and the analyst) and heightens the chances that the analyst will misinterpret the panel. The compromise may be to encourage guidelines panels to work systematically toward incorporation of cost-effectiveness analysis into their processes.

Again, ideally, those estimating costs for specific health care services or procedures would examine costs and health outcomes with the five questions below in mind.

1. What evidence suggests that the services are likely to affect outcomes for the condition or intervention being considered?

2. What groups at risk are most likely to experience benefits or harms from the proposed course of care and its side effects?

3. What is known about the effects of different frequencies, duration, dosages, or other variations in the intensity of the intervention?

4. What options in the ways services are organized and provided (for example, size of institution, type of personnel used, experience of personnel, volume of service provided) can affect the benefits, harms, and costs of the services?

5. What benefits, harms, and costs can be expected from alternative diagnostic or treatment paths, including watchful waiting or no intervention?

Unfortunately, for the vast majority of treatment decisions, developers of guidelines will find that answers to these questions are in short supply. There are several reasons why this is true. First, scientific evidence about benefits and harms is itself incomplete, as has been noted elsewhere in this report. Second, basic, accurate cost data are scarce for the great majority of clinical conditions and services. Third, data on charges may be available, but many significant analytic steps and assumptions are typically required to treat charge data as cost data. Fourth, techniques for analyzing and projecting costs and cost-effectiveness are complex, evolving, and not readily applied by novices. Fifth, and most significant for this discussion, developers of guidelines have, for the most part, not considered costs as a relevant, ethical, or practical subject for their deliberations. In third and fourth areas, further research and development to improve techniques for cost-effectiveness analysis is an important need.

Some guidelines do provide information on costs, but this practice is not yet common. Even the guidelines in *Common Diagnostic Tests* (Sox, 1987, 1990) and *Common Screening Tests* (Eddy, 1991a), compilations that stress in their prefaces and elsewhere concerns about excessive costs, do not uniformly provide information about the cost-effectiveness of different tests used under different circumstances. Likewise, the U.S. Preventive Services Task Force discusses the cost implications of some but not all of the services covered in its 1989 report. Still, the analyses presented in the first two volumes cited here and under way at AHCPR and elsewhere should serve as models for other groups.

Should Developers of Guidelines Go Further?

Explicit Judgments about Cost-Effectiveness

Providing information about costs does not guarantee that such information will be used—even now, after years of growing desperation about the escalation of health care costs. This gap between availability of information and action on that information led the committee to consider a recommendation that guideline developers include cost-effectiveness as an explicit criterion for *judging or recommending* what constitutes appropriate care. Judgments of this kind are made to some degree now, but the role that costs play in such judgments may not always be clearly described in guidelines or related materials.

After much debate, and with some vigorous dissent, the committee concluded that initial developers of clinical practice guidelines need not use economic or cost criteria as explicit bases for recommendations on what constitutes appropriate care for particular clinical problems. Put differently, although guidelines should be accompanied by projections of health outcomes and costs, the specific recommendations for clinical practice can stand on sound assessments of clinical evidence and carefully derived expert judgment.

The committee is *not* saying that judgments of cost-effectiveness should be or can be avoided. Governments, health benefit plans, health care providers, and others must make such judgments, although they may not always do so explicitly and rationally. The committee also is not saying that developers of practice guidelines should *never* make such judgments. In particular, when those developing or cooperating in the development of guidelines are also the intended users, judgments of cost-effectiveness may be sensibly integrated into the process. Thus, HMOs, hospitals, and others may weigh costs against expected benefits in making judgments about drug formularies, equipment purchases, testing protocols, and other matters.

The committee decided not to insist that guideline developers employ cost-effectiveness as a decisionmaking criterion for two reasons. First, committee members could not agree that guidelines developers were, from a policy perspective, the right source of authoritative judgments about cost-effectiveness, and several feared that such judgments would complicate the resource decisions of government policymakers, health plan managers, and others. Second, committee members could not agree that their recommendations should go beyond the demanding standards for guidelines that they had already formulated.

Given the present state of guidelines development, adding information about costs will be both a major contribution and a major challenge. Developers of guidelines are, for the most part, still struggling with relatively meager financial resources, scarce data, limited methodologic capacity, unpredictable political support, professional hostility, and a short and largely unevaluated record of performance. Even the presentation of cost information has the potential to undermine the clinical judgments presented in guidelines if potential users think cost considerations are driving the recommendations about clinical care. Still, the committee believes that the effort is important if guidelines (and the discussion accompanying them) are to be useful to decisionmakers.

In any case, whether developers of practice guidelines only provide cost estimates or choose also to make recommendations based on cost-effectiveness considerations, they must involve individuals with relevant expertise in cost-effectiveness analysis and cost projection in the development process. Further, they should disclose the role that cost information played in their judgments so potential users can assess the extent to which that information drove specific recommendations. Finally, developers of guidelines should, to the extent practicable, specify the settings, payers, and patient groups for which the guideline is being developed or for which it is appropriate.

A Modest Proposal

Even when guideline developers choose not to employ cost-effectiveness as a criterion in formulating statements about appropriate care, they may still be able to state recommendations in ways that help practitioners, patients, and policymakers reach decisions in the face of constraints on individual or system resources. Specifically, they can clearly identify how compelling is the case for particular services or courses of care under particular clinical circumstances. The strength of the scientific evidence (and, secondarily, the strength of the expert consensus) and the nature and importance of the projected health benefits and harms are the central elements in this process.

Depending on available scientific evidence and expert consensus about alternative courses of care, developers of guidelines have several options in formulating statements about appropriate care. Some of these scenarios may be relatively theoretical and rare, but they highlight the ways in which recommendations may relate resources and outcomes.

• In triage situations (such as battlefields or emergency departments overwhelmed by local disaster) in which personnel, space, time, and other resource limits are critical, fixed, and immediate, guidelines exist to help practitioners determine when to provide or to withhold care based on comparisons of expected net benefit to individual patients. This is a generally understood point but worth restating in this context.

• If the existence or importance of benefits and harms of a familiar service or technology is unclear, guidelines might state that practitioners can forego that particular intervention and still be considered professionally prudent. This gives decisionmakers more leeway to consider cost factors. (In today's economic climate, *new* technologies may be held to a stricter standard that requires more definitive information and arguments about benefits, harms, and costs.)

• If evidence is sufficient to support several treatment options that have similar costs but different mixes of risks and benefits, respect for patient preferences generally would warrant informed patient choice. If costs of these treatment options differ, guidelines can illuminate but not answer the question of whether patients or third parties should be responsible for the costs of the more expensive option. They certainly cannot dictate what a patient's preference should be for different combinations of risks and benefits.

• If evidence indicates that alternative courses of care differ greatly in cost but produce health outcomes and side effects that are similar clinically and that are experienced similarly by patients, then it is reasonable (some would say ethically required) for guidelines to make a judgment based on cost-effectiveness and recommend explicitly that the less costly alternative be routinely used. A case in point might involve appropriate antimicrobial agents for common upper respiratory infections. Newer-generation antibiotics (or broad-spectrum agents) are likely to be more costly than older (or narrower spectrum) products. When no *marginal* therapeutic benefit is to be expected from newer or more complex agents, guideline developers may quite reasonably recommend the less expensive agents.

Even when developers of guidelines do not factor costs directly into their recommendations, they or their sponsoring organizations might still regard the publication of guidelines as an opportunity to present opinions or recommendations based on costs. For example, when the *Annals of Internal Medicine* and other professional journals publish a set of guidelines, an editorial or guest commentary could consider how providers and financers, taking resource constraints into account, might act on the guidelines.

The next sections of this chapter approach the question of what is worth doing or recommending from somewhat different perspectives. The first involves the patient as decisionmaker and the conditions for informed consent. The second relates to the physician as decisionmaker. Each discussion attempts to suggest how the "compelling case" approach outlined in the introduction to this chapter may be helpful.

THE PATIENT AS DECISIONMAKER: WHAT IS INFORMED CHOICE?

Good medical care requires that decisionmaking be shared, to varying degrees, between practitioners and patients. This message comes from (1) accumulating research on outcomes and effectiveness of health care, (2) case law on the issue of informed consent, and (3) the consumer movement of the past 30 or so years. In supporting shared decisionmaking, guidelines may serve as a basis for physician communication with patients or as a starting point for informational materials prepared specifically for patients and consumers (or their families or other representatives). The following discussion looks first at questions typically raised under the rubric of "informed consent" and then turns to some issues often considered under the heading of "patient preferences."

Informed Consent

Patient communication and information can serve at least three objectives. One is to help patients choose among possible strategies for managing health care problems (or, less obviously, to select among health insurance plans). A second is to encourage specific changes in a patient's health-related behavior. A third, as described in Chapter 5's discussion of risk management and medical liability, is to reduce the liability risks associated with poor communication and the disappointment that can result from unrealistic patient expectations.

Since the early 1900s, an evolving body of case law related to the crime of battery (touching without consent) has promoted ever-increasing attention to physician responsibilities for communicating with patients about the risks and benefits of proposed care and for obtaining informed consent to surgical procedures and similar interventions (Faden and Beauchamp, 1986; Mazur, 1988; Brennan, 1991a). The term *informed consent* itself dates from a 1957 California appellate court decision in *Salgo* v. *Leland Stanford Junior University Board of Trustees* (154 Cal. App. 2d 560 [1957]); since then, courts have been trying to define what informed consent means and what it requires. In some states, the standard for judgment is whether a physician has disclosed what other physicians in good standing would disclose; in other jurisdictions, the standard is what a reasonable person in the patient's situation would want to know.[6]

Presumably, this judicial stimulus has increased the flow of information to patients, but current institutional procedures for informed consent seem intended, to a very considerable degree, to fulfill legal requirements and protect institutions from liability (Kapp, 1989; Hillman, 1991; Povar, 1991). This role is important. Nonetheless, a narrow, legalistic interpretation of the concept should not obscure the potential for informed consent to act as a vehicle for fulfilling patient preferences and improving the quality of care.

The President's Commission for the Study of Ethical Problems in Medicine and Biomedical and Behavioral Research (1983) noted that "although the informed consent doctrine has substantial foundations in law, it is essentially an ethical imperative [and] . . . a process of shared decisionmaking based upon mutual respect and participation" (p. 20). The commission further argued that education and training, rather than judicial dictates, are the preferred vehicles for improving how physicians and others provide patients with the information they need. A focus on legal requirements can distract practitioners and institutions from the challenges that face profes-

---

[6]In England, the House of Lords (which, in the form of its 15 Law Lords, acts as the final appeals court) has explicitly rejected the "North American standard of informed consent," in particular, the reasonable or prudent patient standard. One opinion in a 1985 case described the prudent patient as a "happy abstraction," a "fairly rare bird" not readily found in "his natural habitat on the Clapham omnibus" (cited by Miller, 1987, pp. 175-176). Closer to home, a distinguished general and thoracic surgeon commented that he could get informed consent only from another general or thoracic surgeon who performed the same procedures. In this framework, even the idea of informed consent from patients, including physicians in other specialties, is at best an abstraction because of the unbridgeable gap in knowledge and experience.

sionals in making information useful to patients. Adding to the difficulties in this regard is that the ability of patients to comprehend and act on information may be compromised by emotional stress, psychiatric illness, intellectual limitations, financial constraints, and language and other barriers (Hillman, 1991; Povar, 1991).

These concerns noted, legal experts stress that informed consent does not exist by virtue of signed forms. If written (or oral) consent lacks real understanding, such empty agreement does not preclude liability. Put another way, legal requirements are consistent, rather than in conflict, with the ethic of informing patients, sharing decisionmaking, and respecting autonomy.

As developers of guidelines become more cognizant of how variations in outcomes are perceived by patients and more specific about the risks and benefits of alternative courses of care for particular clinical situations, the guidelines they develop should provide a better base for patient information and decisionmaking. Several challenges must be faced, however, in moving from initial guidelines documents, which are generally directed at clinicians, to patient-friendly guidelines and information. One challenge is the translation of risk-benefit analyses into messages that will register with patients both intellectually and emotionally. Considerable research has demonstrated the difficulties involved in creating realistic public appreciation of different kinds and levels of risk (National Research Council, 1989). Another challenge, consideration of patient preferences in the construction and use of guidelines, raises both technical and policy issues.

Patient Preferences

In the past few years, health services researchers have made clinicians and others increasingly aware that patients may vary in their preferences for different outcomes of care and that clinicians may perceive these preferences inaccurately (Wennberg et al., 1988; Mulley, 1989, 1991; Kaplan and Ware, 1989; Wennberg, 1990). That research has raised important questions about how to identify patient preferences, how to incorporate information about patient preferences into practice guidelines, and how to help patients make informed determinations about their preferences.

Reflecting a traditional emphasis on practitioners' obligations, discussions about health care decisionmaking and patient preferences may not consider the ethical obligations and personal capacities of patients. On the one hand, the individual's personal and social responsibility for his or her own health behavior and choices may be ignored. On the other hand, how variability in individual intellectual, emotional, and other capacities may affect—and limit—patient decisionmaking is a consideration sometimes lost in more theoretical discussions of patient preferences.

For developers of practice guidelines, incorporating patient preferences presents several challenges (Eddy, 1990d, 1991c). Guidelines developers will not have available much empirical evidence about patient preferences, lifestyles, and attitudes about different kinds of risks as these factors relate to specific clinical conditions or to health care generally. Securing such information will be expensive, even if the effort is aimed at the typical patient rather than the idiosyncratic patient whose preferences and behaviors may pose the greatest problem for clinicians. Further, how preferences or behaviors might or might not be accommodated in light of clinical evidence and judgment may raise significant ethical or policy questions that go beyond the expertise and responsibility of those participating in the development of particular guidelines (Granneman, 1991). This is not to say that guidelines should ignore the challenges of such behaviors and choices. Rather, it is to say that guidelines are unlikely to deal comprehensively with the totality of personal behavior and choice.

Yet even if guideline developers and users become adept at identifying and recognizing patient preferences, problems will remain for decisionmakers. Respect for patient autonomy does not dictate that physicians must always act to help patients or their families implement their preferences (Brett and McCullough, 1986; Povar, 1991). The controversy over continued care for patients in persistent vegetative states is a dramatic illustration. Patient demands for unindicated antibiotics are a routine but still troublesome problem.

Patient preferences may conflict with practice guidelines in at least three general ways, and these conflicts may raise minor to significant ethical questions. One kind of conflict exists when a patient demands care that appears not to be indicated according to a guideline involving the condition or service in question. Such a situation is least troublesome when the patient wanting the nonindicated service is willing and able to be responsible for any additional costs of providing it, is exposed to little or no risk, and imposes little or no burden on society. An example might be a low risk diagnostic test that is otherwise not indicated and that is paid for not by a third party but by the patient.

Other conflicts may involve patients who do not wish to receive care that is clinically indicated. For example, an athlete might prefer to play with an injury that normally would require rest, medications, or surgery. Another instance is the patient who refuses chemotherapy because the low expected benefit of such treatment (in her specific case) does not sufficiently outweigh (for her) its likely and unpleasant toxic side effects. Assuming that these patients have been fully informed of the possible consequences of exercising their preferences (such as a further disability injury or a shorter life expectancy), the two situations would also appear to offer little concern on ethical grounds. They do imply, however, that greater weight has been given to patient autonomy than to some larger professional or social judgment of what is appropriate care.

More troubling are conflicts between a patient's preferences for care and a guideline when a third party (e.g., government, an employer, an insurer) is expected to absorb the additional costs if and when unindicated care is rendered. To the extent that third parties themselves use guidelines to inform utilization review and reimbursement decisions, they reduce the opportunities for patients to shift costs for unindicated care from themselves to others. However, to the extent that patients and physicians misrepresent clinical information in order to secure payment, the ethical problem is compounded.

Information, Preferences, and Policy: The Need for Guidelines on Patient Information and Informed Consent

The potential tensions among patient preferences, requirements for informed consent, and policies to contain health care costs are several. Even if policymakers somehow resolve questions about what care should be covered by private and public health benefit plans, other questions related to the provision of appropriate *information* remain.

• Do all physicians have an equal responsibility to provide information about services that may have some benefit compared with alternative care, even when the more beneficial services are not available under the financing system or in the delivery setting in which they practice? If the answer is no, what information can be omitted? Under what circumstances?

• More specifically, by enrolling in certain types of health plans, should patients forfeit their right to information—at the point of service—about treatment options of some benefit that are not (or may not be) covered by the plan? If so, is such a forfeiture absolute, or is it conditional on the provision to patients of clear advance warning that such limits may be applied?[7] If the latter, who is responsible for that advance warning—government, an employer, the health plan, or the practitioner? How detailed should the warning be with respect to how limits are set and which specific

---

[7] As noted in Chapter 5, health insurance contracts typically disclose certain kinds of restrictions. These restrictions may take the form of excluded services (e.g., cosmetic surgery), services limited by frequency (e.g., 20 mental health outpatient visits), or coverage that is conditional on patient compliance with preprocedure review and other utilization management requirements. The kind of disclosure considered here could involve a general statement that the plan reserves the right, for example, to apply certain practice guidelines or to employ a drug formulary. At one extreme, disclosure of *specific* protocols could be required. Alternatively, guidelines developed by specific organizations or according to specific criteria could be referenced (Havighurst, 1990b). Statutory and case law are still evolving in this area (Miller, 1991).

treatment options are not available (taking legal, organizational, and other practical issues into account)? Should the warning meet certain readability standards (e.g., eighth-grade reading level)?

• What about government policies that forbid the provision of information, for example, on abortion or that require the provision of specific information, for example, on fetal development? What can and should practitioners do if they believe the regulations are scientifically or ethically improper? What proper role should government or other payers have in dictating what practitioners must and must not say to patients (Annas, 1991)?

The following discussion considers these questions only as they relate to the provision of information and the contribution that developers of guidelines might make in resolving these issues.

Provision of Information under Condition-Specific or Treatment-Specific Guidelines

This committee believes that developers of guidelines can do more than they do now to help practitioners define their responsibilities to provide information to patients. By describing the strength of the evidence for a particular guideline, estimating and assessing outcomes in terms that are relevant to patients, and more generally depicting how compelling is the case for different courses of care, they may guide judgments about how compelling are practitioner responsibilities for providing information and recognizing patient preferences. For purposes of illustration only, one possible hierarchy of obligations is outlined below. It is not endorsed in its entirety by the committee, in part because the assumptions about existing information are quite heroic.

First, when evidence and consensus are very strong, responsibilities to provide information likewise should be strong. This precept generally would hold even if the information concerned a service that was not available or not covered by insurance. A relatively obvious example is immunizations, which traditionally have not been covered by indemnity health plans but which clinicians routinely recommend, provide, or arrange for from public programs or other subsidized services. A more difficult case involves expensive services such as kidney transplants or dialysis, which some financing programs implicitly or explicitly ration on budgetary grounds.[8]

---

[8] In Britain, the limiting of these services for patients over 55 years of age may have been facilitated by (and may also have contributed to) that nation's relatively weak medical and judicial interpretation of informed consent requirements (Miller, 1987). Lacking information about treatment options and their expected outcomes, patients are in a poor position to question or change the course of care prescribed by their physicians. They are also not well situated to understand or challenge the policies of health insurance plans that may shape physician decisions.

Second, when evidence is sufficient to support several treatment options with different mixes of risks and benefits, respect for patient preferences generally would prescribe the provision of adequate information to allow informed patient choice. Whether such a choice could be implemented (in particular, paid for by other parties through health insurance or subsidized service delivery programs) is a question that guidelines themselves can illuminate but not answer.

Third, when both evidence and consensus are unclear or nonexistent, the provision of information could be balanced against other factors such as time constraints and financial incentives. That is, if guidelines state that no evidence or strong consensus supports a particular course of care, practitioners face no compelling ethical (or legal) responsibility to provide information about that option.

General Guidelines for Patient Information

The committee also believes that a set of general guidelines for patient information and consent may need to be devised to supplement condition- or treatment-specific guidelines, on the one hand, and legally oriented patient consent forms, on the other. Such guidelines would discourage an unsophisticated, narrowly legalistic approach to informed consent and confront the limitations of common mechanisms of disseminating information to patients (Green, 1991; Hillman, 1991; Povar, 1991; Siu and Mittman, 1991). They would be intended to provide specific assistance to clinicians, institutions, payers, patients and their surrogates, and any other involved parties in determining the types of information that should be provided to satisfy practical, ethical, and legal standards of care. Further, any broad set of information and consent guidelines would need to be relevant for (a) different kinds of care provided to (b) different kinds of patients in (c) different delivery systems and settings, given (d) different levels of certainty about the benefits, risks, and costs of care.

General guidelines on patient information and informed consent should be developed by a systematic process. Compared with processes for developing condition- or treatment-specific guidelines, the process for developing general information guidelines will involve somewhat different challenges and greater ambiguity. It is likely to call for greater consideration of ethical and perhaps other nonclinical factors in determining recommendations, demand more effort to define conceptual and operational measures of nonclinical benefits and risks, and require less specificity with respect to the vast number of individual patient situations that are likely to be encountered. These characteristics imply a more inclusive development process involving, among other things, more representation of health care purchasers and third-party payers, consumers and patients, and the legal profession.

Once formulated, general patient information and consent guidelines would apply to broad categories of patient care, unless they were specifically modified by condition-specific guidelines.

THE PHYSICIAN AS DECISIONMAKER: WHAT CARE IS REQUIRED?

Good guidelines will be welcomed by physicians and other health care professionals. Nonetheless, such guidelines may still present practitioners with ethical problems. One committee member noted that he receives materials labeled "guidelines" that call for a great range of services. His first question is whether any particular set of guidelines are, in fact, sound statements of what he really ought to do or recommend to preserve or improve his patients' health; his second question is whether practically he *can* do everything that is recommended; his third question is what hassles he may expect from payers, patients, or others if he does (or does not) follow the guidelines.

This physician's questions reflect the broader world of medical practice. Clinicians constantly make decisions and recommendations—some routine, some involving life and death—in the face of limited knowledge, time constraints, complex and unpredictable human behavior, and conflicting and even unreasonable messages from payers, courts, and others about the obligations of clinicians to patients and society (Morreim, 1989; Brook, 1991). The dilemma these conflicting pressures create is not always thoroughly appreciated by those outside the profession. That physicians are paid well does not negate the very real strains they may experience in juggling patient, payer, legal, and professional expectations, pressures, and disagreements.

To varying degrees, guidelines can help physicians and others by identifying how compelling is the case for particular services or courses of care under particular clinical circumstances. To further alleviate some of the strains on clinicians, some members of the committee argued strongly that developers of guidelines should specify the minimum (or basic or necessary) care required for each clinical problem or service they address. Such specifications would, in a sense, be intended to describe a "safe harbor," a statement of what physicians ethically and legally would be expected to provide to their patients. Negligence would be implied if they did not provide or at least recommend this minimum level of care.

Most committee members viewed this argument with sympathy, but the group ran into semantic, philosophical, and technical problems that prevented a clear consensus in the area. Nonetheless, the committee wanted to present some thoughts about how these issues might be debated.

One point quickly became clear in the committee's discussions. That is, although the issue of minimum, necessary, or basic care was first raised to the committee in the context of clinical practice and involved ethical, legal, and practical concerns beyond third-party payment, the issue is most identified with controversies about what health insurance plans should cover. For some years, insurers, clinicians, and health services researchers have argued about what care is medically necessary or appropriate and who should make such judgments. That argument is taking on new intensity and significance as proposals for health care reform call for a package of basic benefits to be defined and used more or less uniformly by public and private health insurance plans.

More Definitions

Adjectives such as "necessary" and "basic" are quite common in everyday language, but they also have certain specialized uses that may be inconsistent with each other and with what might be termed ordinary usage. The result is a sizable opportunity for misunderstanding and failed communication. What follows is a brief review of definitions and perspectives intended to illustrate this point.

Dictionaries[9] describe something that is **necessary** as being "of an inevitable nature," "compulsory," "absolutely needed," "required," "essential," "indispensable," "vital for the fulfillment of a need"; it is something "that cannot be done without" or that is "determined by force of nature or circumstance." **Appropriate** means what is "especially suitable or compatible, fitting," "suitable or fitting for a particular purpose; proper," or "specifically fitted or suitable." What is **indicated** may be "necessary" or, less strongly, "advisable" or "suitable." That which is **basic** is "fundamental," "essential," "constituting the starting point," "primary," or "of lowest rank." A **minimum** is the "least quantity assignable, admissible, or possible" or the "least amount attainable, allowable, or usual."

The term *medical necessity* appears to have arisen several decades ago as newly developing health plans sought to limit payment or reimbursement to only that care that was medically necessary for the diagnosis and treatment of a condition, illness, or injury.[10] However, not all insurance programs employ the term in contracts and elsewhere, and not all programs that use the term actually define it. When definitions are provided, they vary considerably (Helvestine, 1989).

---

[9] The definitions here are drawn from Webster's *Ninth New Collegiate Dictionary*, the *Random House Dictionary of the English Language*, and the *Compact Edition of the Oxford English Dictionary*.

[10] This terminology inspired the name and the purpose of the original Blue Cross Medical Necessity Program, which was described in Chapter 2. The fact that the American College of Physicians, which was asked by Blue Cross to assist in assessing medical necessity, named its program the Clinical Efficacy Assessment Program suggests that the medical profession was not completely comfortable with the former term, at least in this context.

The least restrictive definition seems quite simple: medically necessary care is the care a physician provides or prescribes. This definition excludes payment for nonmedical treatments such as faith healing but otherwise defers to the physician. Medicare regulations go a little further, referring to care that is safe and generally accepted by practitioners. Those health plans that use Value Health Sciences systems may be adopting, implicitly if not explicitly, the RAND definition of appropriate care—that is, that the medical benefits of a service exceed medical harms by a sufficient amount to make the service worth providing. In any case, despite the shift by insurers away from unfettered physician discretion in determining medical necessity, the actual interpretation of medical necessity seems to fall between the dictionary meanings of necessity and appropriateness rather than to follow the definitions of the former. A fuller examination would likely show that interpretations vary considerably; for example, newer technologies may well be treated more strictly than older technologies, and matters of site and timing of care may be subjected to more questions than the matter of whether to provide that service at all (IOM, 1989a).

The RAND definition of appropriateness is useful to cite because it more readily prompts the question that underly all the definitions: How much benefit is enough for care to be rated as appropriate (or necessary)? Is it any possible marginal benefit? Is it what physicians say is an important benefit? Is it what an individual patient or the average patient thinks is enough benefit? Any such judgments and distinctions are highly subjective and reflect, in part, the different concerns or interests of different parties.

At least six special concerns seem to be discernible in discussions that employ the terms defined above.

• **The public or private insurer perspective.** It asks, What health services should we pay for? What services will courts say we must cover?

• **The professional liability or risk management perspective.** It asks, What care will the courts hold practitioners responsible for providing or recommending?

• **The perspective of the ordinary person.** It asks, Am I going to get the care I need and want? Will it be paid for?

• **The evidence- and outcomes-based perspective.** It asks, What does science say about what works, and how convincingly does it say it?

• **The conservative style of practice perspective.** It asks, When is intervention required rather than watchful waiting?

• **The ethical perspective.** It asks, What does justice or decency require society to assure its members?

These concerns are by no means mutually exclusive, but neither are they identical. Moreover, within the context of a single perspective, different attitudes can be distinguished about what constitutes a sufficient case for medical intervention.

Adding further to the confusion about adjectives such as necessary, basic, or minimum is the fact that the noun *care* is sometimes not clearly distinguished from such terms as *coverage* or *benefits*. The latter refer not to health services per se but rather to payment for services under the terms of a health benefits plan.

In conventional insurance terms, one is insured against a financial loss caused by some peril; in the case of health care, the loss is the money spent for medical services incurred as a result of illness or injury. The benefit is what the insurer contributes to meeting those losses. Losses and benefits are ordinarily specified in considerable detail in insurance contracts, which may restrict benefits to certain settings of care, types of practitioners, medical conditions, and so forth. "Health care benefits" clearly are not the same as the "benefits of health care" in that some covered care may not be beneficial and some beneficial (necessary or appropriate) care may not be covered. Cases in point involve the not uncommon exclusions of coverage for immunizations, blood products, and dental care; Medicare also excludes outpatient prescription drugs.

In discussions of broad principles for health care delivery and financing, the term *basic benefits* clearly has a variety of different meanings (Veatch, 1991; Hadorn and Brook, 1991; see generally the May 15, 1991, issue of the *Journal of the American Medical Association*). Some meanings are implicit, some explicit. Some are consistent with the common meanings associated with the term *basic*, that is, something that is "essential" or "of lowest rank," "primary" or "constituting the starting point." Other meanings are not in line with common usage and may even be misleading. Among the varied conceptions of basic benefits are the following.

• By their listing of basic benefits, some health care reform proposals seem to mean simply the ordinary kinds of health care services, settings, and providers covered in the typical (middle-class) health plan. Basic in this sense dates back to early health insurance (primarily Blue Cross) terminology that described fully covered hospital and physician services as basic and other services as supplemental. The term *standard benefits* might be a better label for this conceptualization of a benefits package.

• Other discussions suggest that a basic benefits package is an "urgent care" or perhaps "bare bones" package aimed primarily at the kinds of illness or injury that produce significant expenditures (e.g., above a relatively high deductible) but not necessarily catastrophic expenditures (e.g., more than 30 or 60 days of hospital care).

• In contrast, some appear to see basic benefits as those involving preventive and primary care services that have relatively low unit prices and simple technology (e.g., immunizations, well-baby care).

• A few conceptualizations start with the relatively broad range of services now covered by most health plans but then attempt to limit coverage to "effective" services based on considerations of evidence, cost, importance to individuals, and social value.

This last perspective is reflected in some broad proposals for reforming this nation's health care financing and delivery system (see Chapter 8). This perspective also is reflected in Oregon's Basic Health Services Act, which directs a revision of the state's Medicaid program (Eddy, 1991d; Granneman, 1991; Hadorn, 1991c). The legislation calls for services to be ranked by priority and then covered in order of ranking until the program budget is exhausted. The commission charged with setting priorities has employed town meetings, quantitative analyses, subjective judgments, and various other processes to generate information about costs, outcomes, and individual preferences for particular outcomes. It has then used this information in setting and revising priorities. Arguing for an alternative but still comprehensive approach, Hadorn and Brook (1991) would rely solely on judgments of health benefit excluding judgments of cost-effectiveness. Under their approach, a basic benefits package would cover only services that provided significant net health benefits; these services would be not just effective, beneficial, or appropriate but "necessary to a minimally decent life."[11]

Clearly, terminology in this area is confused and fraught with ethically and politically sensitive connotations that intensify the impact of any misunderstandings. For convenience in considering practical and policy issues, the next section of this report employs the term *minimum care*, a term the committee thought carried less policy or political history than the others discussed above. Minimum care in this discussion is not a matter of requiring high deductibles and cost-sharing in health insurance plans but involves what specific services are covered by such plans.

Practical and Policy Issues

Even if a term such as *minimum care* is agreed upon, many difficult operational and policy questions confront efforts to specify just what constitutes such care. One practical issue is whether to attach the term *minimum* only to those individual elements of care that are strongly based in

---

[11] An earlier proposal by Brook (1991) seems to be less restrictive, although it, too, does not include an explicit role for judgments of cost-effectiveness. In this formulation, necessary care is care that "(1) is appropriate (medical benefit exceeds medical risk); (2) produces important benefits to the patients receiving it; and (3) would be considered improper for physicians not to recommend to the patient. It would disturb both primary care physicians and specialists if it were not provided" (p. 3000). Brook notes that these principles are easier to state than to apply and argues that their application must occur within a broader context of decisions about the shape of health care in this country.

scientific evidence and that developers of guidelines can, indeed, describe as required under most circumstances.

This evidence-based approach to defining minimum care has serious limitations. For many conditions for which no strong evidence exists, no specific care could be deemed to be required, even though the alternative— no intervention at all—might be inconsistent with available evidence or strong expert consensus. The blood transfusion example cited in Chapter 1 is a case in point; no direct evidence exists about the precise threshold at which transfusion is indicated, but no one would counsel that transfusions are not required at some point to avoid death or injury in a variety of situations. Similarly, most screening guidelines acknowledge that even when research supports a particular screening service, the evidence is unlikely to speak to the particular interval for screening. An equally serious problem was noted in Chapter 1: scientific evidence is not likely to exist for a great many of the combinations of clinical problems and characteristics that patients bring to clinicians in the real world.

Minimum care would probably need to be defined as a constellation of services, for example, the least number of services (or options) for managing a condition that could be supported by strong expert consensus and that was consistent with available scientific evidence. Unfortunately, trying to draw lines around sets of services will be an even more subjective and controversial process than trying to draw the line for or against a specific intervention. Efforts to assess patient preferences and reflect them in global coverage policies (as attempted in Oregon) have been criticized as inherently unable to deal adequately with variations in individual needs and values (Granneman, 1991).

Efforts to define minimum care and set priorities for insurance coverage across the entire array of existing health services may run into additional challenges not faced by more incremental strategies. Collecting and analyzing information and making objective and subjective comparisons involving thousands of services and combinations of clinical circumstances constitute such a monumental undertaking that simplifying strategies inevitably arise. These strategies—for example, grouping services together in broad categories—may be methodologically flawed and may compromise the resulting judgments (Eddy, 1991d). Although the defects may be fixable in principle and the fixing may be doable for a limited number of services, it is not clear that they are feasibly applied comprehensively to all or even most services.

An alternative, incremental approach would concentrate on "ruling out" ineffective services rather than "ruling in" only effective ones. It would focus on such "targets of opportunity" as new and emerging technologies, obsolete services, services characterized by wide practice variations or thought to be overused or misused, and services that otherwise are of keen interest to policymakers, practitioners, and patients. This is essentially the approach now employed by Medicare and other payers. Some members of the committee believe that incremental approaches are the only workable ones (albeit in need of more serious commitment of resources than available now); comprehensive strategies promise far more than they can deliver—technically, administratively, and ethically. In this view, the Oregon initiative is a valuable exercise but not a policy model.

In addition, some worry that efforts to define minimum care would become an operation to describe not a floor beneath which care should not fall but a ceiling beyond which it should not rise. They also fear that such distinctions will preclude "excellent" care or will compromise a physician's sense of responsibility for a particular patient whose circumstances might justify more or different care. Whether other-than-minimum care should be defined as excellent care, however, raises questions about whether excellent care is to be distinguished by better expected health outcomes, better accommodation of patient preferences, or something else. More care, in and of itself, is not necessarily better care, although it certainly may be.

Other important questions face any effort to identify a constellation of minimum services. For instance, whose "minimum" is at stake? Whose perspective—that of an individual or a population, or of a practitioner, patient, or policymaker—should govern in establishing that minimum? Should the same minimum apply for all purposes? For example, should the same minimum determine what care is to be insured (or made available to all) and, at the same time, serve as the standard for determining negligence? Should people be required to receive minimum care in some circumstances or risk losing insurance or other benefits, as has been suggested recently for welfare recipients or others in Delaware and Maryland (Goldstein, 1991; Robb, 1991)? Can any single process for defining minimum care accommodate the differences in incentives among systems of care, for example, fee-for-service and capitated systems (Granneman, 1991)? Should the same minimum apply to those covered by Medicaid and those covered by employment-based programs? Considering the different circumstances of the "average" poor person in the United States and the average individual in an impoverished developing country, will the definition of minimum care be bound as much by culture and resources as by evidence?

Opinions clearly differ on these issues and reflect complex differences in value judgments. Some argue that those who advocate explicit identification of minimum or basic care must be prepared to accept that minimum for themselves in, say, a basic insurance benefit package provided or subsidized by government or employers. Others disagree. Furthermore, some who agree about the basic package for subsidized insurance disagree about whether it would be unethical for them to supplement the package by paying for additional care that others might want but are unable to afford. Finally, whether one has to resolve these ethical questions before arguing for statements of minimum care is itself a matter of dispute.

A final point: what started out as a committee discussion of minimum care from a clinician's perspective became a discussion of minimum care from an analyst's perspective. The results of an effort to define minimum care for public and private health plans might make it easier for physicians to predict what care would be paid for; however, it is likely to leave unresolved (or to complicate) a variety of other ethical, practical, and legal issues that concern clinicians.

What Should Developers of Guidelines Do?

Given the terminological, practical, and ethical problems raised by the issue of minimum care, the committee confronted this fundamental question: Can and should the (relatively) fragile enterprise of guidelines development be expected to take on extremely sensitive and highly complex issues of "valuation" of health care services for society at large? After extended debate, the committee concluded—with some dissent—that the answer is no. It is *not* prudent to recommend that guideline developers uniformly state the minimum, necessary, or basic level of quality care for every clinical problem or service for which guidelines are formulated. However, guideline developers should attempt to describe the incremental benefit associated with particular courses of care.

Some developers of guidelines may be technically, ethically, and politically positioned to propose minimum care for a limited set of clinical problems, but many others do not now and may never wish to assume this responsibility. More fundamentally, developers of guidelines do not appear to this committee to be the appropriate locus for declaring what is minimum or basic care insofar as those decisions apply to third-party payment or broader resource allocation policies. Demanding that guidelines developers be explicit about "minimums" may undermine the credibility of the entire process, make the evaluation of the science base extremely vulnerable to political biases, and reduce the process, in the view of some, to an exercise in defining "two-tier" health care.

The committee does wish to express its discomfort with the terminological confusion, even sloppiness, surrounding the use of such phrases as "medically necessary care." This discomfort does not stem from a desire for linguistic perfection. Rather, it arises from concerns that very important decisions are being made on the basis of poorly defined criteria, a process that will result in inconsistent and often conflicting judgments that, in turn, will induce confusion, hostility, and, ultimately, inequity.

SUMMARY

Management (if not resolution) of the tensions discussed in this chapter concerning ethics, costs, and information will depend on decisions about how health care is to be financed and delivered in the future. Developers of guidelines can illuminate debates over various individual and collective interests by presenting evidence, analysis, and expert judgment about the risks, benefits, costs, and patient preferences associated with alternative courses of care. Well-developed, evidence-based guidelines that are specific, logical, clearly explained, and accompanied by projections of health and cost outcomes (to the extent possible, given the dearth of this kind of information) can and will be incorporated in quality, cost, and liability management programs. Their incorporation, in turn, will provide powerful support for the consistent application of such guidelines in actual clinical practice.

Nonetheless, differences in philosophies, resources, attitudes toward risks, and other factors will ensure some inconsistency and dispute. Clinical experts and decisionmakers may argue among themselves about how to interpret weak or conflicting scientific data, how to estimate and weigh benefits, harms, and costs, and how to resolve questions of individual versus collective perspectives. Further, pure objectivity and perfect rationality may exist in the realm of theory but not in the world of real human endeavors. Decisions to use or not to use particular guidelines may consciously or unconsciously reflect economic considerations, inclinations toward "conservative" or "aggressive" styles of practice, and other factors. This is one reason that the committee places such emphasis on the attributes of good guidelines—they should reduce the opportunity for important but unacknowledged values or biases to affect the formulation or application of guidelines.

The committee judged that it is not now strategically or tactically prudent to impose on all developers of clinical practice guidelines the task of explicitly recommending what care is warranted on economic as well as clinical grounds. Nor should guideline developers be uniformly expected to declare what services constitute the minimum or required care for a clinical problem. As important and necessary as these judgments may be, developers of guidelines for clinical practice need not take on this responsibility.

A fundamental reason for this position is that users rather than developers of guidelines carry the actual responsibility for deciding how to deploy resources and how the projections of health and cost outcomes offered by guidelines relate to their specific circumstances and objectives. A second, practical reason for the committee's position is that developers of guidelines may be nearly overwhelmed in responding to the expectations already laid out for them in this report and elsewhere. In the committee's view, it is important that they concentrate on these tasks and show that they can build a credible foundation for better decisions by practitioners, patients, and others. The next chapter pursues this point.

7

Evolution in Procedures and Methods for Developing Practice Guidelines

You didn't tell me I'd spend all my time plowing up snakes.

Chair of an AHCPR guidelines
development panel, 1990

Involvement in the development of clinical practice guidelines is a learning experience that has both positive and negative features—as suggested by the above comment from one participant in the process. Involvement in implementation likewise provides lessons that are relevant to the process of developing guidelines. In examining the practical, technical, and policy questions about guidelines implementation and health care reform raised in the preceding chapters, the committee concluded that it needed to underscore the point made in Chapter 2: Planning for successful implementation begins with the development of guidelines. In the future, guidelines developers should give more and earlier attention to what will make guidelines practical and credible. This kind of early consideration will require both improvements in technical methods and greater sensitivity to how guidelines may be appropriately integrated into information systems, quality assurance programs, liability decisionmaking, and cost-management efforts.

Fortunately, accelerating professional, governmental, and other involvement in the guidelines enterprise is reflected in two phenomena: the sheer amount of effort now seen and the increased focus on improving the development process and its products. This expansion of the field shows itself in several ways. Among them are the following:

• maturation and specification of formal procedures and structures for guideline development;
• growing appreciation of the complexity and importance of involving the appropriate kinds of individuals in guideline development; and

163

• increased concern about competing and conflicting guidelines, locally adapted guidelines, and transformed versions of guidelines (such as medical review criteria).

More generally, experience with guidelines development is highlighting two rather different (but not mutually exclusive) emphases in or orientations to the process of guidelines development. One approach stresses the significance of the science base for guidelines and the use of quantitative modeling in systematically estimating and comparing outcomes. The other approach stresses professional judgment in areas in which the science base is weak or nonexistent.

This duality need not and should not be seen as an unbridgeable dichotomy. Professional judgment must be applied to the science base, and science must inform professional judgment. When the science base is strong, however, it should not be disregarded in favor of consensus based on customary practice. When consensus is not consistent with the evidence, the case for consensus should be explicitly and persuasively argued.

This chapter begins with a brief discussion of how certain key players in the guidelines arena have evaluated and refined their organizational structures and procedures over the years. Following are several sections that examine persistent issues about methods for developing guidelines, approaches that selected groups have taken in dealing with these issues, and problems that warrant continued attention. A final section discusses the interface of development and implementation as it involves, first, conflicting "national" guidelines; second, local adaptation of existing or emerging "national" guidelines; and, third, formatting and dissemination of guidelines.

The discussion of attributes for review criteria in Chapter 5 and the discussion of cost analysis in Chapter 6 also relate to the theme of this chapter. Although the focus here is on practice guidelines, much of this chapter is also relevant to development of medical review criteria.

GENERAL STRUCTURES AND PROCEDURES

As organizations recognize the demands of developing guidelines in a credible and accountable manner, those entities that plan an ongoing involvement tend to initiate commonly used organizational processes. They create supporting committees, staff positions, procedures, recordkeeping systems, budget justification mechanisms, communications links, and eventually, with more difficulty, mechanisms for evaluating performance and results. Certainly, organizational resources constrain what can be established, but if resources are too limited to create and maintain such organizational structures, they may also be too limited to support the development of products consistent with the attributes set forth in Chapter 1.

The following examples indicate some key ways in which guidelines development is evolving. The first considers the early learning experience of the Agency for Health Care Policy and Research (AHCPR); the second and third examples involve one private and one public organization's efforts to evaluate their work and make their products more credible and useful to practitioners; the fourth example focuses on interorganizational cooperation as a way of building both relevance and credibility.

Learning Lessons: The Agency for Health Care Policy and Research

Not surprisingly, given its short existence and its pattern of rather substantial staff turnover (since September 1990, three directors and three contractors), the AHCPR Forum for Quality and Effectiveness in Health Care has found its structures and procedures to be somewhat in flux. Still, the richness and value of the first year's experience with the AHCPR panels should not be underestimated, and the Forum has made a serious effort to evaluate and build on their experience. When the Forum was barely into its second year, the staff organized a retreat to consider what panel participants and staff had learned from its first few guidelines panels. "Lessons learned" about these complex activities included the points below.[1]

First, the work of the guidelines panel chairpersons has proved vastly more demanding than had been originally envisioned. Current panel chairs and AHCPR staff believe that a commitment of at least 25 percent time is needed to handle these activities adequately.

Second, the literature reviews have been more time-consuming and in some senses more costly than expected. The literature searches, reviews, and analyses took as much as nine months from start to finish and cost anywhere from $22,000 to $235,000, evidently depending chiefly on the strategy used for the literature review and the size of the body of work that needed to be included. In some cases, they were also less rewarding than anticipated, owing in part to the difficulty of identifying (only) appropriate journal articles and similar materials through current National Library of Medicine indexing and coding systems.

Third, costs could probably be brought down somewhat if time constraints on the panels could be loosened and if more specific instructions for methodology were available. Trying to meet tight deadlines tends to be expensive. For example, to complete their work on time, some panels employed unnecessarily highly qualified individuals to carry out the literature review; most made extensive use of Federal Express and overnight mail

---

[1] The points cited are based on unpublished materials ("Summary of Responses to a Questionnaire on Guideline Panel Activities and Views") prepared for the AHCPR Office of the Forum by Health Systems Research, Inc., January 24, 1991.

instead of regular mail. Participants in some panels argued for more centralized guidance about, for example, summary tables, schemes for rating evidence, and other details, which might help to minimize costs related to unnecessary "experimenting" in these areas.[2]

Fourth, in general, the procedures for the first round of AHCPR panels were not uniformly helpful to the panels and their chairpersons. Participants in this first staff retreat, however, could not agree on what specifically they might leave unchanged and what they might modify. One area in which consensus did materialize was that a skilled methodologist should assist the chairperson in organizing the literature search, review, and analysis throughout the process.

The variability in views of the panel chairs and others engaged in the agency's early efforts is itself instructive. Certainly, much of the seeming inefficiency of the initial panels can be ascribed to the fact that the Forum was a new unit in a new agency performing a new function with little time for adequate advance planning—under those circumstances, the endeavors may have gone as smoothly as might have been expected. A second retreat may also be scheduled.

As described in Chapter 2, the agency has elected to sponsor some guidelines panels (on otitis media, rehabilitation following stroke, and congestive heart failure) through a contracting mechanism. The contractors are required to recommend chairpersons and approximately 15 members of the panels, according to an explicit set of criteria specified by AHCPR. Among those criteria are relevant training and clinical experience, interest in quality assurance and research on the clinical condition in question, capacity to lead a health care team and to respond to consumer concerns, a broad public health view, *and* a commitment to and prior experience in the development of clinical practice guidelines.

Building a Formal Program: The Clinical Efficacy Assessment Program

The work of the American College of Physicians (ACP) exemplifies the ongoing formalization of professional society efforts to develop guidelines (Morris, 1987; Ball, 1990; White and Ball, 1990). The ACP began its work on guidelines in 1976 in response to a request from what is now the Blue Cross and Blue Shield Association for assistance in assessing medical techniques; the initial effort was consensus based and relatively informal. In 1981, with a grant from the John A. Hartford Foundation, the ACP initiated

---

[2]A consultant to AHCPR prepared an "Interim Manual" as a protocol for expert panels convened by the Forum; although dated October 1990, it was available in draft form earlier in that year (Woolf, 1990a).

a demonstration project, the Clinical Efficacy Assessment Project (CEAP). In 1984, the ACP established CEAP as a permanent program and in 1986 published its procedures for guidelines development (ACP, 1986).

During 1990, the college evaluated the CEAP effort on the principle that "any good policymaking process must be both self-critical and, when called for, self-correcting" (White and Ball, 1990, p. 51). In one innovative step, the ACP convened focus groups to learn more about the utility and significance of its CEAP efforts. The review made clear that the ACP's decade of experience with CEAP laid the groundwork for experimenting with new models for guidelines development and evaluation.

In the 1990s, the college plans to strengthen its program. Among plans for the future are (1) using new methods for assessing data, including patient preferences; (2) revising formats for guidelines; (3) making draft guidelines available on line for a network of members who will pretest the guidelines and then measure patient outcomes when the guidelines are used according to specific protocols; (4) starting a formal convening activity to involve multidisciplinary groups in the development of guidelines; and (5) developing a systematic and perhaps new way of updating guidelines (Linda White, ACP, personal communication, August 1991). The ACP is also working with researchers at Johns Hopkins Medical Institutions to survey ACP members about their knowledge, perceptions, and use of guidelines. Finally, the ACP has announced plans for a new center to link guidelines development and outcomes research and to try to determine more reliably the use of guidelines by physicians and their utility for these practitioners. In sum, the focus is very much on improving guidelines development and evaluation so that the products of these processes can be more readily and effectively adopted.

Improving Consensus Development: The National Institutes of Health

Over time, government agencies involved directly or indirectly with guideline development have—like professional societies—refined their procedures and methods. One example is the National Institutes of Health (NIH) Consensus Development Conference program, which is administered by the Office of Medical Applications of Research (OMAR, 1988). In the 1980s, OMAR undertook several assessments of the program. Some work was done internally—for example, trials of different mechanisms for running conferences and for disseminating consensus statements (Jacoby, 1983, 1985; Perry, 1987, 1988). Other evaluations were performed by outside parties (Wortman and Vinokur, 1982; Wortman et al., 1988), culminating in a lengthy and rigorous evaluation conducted by RAND Corporation researchers of the content of consensus statements and their impact in terms of different behaviors on the part of physicians (Kosecoff et al., 1987; Kahan et al., 1988; Kanouse et al., 1989).

More recently, an IOM study committee examined OMAR's program and made several recommendations about its structure and functions (IOM, 1990d).[3] The committee called for, among other things, greater emphasis on the concerns of users of consensus statements, with an acknowledgment that the program's fundamental purpose should be "to change behavior toward appropriate use of health practices and technologies" (p. 1). Other issues that the committee addressed were topic selection; better collection, analysis, and use of scientific data before a given conference; attention to dissemination strategies; continued experimentation and self- (or outside) evaluation; and appointment of an external advisory council to assist OMAR in setting its agenda. Again, the objective of these recommendations was to make consensus statements more usable and useful.

Interorganizational Cooperation: Medical Societies and Others

Moving beyond the internal use of multidisciplinary processes, several organizations are looking for opportunities to join formally with other groups in cooperative efforts. To date, collaborations appear to involve mainly physician organizations, although a few involve nonphysician professional groups, research organizations, and payers.

One notable effort aimed at training guidelines developers rather than developing guidelines per se has been sponsored by the John A. Hartford Foundation and the Council of Medical Specialty Societies. Activities have included a training course in which specialty society participants developed guidelines and an introductory manual for developing guidelines (Eddy, 1991c). Reflecting the challenges faced by those who work across specialty lines, workshops on resolving interspecialty conflicts have been another feature of this initiative.

Organizational cooperation, whether within or across professional boundaries, can serve several aims. They include the following:

• greater efficiency through pooling of resources and expertise for methods development, training, and problem solving;

---

[3] In addition, in 1989 the IOM organized a workshop on international consensus development programs in conjunction with an annual meeting of the International Society for Technology Assessment in Health Care (IOM, 1990g). A group of workshop participants developed a lengthy set of recommendations about strengthening such programs. Procedures and methods figured prominently in those recommendations and presaged many of the points made by the IOM practice guidelines study committees. For example, these recommendations concern documentation, use of the best available scientific evidence (including meta-analysis where possible), monitoring and review to determine if recommendations need to be reassessed, and attention to information dissemination and evaluation at the outset of development.

- learning from shared experience;
- better anticipation of user circumstances and concerns; and
- development of commitment and support for implementation from individuals with varied professional and institutional affiliations.

One complex effort involving the American Medical Association (AMA), the RAND Corporation, and a consortium of academic medical centers has already been cited in Chapter 2. This effort has been multiorganizational less in its individual components—indicator construction, guidelines development, and guidelines testing—than in its attempt to create planned links among these activities. The complexity of coupling organizations (not just individuals from different disciplines) has made this project quite difficult to negotiate, execute, and maintain.

Two other multiorganizational efforts led by the AMA were also noted in Chapter 2: the Specialty Society Partnership, involving the AMA and 14 national medical specialty societies, and the Practice Parameters Forum, comprising national medical specialty and state medical societies. Two major objectives of the AMA and the groups working with it have been to devise criteria for judging the soundness of the process for developing practice parameters and then to establish a process for judging specific parameters according to these criteria and perhaps endorsing those that pass (AMA, 1990a). The first criterion is that guidelines should be developed by physician organizations. Reflecting the weight that most professional organizations place on individual professional judgment, the AMA's assessment effort concentrates on process and documentation; it assumes that expert health professionals will have ensured that guidelines correspond to scientific knowledge.

The long-standing collaboration between the Blue Cross and Blue Shield Association and the ACP has produced two seminal handbooks: *Common Diagnostic Tests* (Sox, 1987, 1990) and *Common Screening Tests* (Eddy, 1991a). These handbooks include papers that systematically analyze research, project outcomes, estimate cost-effectiveness, and recommend practices based on the strength of the evidence concerning each test. Each handbook concludes with summary recommendations (guidelines) intended to aid health benefit plans in making coverage decisions. The first handbook prompted considerable furor: it was hailed by the health services, technology assessment, and quality assurance communities and decried by at least some members of the practice community. Criticism soon gave way to acknowledgment of its major contribution to more effective and appropriate clinical decisionmaking, and the major charge that has been made against the second edition is that not all the groups that wanted to be involved in its development were included.

Several other collaborative efforts can be cited. For example, the ACP, the American Academy of Ophthalmology, and the American Diabetes

Association are cooperating on guidelines for management of diabetic retinopathy. The American College of Cardiology and the American Heart Association have had an ongoing collaboration for the past decade. This arrangement has produced nearly a dozen guidelines, which have been published in the *Journal of the American College of Cardiology* and in *Circulation*. The most recent have been for coronary artery bypass graft surgery and for implantation of cardiac pacemakers and antiarrhythmia devices; future guidelines are planned for cardiac catheterization and cardiac catheterization laboratories, electrocardiography, chest pain management in the emergency room, and cardiac radionuclide imaging (a revision of a guideline released in 1986).

PERSISTENT QUESTIONS FOR THE DEVELOPMENT PROCESS

Participation in the Process

As the guidelines development process evolves, more attention is being paid to who takes part in the process, when and how they participate, and what such participation should achieve. This interest reflects both the increasing sophistication of sponsors and the increasing visibility of the process and its products. Several persistent debates about participation can be identified, although the general trend seems to be to expand the scope of involvement. This subsection briefly reviews participative patterns to date; the next subsection addresses points about the development process from a more methodologic stance.

Creating Guidelines Panels and Selecting Panel Members

One issue related to panel selection is whether organizations assemble panels for each guideline or create standing groups. OMAR (for the NIH Consensus Development Conferences) and AHCPR establish independent panels for each guideline. RAND similarly creates a new panel for each technology, procedure, or condition for which it develops appropriateness indicators. By contrast, the Canadian Task Force on the Periodic Health Examination and the U.S. Preventive Services Task Force (USPSTF) have stable, standing panels and expert consultants and engage in a continuous process of revising previous recommendations and addressing new topics. The ACP process occupies the middle ground, with a standing oversight committee but selected experts who are engaged to develop guidelines on specific topics. Although no evidence exists on the subject, it is likely that each strategy is appropriate for different circumstances.

Principles for selecting members of guidelines panels differ along two major dimensions: (1) the generalist-specialist dimension and (2) the physician-nonphysician dimension. The former dimension has been a major concern of physician groups and involves three subdimensions: primary care versus specialist physician, community-based versus academic physicians, and specialists in related fields (for example, the role of a cardiologist in guidelines developed by thoracic surgeons). Questions of expertise and turf are not the only limiting factors: any group tends to find it easier to organize, communicate with, and rely on its own members than on nonmembers.

The second dimension of selection—physician-nonphysician—is debated by most groups that engage in guideline development. It tends to dissolve into two questions: Should other clinicians and health professionals, such as nurses, therapists, health educators, and nutritionists, be involved, and if so how and how much? Similarly, what should be the role of patients and consumers, payers, administrators, and public officials?

Beyond these groups, any number of other types of interested parties and experts may wish or need to be involved in the development of specific guidelines. Among those who might be considered, in the former case, are representatives of voluntary patient and disease groups or representatives of affected provider associations (e.g., hospital or home health agency associations). Involvement in the latter case might comprise expert clinical consultants, expert consultants in other disciplines (economics, law, outcomes measurement), and other methodologists (e.g., those skilled in meta-analysis).

The great majority of specialty organizations apparently rely on expert panels composed entirely of physicians in that specialty. Exceptions to this rule include AHCPR panels, which include primary and specialty physicians, nurses, selected allied health disciplines as appropriate, and consumers. NIH Consensus Development Conference panels may include Ph.D. researchers in addition to physicians and other types of clinicians. Similarly, RAND panels for developing appropriateness criteria and some ACP panels have gone beyond the specialty-specific approach. Site visits for this study suggested that institutional providers (e.g., hospitals, HMOs) that develop guidelines for internal use also are more likely to include different types of clinicians and health professionals.

Selecting Reviewers of Draft Guidelines

Identification of reviewers for sets of draft guidelines is another area in which groups may differ substantially in how they select participants—assuming that they have a process for reviewing draft documents at all. Debates about physician and nonphysician involvement tend to reappear at this stage. Nonetheless, whatever the position of an organization with respect to composition of guidelines panels, it tends at this stage to broaden its range of participants.

The USPSTF, for example, sent its recommendations and draft background papers for review by more than 300 medical, public health, and "other" experts, including individuals in government health agencies, the U.S. Public Health Service, academic medical centers, and medical organizations. The recommendations were revised if a reviewer

> identified relevant studies not examined in the report, misinterpretations of findings, or other issues deserving revision within the constraints of the Task Force methodology. The format of this [the Task Force's] report was designed in consultation with representatives of medical specialty organizations, including the American Medical Association, the American College of Physicians, the American Academy of Family Physicians, the American Academy of Pediatrics, the American College of Obstetricians and Gynecologists, the American College of Preventive Medicine, the American Dental Association, and the American Osteopathic Association (USPSTF, 1989, p. xxxvii).

The AHCPR guidelines are a special case because they are the products of nongovernmental panels supported with federal funds. The government's internal review of the guidelines examines only the process by which they were developed; an elaborate external review and pilot-testing process is being implemented to consider the soundness of the guidelines themselves. For the guidelines to be developed through the contracting mechanism, *four* drafts of guidelines are required. The third draft will be reviewed by an outside group of "peer reviewers," and the fourth (that is, the version produced after the peer review process) will be subjected to pilot-testing. Based on comments from the pilot-testers, a fifth and final version of the guideline is to be submitted to AHCPR.

Increasing concern about the practical needs of professionals is reflected in the recent activities of the American Society of Internal Medicine (ASIM) and its Internal Medicine Center to Advance Research and Education (IMCARE, 1990; Simmons, 1990). The center has created an innovative Guidelines Network that will not develop guidelines but instead organize network internists to review, upon request, the guidelines of other organizations. The intent is to provide greater insight into how well a guideline may work in clinical practice. For guidelines developed by a subspecialty but intended for use by all internists, network members offer broad-based feedback beyond the subspecialty.

More than 400 internists nationwide, including physicians in general and subspecialty internal medicine, have contacted the network about being volunteer reviewers. Furthermore, to broaden participation, internal medicine-related organizations are being asked to suggest additional volunteers. Although network members are primarily ASIM members, ASIM membership is not a requirement. IMCARE plans to establish an advisory panel on an annual basis; 1991 appointments were announced in March (IMCARE, 1991).

The IMCARE guidelines network is informing AHCPR and other organizations of its availability to aid their guideline development or evaluation efforts. One early activity of IMCARE involved this IOM project. Specifically, the center staff organized an evaluation of the IOM's draft guidelines assessment instrument, which appears in revised form in Appendix B. That review produced 65 useful responses (and an overall summary) in a relatively short turnaround time.

Another review strategy is typified by the ACP's practice of publishing background papers and policy statements in the *Annals of Internal Medicine*. This opens the analyses and guidelines to very broad professional and scientific scrutiny. In general, the ACP has instituted a sort of "due process" by seeking the opinions of any agency, group, or individual with a potential vested interest.

Updating Existing Guidelines

"Scheduled review," one desirable attribute for practice guidelines, asserts that guideline documents should state when a guideline ought to be revisited and what information would trigger a detailed review and possible change in or withdrawal of the guideline. Generally, such statements put users on notice that the developer group may not or will not stand behind the guideline in its current form once the deadline has arrived. Given the acute sensitivity of professional organizations to advancing medical knowledge, the need for such a review process appears to be well understood, although in practice it may be implemented to differing degrees.

The General Accounting Office's (GAO, 1991b) survey of medical specialty societies found that most of the groups had discussed a process of periodic review and updating of guidelines but that not all had begun (or had even begun planning) such a process. Of those societies with plans or programs, seven planned annual reviews and one planned a 10-year review with earlier revisiting of the guideline if the need was clear. One society invokes a "sunset" provision by stating that guidelines will expire after 3 years and must be rewritten (unless they have been revised in the interim). As organizations continue to formalize their guidelines development activities, a typical goal is to establish a formal review process to determine if and when guidelines need updating or other action.

Formal updating activities can involve specifying a target review date when a guideline is first proposed and reinstating a former guidelines panel or appointing a new one. Alternatively, a periodic or rolling review process can be established that routinely covers all guidelines. The Canadian Task

Force, for instance, reconvened in 1982, 1984, 1986, and 1988 to revise recommendations and evaluate new topics (USPSTF, 1989, p. xvi). A much lower level of activism is pursued by many organizations, which simply include in their guidelines a statement to the effect that the guidelines should be, or may need to be, modified as more information becomes available.

At a presentation to the committee in early 1991, J. Jarrett Clinton, the AHCPR administrator, noted that the AHCPR Forum expects that updating of at least some of its guidelines may be needed as often as every year. The Forum does not plan to conduct "continuous" review and updating but rather to institute a "regular" procedure. Overall, it aims to produce dozens of guidelines, resulting in a large family of guidelines; at some point, however, it will not be able to grow and simultaneously continue to revisit the entire set of guidelines, so some priority setting will have to be done and choices about updating will have to be made. In the meantime, the Forum expects to implement a form of scheduled review either by asking panels to state when their products should be revisited or by bringing the panel back to see how much has changed and to decide and recommend what to do. In some cases the difference between what would be needed for a new guideline and what exists in the current one might be sufficient to prompt the Forum to create a new panel.

These updating procedures can ameliorate but not resolve the dilemmas that arise if a guideline has not been revisited or revised, particularly if such a guideline has been accorded any special legal or regulatory status. Some believe that the idea of dating or withdrawing guidelines or otherwise implementing scheduled review procedures puts physicians and other clinicians in an impossible situation—using "definitive" guidelines one day and "expired" ones the next. Others contend that the dilemma of what authoritative information is available and should be used is precisely the situation health care providers find themselves in today. Arguably, definitive guidelines, even if they expire at some point, would be an improvement on today's environment.

AREAS FOR METHODS RESEARCH AND DEVELOPMENT

Several issues in particular appear to the committee to be worth further investment in methodological research and development. These issues involve the selection of topics for guideline development, processes for securing expert judgment and consensus, ways of assigning weights to the scientific evidence, outcomes measurement, techniques for determining and incorporating patient preferences, and means for identifying and evaluating inconsistencies and conflicts among guidelines on the same topic. The suggestions in the sections that follow reinforce the committee's general point that the methods and processes used in guidelines development can significantly affect the credibility and utility of guidelines and the extent to which guidelines can achieve the objectives discussed in Chapter 1. Chapter 6 has already noted the need for further technical work to advance the field of cost-effectiveness analysis.

Topic Selection

The demands of guideline development on sponsor resources and the huge array of interesting topics make the identification of priorities and the selection of topics an inevitable and important issue. Any effort to establish a systematic process for these tasks faces certain questions of methodology. In particular: (1) Should the focus be chiefly on clinical conditions (broad or narrow diagnoses, illnesses, symptoms, or complaints) or on specific technologies (broadly defined to mean invasive or noninvasive procedures, medications, devices, and specific medical, nursing, or other health care practices)? (2) Should the priority-setting strategy rely more on expert opinion or quantitative data?

The Omnibus Budget Reconciliation Act of 1989 (OBRA 89) contained a fairly typical statement of broad criteria for selecting topics for guidelines development, at least for AHCPR assignments. These criteria seem to favor clinical conditions over specific technologies but take no explicit stand on expert opinion versus data. Per OBRA, AHCPR, in selecting topics, should consider practice variations, the potential for improving outcomes, and Medicare expenditures and program needs.

Many organizations list two criteria among their own priorities. One is the frequency of use of an intervention or the prevalence of the condition, and the other is the cost (to the nation or to a specific organization) of caring for that condition (or, possibly, using that technology). These criteria seem to stress quantitative data, perhaps assuming the use of expert opinion.

Even when explicit criteria are publicly stated, the process of choosing topics often remains relatively casual and uninformed by systematically collected, quantitative data. Choices may be posed and decisions made by program staff or oversight groups based on subjective judgments of what would be useful and what could actually be done, given the organization's resources.

Sometimes, topic selection is complicated by outside influences or interests. A case in point is the NIH Consensus Development Conferences. Topic selection in this case is made more difficult by OMAR's need to interest, or be responsive to, individual institutes within the NIH complex. Those institutes may well have their own criteria for topic selection, and they vary in their preferences for a focus on clinical conditions and a focus on technologies.

Paralleling the processes for developing guidelines are two "competing" ways to set priorities for guideline development: consensus methods and quantitative (or modeling) approaches. These methods are marked by quite different techniques that are likely to produce different results (IOM, 1990j).

The consensus approach to priority setting synthesizes the judgments of a group of experts who have been asked to identify topics and rank them. In its ideal form the group would be well balanced in terms of the professional disciplines and characteristics of its members (as recommended for other aspects of the guideline development process), although this form of topic selection probably achieves the ideal only rarely, if ever. Consensus processes vary considerably in the extent to which they employ explicit criteria to guide judgments.

Phelps and Parente (1990) and Eddy (1989) have both described formal modeling approaches that rely heavily on quantitative data to inform priority setting. These approaches, too, have their drawbacks: they are necessarily limited by the availability and quality of data, especially data on important but difficult-to-quantify criteria, and by the degree to which assumptions are explicit and reasonable.

In general, a good—and attainable—priority-setting process would attempt to establish explicit criteria for rating potential topics for guidelines or related assessments and to apply the criteria using available data; it would also include the systematic use of consensus methods when data were unobtainable. Further research, however, is needed.

The IOM is presently engaged in a follow-on study to its earlier pilot project (IOM, 1990j) of setting priorities for technology assessment and reassessment. The study is based on directives in OBRA 89 and funded by AHCPR; its charge is to advise the agency's Office of Health Technology Assessment (OHTA) on processes and criteria for priority setting. Among the criteria to be considered are the potential for an assessment to change health outcomes, the extent of variations in practice styles, the prevalence of a condition (or rate of use of a technology), the burden of the illness (for example, in terms of quality-adjusted life expectancy), costs (including total annual outlays for the condition or the technology), and various ethical, legal, and social issues. A report on IOM's proposed model and its relevance for both OHTA and other organizations that perform technology assessment was published in early 1992 (IOM, 1992).

Expert Panel Processes

A second major area for empirical investigation involves mechanisms for identifying and convening expert panels and similar groups and for deriving statements of expert judgment or consensus (Fink et al., 1984;

IOM, 1990g; Lomas, 1991). Group judgment techniques (e.g., pure and modified Delphi approaches, nominal group techniques) and related group-oriented activities (e.g., focus groups) have many uses beyond guideline development; some of these uses include technology assessment, consensus-building in areas outside health, sales and marketing, and the like.

Despite the long history of these approaches (some date back decades), many questions still remain about their reliability and effectiveness. For example:

• *What is the optimal size of a group?* Depending on its procedures and objectives, an expert panel might have as few as 8 members (a small panel) or as many as 18 (a large one). It would be a mistake to organize a large panel and expect it to function well according to small-panel procedures. Group size affects group dynamics; the potential effect of group size on judgments and on group commitment to those judgments needs to be considered.

• *How should members be identified and appointed?* Is it better to rely on personal networks and acquaintances to identify respected clinician leaders in a particular area, or to use nominations from professional associations and societies? Additionally, is it important always to have geographic and other demographic or professional diversity (e.g., practitioners from all regions of the country; rural, urban, and inner-city workers; representatives from fee-for-service and prepaid systems; experts from academic centers and from private practice)? How is the threat of bias or conflict of interest to be balanced against the need for experience and expertise?

• *Who should lead the panel?* Among experts in group judgment techniques, debate still arises as to whether physician groups should be led by a physician or by a nonphysician facilitator. (The same issue arises for guidelines related to conditions or technologies involving nonphysician health professionals.) For any given guidelines development effort, the physicians who are candidates for the role of group leader may or may not be good facilitators and may or may not have biases that, whether spoken or not, would unduly shape group processes. On the other hand, a skilled nonphysician group leader may or may not be able to command respect from physician panel members and may or may not be sufficiently well versed in the clinical issues to recognize when problems are emerging or when clinical preconceptions are unduly influencing the discussion.

• *How should the deliberations and decisionmaking of expert panels be structured?* Various evocatively named approaches have been tried—for example, the "town meeting," "science court," and "science conference"—and both mail and face-to-face processes for defining questions and evaluating alternatives have been used (Lomas, 1991). Little research is available on the impact of different procedures on panel decisions. Even the question of how to define consensus (e.g., through informal means or formal votes, using percentages or scaling techniques) has not been subject to much, if any, empirical testing. Similarly, the consequences of different strategies (e.g., explicit versus implicit) for defining and reaching consensus are not well documented.

Evaluating Scientific Evidence

The third set of methods issues involves techniques for assessing, rating, and combining scientific evidence. Guidelines developers normally must weigh the soundness and relevance of both direct and indirect evidence, evidence generated by processes of varying degrees of rigor, and studies that differ in design details and findings (Eddy, 1991b).

Problems tend to be most explicit for meta-analysis and related information-synthesis activities, for which investigators must formally combine information from (often completely) dissimilar articles and publications.[4] Mulrow (1987) and Thacker (1988) both provide useful introductions to meta-analysis and ways to combine evidence of differing types and quality. Thacker cautions that although meta-analysis is more explicit than traditional methods of narrative review of the literature and has other advantages, it may impart an "unwarranted sense of scientific validity" (p. 1688) of which consumers of such reviews (particularly those unfamiliar with the limitations of the statistical methods) need to be wary.

Most guideline developers do not elect to employ such complex techniques for weighting and synthesizing evidence, and many do not use any explicit approach. One simple but explicit rating scheme was pioneered by the Canadian Task Force and slightly adapted by the USPSTF (1989). This approach gives the greatest weight to information from randomized controlled trials (RCTs) and the least weight to simple case reports. It can also be criticized, however, for effectively placing more emphasis on poorly conducted RCTs than on well-done case-control or other quasi-experimental studies; in addition, the weighting scheme itself is an arbitrary one. More flexible but less arbitrary weighting schemes have been proposed and compared with more conventional approaches (Eddy, 1990k); one problem with

---

[4] Meta-analysis, a quantitative method to combine data, has several advantages over traditional narrative analyses of the literature on a clinical topic. In particular, it is a means for estimating the magnitude of effect of a given clinical intervention in terms of a statistically significant effect size or an odds (probability) ratio. More qualitatively, it forces those doing the literature analysis to think systematically about several aspects of the studies being reviewed and the data being pooled. The literature about meta-analysis (both substantive and statistical) has grown considerably in the 15 years since the term was first coined (Glass, 1976). Authoritative works include Hedges and Olkin, 1985; L'Abbe et al., 1987; Sacks et al., 1987; Oxman and Guyatt, 1988; and Berlin et al., 1989.

these schemes, however, is that they are technically demanding. Notwithstanding that systematic clinical evidence is relatively limited and typically flawed in some respects, it is nonetheless important to find feasible ways to make the best use of that evidence.

Patient Outcomes

A fourth area of methodologic concern focuses on means of improving knowledge of patient outcomes, interest in which accelerated at about the same time but somewhat independently of the growing interest in guidelines development.[5] IOM committees concerned with practice guidelines and with related issues (quality of care, effectiveness research, disability) have been particularly strong proponents of incorporating patient outcome information into clinical practice guidelines. Their recommendations are based on a broad conceptualization of outcomes that involves several dimensions of health status and health-related quality of life, especially those of direct importance to, and reported by, individual patients or their family members.

In this conceptualization, the dimensions of health status include survival and life expectancy, symptom states, physiologic states, physical function states, emotional and cognitive states, perceptions about present and future health, and satisfaction with health care. The last six of these seven domains of health status are particularly significant for guidelines aimed at conditions that are not life-threatening.

The field of health status assessment is becoming well established in the health services and health policy research arenas. (For a sampling of this literature, see Bergner, 1985; Lohr and Ware, 1987; McDowell and Newell, 1987; Lohr, 1988; Patrick and Erickson, 1988; Lohr, 1989; Mosteller and Falotico-Taylor, 1989; Tarlov et al., 1989.) In OBRA 89, Congress gave AHCPR the legislative mandate to conduct effectiveness research, chiefly through the Patient Outcomes Research Teams (PORTs) program described in Chapter 2. Acceptance and application of health status assess-

---

[5] The Health Care Financing Administration (HCFA), with the guidance of former administrator William Roper, is generally credited with giving outcomes and effectiveness research a major boost through its proposed effectiveness initiative (Roper et al., 1988; IOM, 1990e). Paul Ellwood's Shattuck Lecture (1988) is also recognized as a major influence. (The Inter-Study Outcomes Management System, a private initiative stimulated by Ellwood, was described in Chapter 4.) Also widely cited is the work by John Wennberg and his colleagues on practice variation (Wennberg and Gittelsohn, 1973, 1982; McPherson et al., 1982; Wennberg, 1984) and on outcomes of open and transurethral surgery for benign prostatic hypertrophy (BPH) versus "watchful waiting" (Wennberg et al., 1987, 1988; Barry et al., 1988; Fowler et al., 1988; Greenfield, 1989). HCFA's controversial efforts to produce hospital-specific mortality rate data on Medicare patients were an early attempt to provide the public as well as health care institutions with information on patient outcomes (Brinkley, 1986; HCFA, 1987-1991; Jencks et al., 1988a,b; Chassin et al., 1989).

ment methods are also increasing in biomedical and clinical investigation (Wenger et al., 1984; Mor, 1987; Luce et al., 1989; Spilker, 1990). This work is not very well known to the practice community, however, and information it has assembled has not yet permeated the guideline development process.[6] The GAO survey of medical specialty societies (1991b) found that some but not all guideline developers believed that outcome information should be incorporated in guidelines.[7] How to do so remains a significant challenge to guidelines organizations, as reflected in a recent essay by Mulley (1991).

Several knotty problems can be cited. First, the significance, value, and validity of health measures based on patient self-reports have been questioned. Second, little empirical evidence exists because broad health status measures have not been widely used in clinical trials or technology assessments until recently. Third, amassing information on outcomes of all reasonable alternative courses of care is difficult, although information may be available on a specific intervention. Fourth, the unrepresentative populations used in most clinical trials limit the generalizability of findings to other populations such as women and minorities. This committee hopes that its strong stand on the need to incorporate estimates of patient outcomes will lead to more use of outcomes measures and further work to overcome their current limitations.

Patient Preferences

Chapter 5 discussed patient preferences in the context of concerns about ethics, costs, and informed decisionmaking and noted the difficult conceptual and policy challenges this topic presents to developers and users of guidelines. A particular problem involves the weight to be given to patient preferences. Judgments may vary depending on the nature of the expected benefits and harms, their various probabilities of occurring, the degree to which patients truly understand the information presented to them, and the locus of responsibility for payment.

In addition to conceptual and policy challenges related to patient pref-

---

[6] In September 1991, the IOM convened a conference on advances in health status assessment that focused heavily on the use of health-related quality-of-life measures in clinical practice and clinical settings. The papers and discussions were aimed more at the practice community than at the research or policymaking community; the proceedings will be published in mid-1992 in *Medical Care* (Lohr, forthcoming). A landmark set of papers concerning quality-of-life measurement in surgery has also appeared in the *Journal of Theoretical Surgery* (Neugebauer et al., 1991).

[7] The most ambitious project cited in the survey involved a society that proposed to estimate outcomes and to conduct the work necessary to assess actual outcomes over a three- to five-year period.

erences, various practical difficulties arise for those seeking to apply guidelines in everyday practice. One approach is to incorporate patient preference "decision nodes" into algorithms and protocols that are devised from guidelines documents. These points would highlight for physicians and other caregivers points at which options for diagnosis and management should be discussed with patients or families and their preferences for particular options elicited.

An approach that focuses on how rather than when to elicit patient preferences involves the interactive videodisc technology developed at Dartmouth Medical School (Wennberg, 1990). Progress has been greatest on a videodisc for BPH; others on breast cancer and low back pain are under way. A patient sees, from the videodisc, a narrative about the main treatment options (a form of "guideline") and possible outcomes and complications (benefits and risks of those options). Because the information is presented in an interactive medium, it puts the patient in an active role and tailors the information presented to that patient's status, taking into account such factors as age and symptom severity.

The issue of patient preferences will stimulate further methodological development, research, and debate on at least three fronts. First, what are the best techniques for eliciting preferences? Second, what information and other conditions are required for informed and rational statements of preference? Third, what are the technical and policy issues in quantifying individual preferences (utilities) and aggregating preferences for purposes of making judgments about what care is appropriate (Mulley, 1989; IOM, 1991a)? Still, as much as methodological improvements and more research are desirable, they will not resolve policy debates about what preferences should be supported through coverage under public or private health plans and what should be the financial responsibility of the patients.

Conflicting or Inconsistent Guidelines

As the examples and discussion throughout this report make clear, the guidelines enterprise is a singularly pluralistic one. Furthermore, although the topics that might be addressed (clinical conditions, or technologies, or both) are nearly endless, the ones that tend to surface more frequently are those that affect large numbers of individuals, that have large costs associated with them, or that are mired in uncertainty or controversy. As a consequence, more than one group may well be working on guidelines on similar topics. Furthermore, these groups may take different approaches to the methodological issues discussed above, and some may apply cost-effectiveness or other criteria that others do not apply in making recommendations. This pluralism makes it likely that different groups will produce somewhat different and perhaps inconsistent and conflicting guidelines.

The extent to which inconsistent guidelines are "a menace and an obstacle to improved care" as argued recently (Hinterbuchner, 1991, p. 5) rather than tolerable or possibly desirable depends on the reasons for inconsistencies. One approach to identifying and understanding inconsistencies and weaknesses in specific guidelines has been developed by Margolis, Gottlieb, and their associates (1991). This method, which they call algorithmic analysis, focuses on the completeness and consistency of clinical practice guidelines taken individually and in comparison.[8] Hayward and his colleagues (1991) also have systematically compared several guidelines for preventive services.

Both sets of investigations found inconsistencies and conflicts in the guidelines they examined. Some guidelines were simply more complete, internally consistent, and specific than others. Other inconsistencies appear to reflect implicit or explicit differences in attitudes about the use of expert judgment, the risk of false-positives, the importance of costs, and other matters. Finally, some of the differences reflect the impact of new evidence that has appeared in the intervals between publication of different guidelines; for example, between the publication of the first and second asthma guidelines studied by Margolis and coworkers, the recommended sites of care for many specific problems had shifted from inpatient to outpatient settings.

Some committee members argued, when conflicting guidelines are encountered, for deliberately seeking areas of consistency, on the grounds that the stronger, more defensible points will be found there. Others on the committee noted that for certain conditions or technologies about which the science base is limited, conflicting guidelines may not necessarily be "wrong."

---

[8] In one test of this method on multiple sets of guidelines for measles immunization, breast cancer screening, and management of asthma, each set of guidelines was converted from free-text (prose) to flowchart format (the algorithm map) and then restated as clinical rules (if-then statements). The first category of deficiency involved *nonspecific terms and phrases*, which generally were retained in the flowchart. Among these phrases were the following: "mammography every 1-2 years"; "unless medically indicated sooner"; "quarantine measures"; and "supportive care." The second type of problem concerned *nonspecific phrases* that had to be better specified in constructing the algorithm map. Examples included "approximately age 75," which was changed to "age 75"; "at an earlier age," which was modified to read "between age 35 and 39"; and "nurses, nursing and medical students," which became "all employees with patient contact." The third and fourth categories covered *missing items*. Relevant missing items included recommending the teaching of breast self-examination but not recommending a specific frequency; providing overly abbreviated descriptions of contraindications to measles vaccine; and failing to indicate age ranges to which recommendations applied. The fifth category of deficiencies involved *logical inconsistencies that can be regarded as errors*. For example, a student in grades kindergarten through twelfth grade cannot have been born before 1957 despite an evident assumption to this effect in one of the guidelines (presumably the result of a failure to update the guideline).

Sometimes conflicts and inconsistencies will direct attention to critical areas of desirable research to support more consistency and certainty in the future. In other cases, inconsistencies may prompt some groups to consider whether they have declared a position on a matter that might better be treated as a question with only a tentative answer at best. This stance may be psychologically disquieting for those who are accustomed to being (and who are expected to be) definitive.

A challenge remains in how to reconcile conflicting guidelines emanating from two authoritative groups, such as general internal medicine and a subspecialty society. It is particularly germane to certain settings or types of practice that must accommodate both clinical groups—for example, large multispecialty groups or health maintenance organizations. The solution here may be a form of disciplined accommodation in which both guidelines are rewritten in ways that are acceptable to both groups, probably by (1) strenuously seeking areas of agreement, (2) working to make rationales for differences explicit and susceptible to comparison with available evidence, (3) assessing the value of reducing practice variation in accord with the tenets of continuous quality improvement, and (4) allowing options to remain where a case can be made that evidence is inconclusive, professional consensus is split, and variation is unlikely to harm quality of care.

ISSUES AT THE INTERFACE OF DEVELOPMENT AND IMPLEMENTATION

At least three topics are not clearly development or methodological issues in the strictest sense: local adaptation of national guidelines, translation of guidelines into medical review criteria, and formatting and dissemination activities. In each of these areas, those who develop guidelines ought to be sensitive to the needs of users of guidelines so that they do not—through inadvertence, ambiguity, or lack of thoroughness—lead users astray. Conversely, those who are taking guidelines from the development to the application stage should be sensitive to the ideals of credibility and accountability stressed in Chapter 1.

Local Adaptation

Although national efforts to develop guidelines through public and private organizations have received considerable attention, local development and adaptation of national guidelines appear to be both widespread and little examined. This committee does not have extensive documentation of the extent, quality, and impact of local efforts, but it believes there is reason to be concerned about these efforts. The possibility for conflict and inconsistency simply multiplies, if and to the degree that local provider institutions, medical societies, and the like adapt and modify guidelines to make them more locally appropriate or palatable.

Reasons for Local Adaptation

From site visits, anecdotal literature, personal experience, and similar sources, the committee identified many ways in which guidelines developed by national professional societies and other groups may be adapted, changed, or even ignored to serve the purposes of particular groups. Such adaptations are termed "local" even when the adjustments serve a multihospital system, nationwide network of HMOs, or other similar groups.

The reasons for adaptation, which are not necessarily defensible, may involve one or more of the following: (1) weaknesses in the guidelines or their dissemination that have no particular relation to local circumstances; (2) specific local or organizational objectives or constraints; (3) strategic judgments about the need to secure practitioner acceptance; and (4) protection of habit or self-interest. In addition, when local organizations face inconsistent guidelines, their choices will almost certainly lead to departures from one or more of these guidelines. For example, a group might choose to follow the ACP in not recommending a baseline mammogram but then follow the American Cancer Society guidelines for screening every 1 or 2 years for women aged 40 to 49.

Local adaptation might also be done on the basis of a thorough decision analysis of a "national" guideline. Such analysis might clarify how patient care options can legitimately differ depending on prevalence of disease, diagnostic test performance, physician skill level, costs, or other variables that might vary from locality to locality. If the "adapted" guideline were based on such an analysis of a national guideline that made such distinctions, it might then be more easily justified than if it had no such analytic underpinnings.

By contrast, some national guidelines are poorly drafted and give inadequate attention to their applicability to specific patient problems, identification of foreseeable exceptions, and clarity or precision. Thus, hospital medical staff who want protocols to guide treatment of patients with particular conditions may have to "fill in" when guidelines lack the specificity needed to make decisions about individual cases. Although such adjustments may be initiated by local organizations, the rationale need not be organization or community specific.

Other adjustments will reflect local conditions because even generally well-developed guidelines are unlikely to foresee or accommodate all the varying characteristics and objectives of potential users of a set of guidelines. For example, if the prevalence of a problem (e.g., human immuno-deficiency virus infection) in a community or the characteristics of a particular patient population (e.g., mobility of migrant workers) differ dramatically from the situations contemplated by a set of guidelines, some modification in recommended preventive, diagnostic, or treatment regimens may be reasonable.

Similarly, some health delivery systems and institutions may face constraints that are unchangeable in the short term. These constraints might involve regulatory prohibitions, lack of equipment, or shortages of personnel. Such problems may prompt adaptations that define protocols for situations in which care must be provided but the most appropriate course of care is impossible to implement.

Chapter 6 recognized that national guidelines may not incorporate judgments of cost-effectiveness, which some organizations believe they must have to allocate limited resources in a manner consistent with their objectives and environments. Other organizations may seek to apply continuous quality improvement precepts to narrow variations in practice. The result of both these policies may be guidelines that exclude certain options, on the grounds that they are too costly relative to their benefits, or that delineate specific "pathways" or "protocols" that are less variable than those described in a set of national guidelines. A typical example of a narrowing in guidelines occurs when an organization or a public agency (e.g., a state Medicaid program) creates a drug formulary that does not include all of the drugs that are considered reasonable options for treating certain problems. Depending on the extent to which an institution intends to constrain its financial liability for the use of costly but optional forms of care, patient preferences may be accorded greater or lesser weight than they are in national guidelines.

Another rationale given for the adaptation of guidelines is behavioral. Some argue that it is important to secure practitioner (and, less commonly, patient or enrollee) acceptance of guidelines through participation in their adoption. Some departures from national guidelines are viewed as acceptable when it is thought that such variation will lead to the actual use of the most critical elements in guidelines rather than to their rejection. The committee had mixed feelings about this rationale, and this discussion should not be seen as a justification for wholesale or casual departure from well-documented, science-based guidelines for clinical practice.

Finally, generally unstated rationales for local adaptation may be to protect professional habits and local customs for their own sake and to protect economic self-interest by endorsing unnecessary care or care that others could provide as well or more economically. For example, a guideline that did not specifically limit the type of practitioner who could perform certain kinds of eye examinations might be reworked to restrict the practice only to physicians or to particular specialists. Committee members were distinctly unsympathetic to such practices and to rationales for guidelines that were covertly designed to protect habit, "turf," or income at the expense of patients and those who pay for their care.

In short, the main concern here is with fundamental departures from an existing scientifically based, well-documented set of guidelines. Among such changes would be designating certain practices appropriate when national guidelines define them as inappropriate, labeling a practice optional rather than recommended or vice versa, or changing threshold values for making treatment decisions.

When local institutions do adapt national guidelines, one useful step might be for them to notify the originating group and to explain the circumstances that led to their modifications. Whether national guidelines could or should be revised to accommodate or recognize these circumstances will depend on the specifics (for example, the likelihood that the same circumstances will occur more generally). If this process of communication and consideration became established, it would provide an ongoing—if not always systematic—source of feedback for revising and improving guidelines.

Processes for Local Adaptation

Local programs to adapt guidelines vary greatly in the formality of their processes and structures, but they appear generally to be a less sophisticated, less rigorous kind of effort than that endorsed by this committee. One effort located toward the sophisticated, science-based end of this spectrum is the work by Group Health Cooperative of Puget Sound (GHCPS) to develop a preventive care manual for its primary care practitioners. This activity, described in Chapter 6, reflects a specific objective (focusing resources on high-risk groups) and specific organizational characteristics (for example, an enrolled population and integrated patient records). One particular task for GHCPS has been to reconcile or choose from among inconsistent guidelines from different sources, although the materials available to this committee do not fully explicate the basis for different choices.

The less scientific, more behavioral or strategic approach is represented by one of the groups visited by the committee. This organization was developing guidelines or pathways for the care of patients admitted for certain common clinical procedures. Those involved did not employ a systematic process to identify and assess the scientific literature, estimate health outcomes, explain the rationale for the pathway, or document these steps. The pathways were presented as charts to advise clinicians on generally desired practices and to reduce variability in patient care. Although this last process did not incorporate systematic use of the scientific literature on a clinical problem, it was systematic and data oriented in that it identified topics for pathway development based, in part, on the variability in existing practice patterns. Practitioners received periodic reports on how their performance compared with that of their peers and with the pathway.

Within a framework such as that offered by continuous quality improvement, empirical and incremental testing and modification of guidelines may well be appropriate (indeed, even necessary). Such testing may not conform to the highest standards of experimental research design, but it can provide a systematic, practical, and direct means of identifying where guidelines—as well as clinical practice—may need modification. Ideally, this kind of local but systematic information will become part of the broader evolutionary framework for guidelines development and improvement as national and local groups develop communication and tracking mechanisms.

Other local processes may be fairly unsystematic. They involve no analysis of local patterns of care, no explicit formulation of objectives, no literature review, no formal decisionmaking processes, and no documentation of evidence or rationales for decisions. This method might be called a "back of the envelope" approach to guideline development.

Even when the rationale is worthy, this "back of the envelope" approach to adapting or developing guidelines (or medical review criteria) is unacceptable. It offers too much leeway, on the one hand, for uncritical accommodation of local traditions and narrow self-interest and, on the other, for excessive and unwarranted interference with physician-patient decisionmaking.

The Standing of "Adapted" Guidelines

Adaptation processes intended to win physician acceptance of guidelines—the behavioral rationale for adaptation—should be guided and constrained by an expectation that the resulting guidelines and criteria will still be credible in their process, rationale, and documentation. The requirement for systematic and careful procedures applies as well to de novo development activities and efforts to devise medical review criteria. Where carefully developed and documented "national" guidelines exist, local adaptation processes should provide explicit rationales for changes that relate to specific, well-defined local conditions or objectives.

If national guidelines are in one way or another accorded legal stature with respect to malpractice liability (or immunity from liability), then serious attention must be given to the stature of guidelines that are modified to suit local circumstances or preferences and, possibly, to the criteria used to evaluate the quality of care that is rendered. Even if it can be shown that these derivations of existing national guidelines were arrived at through procedures similar to those that produced the original guideline, they may or may not enjoy the same legal stature as the originals. Although the "respectable minority" doctrine described in Chapter 5 could accommodate some differences, it would be troublesome were it to justify departures from guidelines that are based on strong scientific evidence and consensus. Given the evolving views about the relationship between malpractice and guidelines in general, this issue is quite speculative at this time.

Formatting and Dissemination

For the purposes of this report, effective formatting means presenting guidelines in physical arrangements or media that can be readily understood and applied by practitioners, patients, or other intended user groups. Effective dissemination means delivering guidelines to their intended audiences in ways that promote the reception, understanding, acceptance, application, and positive impact of the guidelines. For the purposes of this discussion, effective dissemination presupposes effective formatting, and the discussion centers on the former. Appendix A discusses and illustrates some approaches to formatting guidelines.

Dissemination is in part an answer to the question: "Suppose I want a guideline for something. What do I need to do to find it?" Two broad possibilities exist. First, organizations currently producing guidelines probably have distributed them or related materials, and the questioner may well have filed the documents so that they can be retrieved. Second, the relevant guidelines may have been acquired by a general information resource such as the National Library of Medicine (NLM) and entered into a data base that can be queried on a wide array of topics.

Sponsors and developers of guidelines usually take responsibility for their initial dissemination to major target audiences, often either physicians or nurses. For example, many specialty societies, such as the ACP and the American College of Cardiology, begin their dissemination efforts by publishing individual guidelines in their journals, which all members receive. The GAO survey (1991b) reported that societies also publish in newsletters, the journals of other societies, and other places. For some types of guidelines, particularly for collections dealing with similar clinical issues, the initial step may be direct distribution of the guidelines to members. The American Academy of Pediatrics does this every other year with its Report of the Committee on Infectious Diseases, familiarly known as the Red Book (AAP, 1991). Specialty societies may also distribute guidelines to other societies, to federal agencies, and to selected audiences in the health care and medical education communities. Press conferences and press releases may accompany such publications.

One strength of these kinds of dissemination activities is that they are part of an ongoing process. They have an institutional past and a future that should help build both awareness and acceptance, at least among members of the sponsoring organization and eventually among outsiders as well.

Following initial dissemination steps,[9] guideline developers may proceed with an array of activities such as cooperating with other interested parties in disseminating information to patients or consumers. This is where the second response noted above comes into play. The lay press, patient groups, computerized information systems, and directories may begin to make guidelines more widely available or known to practitioners, patients, and others. As noted earlier, the AMA publishes quarterly update listings of guidelines developed by both the AMA and specialty societies. In addition, publications are emerging that reprint or summarize selected guidelines or otherwise report on the field; the *Report on Medical Guidelines & Outcomes Research*, published by Health & Sciences Communications and now nearing the end of its second year, is an example. The NLM, as described elsewhere in this report, will store, index, and otherwise make available information on practice guidelines, specifically including those from AHCPR panels.

Those involved in the development and use of guidelines are paying increasing attention to a series of strategic "who, what, why, when, and how" questions. Specifically: Who do you want to reach and why? What do they need? How quickly do you want to reach them? What relevant techniques are available, and how do they vary in effectiveness and cost? Answers to these questions will influence some dissemination decisions such as whether to use professional or mass media, direct mailings, or journal publication. The length and complexity of the guideline will also influence the choice of dissemination technique. As noted in Chapter 4, options for dissemination now include a variety of computer-based tools including on-line literature search systems, floppy disks, and CD-ROM disks.

Other decisions will be contingent on a variety of environmental factors. What are the opportunities for dissemination and application within the intended audience? What are the barriers? How can different dissemination strategies be combined and coordinated with other implementation strategies to increase the probability of effective application of guidelines? Answers to these questions will yield ideas about who else will be or should be involved in dissemination, whether it should be a one-time effort or a continuous process, and what resources are needed. Many of the issues raised in the discussion of education in Chapter 4 will apply here as well.

Several specific factors related to dissemination might be considered legitimate and realistic concerns of guidelines developers, even if develop-

---

[9] In addition to publishing guidelines (in various media) and generally publicizing the availability of the guidelines document, disseminating organizations may also respond to requests for and inquiries about the guidelines and undertake similar tasks. Dissemination should also be understood to include any efforts needed to inform users of mistakes ("errata" or corrections, in publishing terms) and to advise users that existing guidelines are being withdrawn or revised.

ers do not actually carry out dissemination activities. Among these are
characteristics of the target audience, timeliness and number of dissemination efforts, and the planned publishing, publicizing, and distribution of the
guidelines. Depending on the combinations of these factors, dissemination
activities might be considered relatively narrow and weak or relatively broad
and robust.

The number of independent dissemination efforts—for instance, a one-
shot announcement or several sequenced activities—may also influence the
eventual result of the impact. Again, developers may need to be aware of
plans in this area so as to be available for comment or interpretation over a
longer or shorter term.

The impact of the guideline might also be affected by the timeliness or
urgency of the dissemination effort. For example, some guidelines might
be rushed into print in a special journal issue or put on a fast-track publication schedule; others may be published in a more routine manner. Developers may need to be sensitive to the significance of their work so that they
can accommodate it to the demands or expectations of such schedules. In
addition, the nature of the publication(s) may have implications for what
guideline developers do (and for their length of service on a guideline
panel). Guidelines may appear in their entirety, as synopses, or both; furthermore, they may appear in different formats and languages.

The AHCPR guidelines are a case in point.[10] As this report was being
prepared, the agency was planning to produce three versions of the guidelines aimed at the professional community: (1) the full technical guideline
plus all documentation (biosketches of panel members, description of the
processes followed, results of the literature review and analysis, recommendations, references, etc.); (2) a shorter version that includes the full set of
recommendations and the entire bibliography; and (3) a pocket-sized, "quick
reference" version that summarizes just the recommendations. (These have
been referred to variously as "Papa Bear, Mama Bear, and Baby Bear" and
the "500-page, 50-page, and 5-page" versions.) The agency appears to be
focusing its broadest dissemination efforts on the shortest version as the one
most likely to be sought out or read, once it has been noticed. For some
topics or conditions that cut across all age groups, these three types of
publications will be produced separately for adult and pediatric populations.
Plans also call for consumer versions of at least the smallest version. Finally, editions of the consumer brochure in both English and Spanish are planned.

At least one of the shorter versions (probably the medium-length one)
will be available through the NLM's on-line capabilities. Those who request the longest (full) technical document from AHCPR's Center for Re-

---

[10] Dissemination activities will be handled by the Center for Research Dissemination and
Liaison at AHCPR, not by the Office of the Forum.

search Dissemination and Liaison will receive it by mail, although whether the Center will make it available free of charge or for a nominal amount is not yet decided. The NLM will probably forward orders for the full document to the Center for handling.

"Version-specific" dissemination plans are still under discussion. The *Journal of the American Medical Association* may publish the announcement of the guideline and the shortest, clinician version of it; AHCPR will encourage relevant specialty societies to announce the guideline as well. Some thought is being given to dissemination of the consumer version through mass print media, such as *Good Housekeeping, Ladies Home Journal*, and the like. Other avenues of dissemination being considered include an 800 telephone number for inquiries (1–800–358–9295); other, more sophisticated marketing strategies are also being explored.

Publicizing the guidelines, as contrasted with publishing them, may be another activity to which developers should be attentive. Public relations and marketing activities in such cases might range from the printing of an announcement of the availability of the guidelines, to a formal press release, briefing, or conference,[11] to announcements broadcast through newsletters, journals, and computer bulletin boards, to even more elaborate strategies and combinations of strategies.

A final set of decisions concerning the distribution of guidelines may have little direct effect on what developers do but may well affect the long-run impact of what they produce. These decisions involve the question of whether guidelines documents (or synopses, or both) are made available free of charge or at some price (and, if the latter, what that price might be). For example, guidelines developed under AHCPR auspices and made available through the NLM may be free of charge except for the nominal charges of the NLM for connection times to the relevant bibliographic and retrieval services.

Dissemination of information or guidelines is by itself insufficient to induce use of that information or to change behavior; indeed, excessive distribution of information to physicians or other clinicians can lead to a significant problem of information overload with no redeeming change in practice patterns or habits. Nonetheless, bringing guidelines to people's attention, and making them available as requested or required, are precur-

---

[11] The production of the first three AHCPR guidelines was accorded such significance that as of late 1991, plans were being developed to convene a press conference at which the Secretary of Health and Human Services would present at least the first of the guidelines (on postoperative pain management). Chairs of the panels and staff of the AHCPR and the Forum would be present, and representatives of relevant specialty societies and professional associations would be invited to give statements concerning at least the aim of the effort and the process followed.

sors to more direct efforts to influence behavior. Recognition of that reality and appropriate planning for dissemination are thus important components of what guideline developers need to do in the future.

Evaluating Impact

If formatting and dissemination operate at the interface at which development begins to shift over to implementation, then evaluation operates at the interface at which the results of implementation are fed back to improve and revise guidelines. Although evaluation of the impact of guidelines is not fundamentally a task for developers, the latter can be presumed to have at least an interest in learning what effects, if any, their work has had. Some groups may, in fact, have sufficient concern about what influence their guidelines are having to carry out various evaluation efforts; others may simply cooperate with outside evaluation activities. This chapter briefly raises the subject, therefore, on the grounds that those in the business of developing guidelines will have concerns about, if not direct involvement in, assessing the effects of their efforts.

As professional societies, public agencies, and others assess their involvement in developing guidelines, they eventually face questions about results. For example, do practitioners, patients, payers, and others even know the guidelines exist? Do they think they are credible and usable? Do they, in fact, use them? How do they affect patient decisions and behavior? Are guidelines having any impact on health outcomes, payment decisions, medical liability, costs, or other factors?

In general, groups have confronted these questions after they have developed several guidelines and have not built evaluation of impact into their programs (Audet et al., 1990). This approach is beginning to change, however, as organizations consider whether their financial and volunteer resources are being constructively used. For example, the GAO (1991b) survey reported that at least four medical societies were interested in evaluating the impact of their guidelines. The ACP self-evaluation of the CEAP activity has already been noted.

Focus groups and surveys are relatively inexpensive means of evaluating results, but they are also relatively weak research strategies in a world where the double-blind randomized clinical trial is the ideal. This report has described one randomized clinical trial involving the use of computer-based reminders for preventive care (McDonald et al., 1984); at least one other similar trial involving hospital admission testing guidelines has been planned (Audet et al., 1990). As noted in Chapter 4, some research has attempted to compare the results of different strategies for informing and educating practitioners about guidelines.

A recently completed but not yet published evaluation sponsored by a large managed care organization examined several questions (Audet et al.,

1990): (1) Does practitioner participation in the process of guideline development affect subsequent use by practitioners of the guidelines? (2) Do guidelines decrease resources utilization? (3) If guidelines do reduce utilization, is it at the expense of quality of care, as reflected in patient outcomes? Preliminary results indicate that "physician generated guidelines codified parsimonious practices, which had a salutary and not negative effect on patient outcomes" (Greenfield, 1991). However, physicians who developed guidelines were no more likely to change practices (for example, to order diagnostic tests more conservatively) than were those who were not involved. The organizational response to these preliminary findings is that involvement in guidelines development is not a sufficient stimulus for change and that they must become part of an integrated quality improvement strategy.

Efforts to evaluate the impact of the guidelines development require both interest and resources. As expensive and methodologically demanding as guideline development is, evaluation of the impact of guidelines is even more demanding. Partly for this reason and partly because the guideline development enterprise is still relatively young, evaluation projects are likely to remain relatively uncommon. To the extent that evaluations are undertaken, they may have more in common with models of program evaluation than with models of clinical biomedical research.

One organization with a clear mandate to undertake evaluation of guidelines is AHCPR. Under OBRA 89, it is required to determine the impact of its first three guidelines on the cost, quality, appropriateness, and effectiveness of health care and to report these findings to Congress by January 1, 1993. As of late 1991, AHCPR's attention was solidly focused on development of guidelines and related medical review criteria; none of the guidelines due by January 1, 1991, had yet been published. Possible activities were still under discussion, and no formal research plan had been made public. (The effort to develop review criteria, described in Chapter 5, includes some provisions for testing their use and impact.) This lack of progress on impact evaluation is not surprising, given the unrealistic deadlines faced by AHCPR.[12]

The agency's 1993 report to Congress will be a status report of activities in progress and planned; with respect to the actual impact of guidelines, some proxy measures (e.g., media citations) may be generated. In addition, lessons learned as the initial guidelines panels pretested their draft guidelines will be a form of impact evaluation. Among the proposed activities

---

[12] The timetable is unrealistic for several reasons. First, the guidelines will probably not have had time to make a measurable impact on health, cost, or other outcomes; this would probably be true even if the first three had been published on schedule. Second, even if the guidelines have fairly immediate effects, the data to document such effects will generally be unavailable. For example, insurance claims or other data showing changes in the use of procedures or practices may not be accessible in the time frame specified. Likewise, data on patient outcomes will take time to collect.

will be a set of internal projects, grants, and contracts with a mix of short- and longer-term objectives—for example, to consider the impact of guidelines for preventive services in inner cities, to investigate the impact of dental surgery guidelines, and to evaluate interactive videodisc technologies to encourage behavioral change (Linda Demlo, AHCPR, personal communication, October 1991).

In its 1990 report, the IOM noted that explanations of policy success or failure, in general, needed to consider the following:

• the validity of the policy premises—for example, the assumption of many policymakers that broader development and use of practice guidelines will achieve significant cost savings;

• the quality of the implementation process—for example, the extent to which information was disseminated or incentives were created for the use of guidelines;

• the existence of countervailing events—for example, court decisions limiting the ability of health care organizations or payers to review the appropriateness of care and then deny either practice privileges or payment for practitioners providing inappropriate care; and

• the nature of supportive or enabling conditions—for example, the breadth of professional interest in the topic covered by the guidelines or a technical breakthrough in access to computer-based information systems.

Even groups that cannot contemplate rigorous evaluation may benefit by considering what would be required to evaluate their guidelines. What would they consider success? What potential adverse consequences should be tracked? What information about the clinical problem, the patient's circumstances and preferences, and the delivery setting should be recorded to permit later evaluation of the processes and outcomes of care? What confounding factors should be considered? Are there intermediate steps that might be usefully monitored? Short of full-scale evaluation, what might users of guidelines do to assess short- or long-term results? Might these users be encouraged to undertake some evaluation on their own or perhaps in collaboration with the guidelines development group?

Some attention to these and similar questions may help developers of guidelines identify previously unsuspected opportunities for evaluation. It may also intensify their interest in finding resources to support evaluation and to refine the way they approach the process of developing guidelines.

SUMMARY

More resources and more systematic procedures do not guarantee good guidelines, but the committee reiterates that guidelines development is a serious enterprise that deserves careful planning and execution. The committee observed several promising efforts at improving structures and processes for developing guidelines, strengthening methods, and incorporating more attention to implementation, evaluation, and revision.

This last step is critical to effective, comprehensive application of guidelines. The attitudes, needs, and circumstances of practitioners, patients, and other users of clinical practice guidelines must be anticipated and considered from the earliest stages of guidelines development, if guidelines are to be applied to achieve their goals. Likewise, evaluation issues—the intended effects of guidelines, means of measuring impact, potential confounding factors—have to be considered when guidelines are being framed rather than dealt with after the fact.

The next, concluding chapter of the report brings together this committee's principal conclusions and recommendations about the clinical practice guidelines enterprise. It does so in some comfort with the progress that the field has made in recent years, taking it as a good omen of the progress that *can* be made on the many conceptual, practical, methodological, and political challenges that still remain.

8

A Framework for the Future

It might be helpful to try viewing our world with both pride and alarm, both tempered by historical sense.

Herbert Muller, 1952

What, then, are we to make of the world of clinical practice guidelines? Gratification, perhaps, over the increasing commitment to develop systematic guidelines and move them into the everyday world of patient care. Concern for the future if too much is expected too soon. And dismay—but not surprise—that little empirical evidence exists about what makes guidelines useful and effective. Nevertheless, some findings, some conclusions, some lessons, some predictions, and some recommendations can be drawn from this study.

In this chapter, the committee responds to the second and third of its charges. It identifies some general strengths and limitations of current structures and processes for developing and applying clinical practice guidelines and then presents a framework for the future development, use, evaluation, and improvement of guidelines. That framework includes, first, a recapitulation of the committee's more specific findings about existing processes for developing and implementing guidelines; second, its recommendations for improvements; and, third, a proposed method and structure for assessing the soundness of guidelines developed by various organizations. The chapter concludes with some recommendations for a research agenda and a few comments on the role of guidelines in health care reform.

WORKING ASSUMPTIONS AND PRINCIPLES

The strongest of the committee's working assumptions was that practice guidelines can help to improve the quality of health care, reduce expenditures for inappropriate and unnecessary services, and increase the value received for this country's spending on personal health care. Individual and organizational behavior are amenable to change; progress is possible. Nothing in the course of this project fundamentally undermined this assumption.

Progress in the development and use of practice guidelines will be accompanied by continuing methodological, technical, ethical, political, attitudinal, and behavioral challenges. Perfect rationality, unswerving ethical behavior, and consistently thoughtful compliance with guidelines lie in the realm of ideals. Scientific knowledge will grow but will always be an incomplete foundation for guidelines. Concerns about costs will always be present. Practitioners and policymakers will inevitably face ethical strains as they try to balance the interests of the individual and of society.

Fortunately, the long history of professional commitment by physicians, nurses, and other clinicians to the good of their patients and to the advancement of clinical knowledge is a critical resource for both the development and implementation of practice guidelines. Public commitment to the support of research and training is another essential component of progress.

As a working principle, the committee accepted that its recommendations must be sensitive to the country's strong tradition of pluralism, despite some negative aspects of that tradition (to be noted shortly). Strong political and cultural traditions favor shared roles and responsibilities for the private and public sectors, although the general inclination is to favor private over public initiative.

GENERAL STRENGTHS AND WEAKNESSES OF CURRENT PRACTICE GUIDELINES ACTIVITIES

Efforts to develop practice guidelines can be characterized, somewhat simplistically, as long-standing or embryonic. Many professional and provider organizations have for many years been creating and applying what they construe to be practice guidelines; for them, guidelines development and implementation is not new. Others focus primarily on "modern" efforts to develop guidelines, which they see as dating back only a decade or so. In either formulation, strong and weak points stand out; they must be understood and either built on or overcome as efforts to develop and apply guidelines push forward.

One caution: it is usually easier to spot problems than successes. The committee notes the limitations and problems in a spirit of identifying opportunities for progress. It hopes that this attitude will help to encourage those interested in better development, use, and evaluation of guidelines. Ultimately, this committee is confident that the history of clinical practice guidelines will be a positive one.

What Are the Strong Points of Current Efforts?

A first strength of current efforts is their pluralism. The commitment of both public- and private-sector resources helps to protect guidelines efforts from real or perceived "capture" by narrow interests. The lack of a dominant model and the existence of multiple, diverse sponsors have encouraged innovation in methods and flexibility to accommodate different potential users. For example, some initiatives have concentrated on new technologies that are of great interest to particular specialties or payers; others have focused on high-volume, low-unit-cost services. Likewise, some efforts aim to guide practitioners through complex clinical problems, whereas others seek practical tools for quality review and payment entities to assess the appropriateness of clinical decisions. By fostering a wider range of development and implementation activities than would be prompted by less diverse sponsorship, pluralism may also facilitate broader understanding and acceptance of guidelines.

A second strength of the guidelines enterprise is simple enthusiasm. Policymakers have endorsed the undertaking, funding is increasing, and how-to-do-it conferences and similar products have been multiplying. Professional and specialty societies are clearly involved to a degree far beyond that observed 2 to 5 years ago. Processes for guidelines development are even seen as mechanisms for defining health insurance and benefit packages in ways that were rarely thought possible just a short time ago.

Third, guidelines are gaining credibility. Expectations about the rigor needed to develop sound guidelines are increasing, and processes for guideline development are beginning to be reshaped. Also growing is professional consensus on two scores: the outcomes of patient care must be more broadly defined and carefully appraised, and the appropriateness of both new and old services must be subjected to more objective, critical scrutiny.

A fourth strength is that researchers, clinicians, educators, and managers are being stimulated to consider how guidelines and other efforts to improve the quality and efficiency of health care can support and complement each other. These efforts include outcomes and effectiveness research, methods for strengthening informed patient decisionmaking, and both traditional and newer techniques for quality assessment and quality improvement.

The above strengths have not emerged from an overarching, deliberate plan. Rather, they are the result of a combination of deliberate strategies (for example, the creation of a guidelines function in the Agency for Health Care Policy and Research [AHCPR]) and the unorchestrated accumulation of many separate organizational initiatives. Part of the message of this report is the dual need to understand and capitalize on these processes and to channel them to better match health care needs.

What Are the Limitations of Current Efforts?

Another part of the message of this report concerns the current limitations and weaknesses of efforts to develop and apply practice guidelines. Some of these drawbacks are the "downsides" of factors mentioned above. Others relate to more general problems inherent in the nation's health care system.

First, pluralism—the involvement of diverse groups in guidelines development—has negative as well as positive consequences. The limited resources for guideline development, use, evaluation, and improvement are inefficiently deployed. Development efforts are fragmented across groups with greatly varying goals, methods, and capacities, and cooperative efforts to develop guidelines that affect multiple specialties and practitioner types are still too atypical. Even if formal priorities have been established, the actual selection of topics for guidelines development seems to be haphazard within organizations and thus across the entire system.

Second, the lack of quality control over methods and procedures is a particularly serious drawback of both national and local processes for developing guidelines. Many national organizations involved actively in developing guidelines and review criteria are moving to improve their programs, but weak procedures and products are common. Methods and procedures for local adaptation of national guidelines and for translation of guidelines into medical review criteria have not been thoroughly documented, but they certainly appear to be subject to equal or greater weaknesses. Potential users of guidelines and review criteria have no ready means to judge the soundness of materials produced by different groups with different approaches.

Third, most guidelines fail in fundamental ways to anticipate the needs of clinicians, patients, and programs to assure quality, control costs, and reduce medical liability. Few guidelines provide any explicit treatment of patient preferences or estimates of the cost implications of their recommendations, certainly not in comparison with alternative practices. In addition, the educational opportunities implicit in guidelines cannot be fully exploited because the evidence and rationale for the guidelines are not presented.

A fourth weakness is that efforts to evaluate the impact of practice guidelines have been limited. Despite widespread interest in guidelines as a tool for improving the quality and cost-effectiveness of care, almost nothing is known about whether they can or do contribute to these goals.

IMPROVING THE DEVELOPMENT OF GUIDELINES

Although this committee intended to focus attention almost exclusively on the implementation of guidelines rather than on their development, it discovered that the application of guidelines was sufficiently dependent on certain characteristics of the development process that revisiting this subject became imperative. In doing so, the committee has stressed several points. First, guidelines developers must do better in anticipating the needs and concerns of potential users. Second, for developers to do this, procedures and methods need improvement. Third, more attention should be paid to the identification and analysis of inconsistencies among guidelines and to the rationales and results of local processes to develop or adapt guidelines. The committee also asked whether guidelines developers should be expected to take on even more demanding tasks by factoring cost-effectiveness into all their recommendations and by defining the minimum level and types of care that should be provided and ensured for all individuals.

Building a Compelling Case for Recommendations

Projections of health outcomes and the costs of achieving those outcomes are absent from most guidelines. Most also lack explicit assessments of the strength of the evidence, the relative importance of the projected benefits and risks, and how compelling is the case for particular interventions. Many of the future directions endorsed by this committee and summarized later in this chapter depend on better performance in these areas.

For potential users to accept the case being made for the recommendations offered in a set of guidelines, other factors are also important and are included among the attributes for guidelines and review criteria identified in Chapters 1 and 5. In varying degrees, practitioners, payers, risk managers, and those involved in quality assurance and improvement perceive that many guidelines fall short in their applicability to real-world circumstances and in their clarity and precision.

The committee recognizes the considerable gaps in empirical information about the natural history of many diseases and conditions, about health outcomes for many diagnostic or therapeutic interventions, and about the costs of providing those (or alternative) interventions. It also recognizes that the development strategy recommended here is highly demanding and that some, perhaps most or all, guidelines will never fully achieve the ideal. Nonetheless, if developers of practice guidelines make serious, persistent efforts in that direction, their products should become substantially more valuable and credible.

Procedural and Methodological Issues Needing Particular Attention

Given its emphasis on evidence, outcomes, and patient preferences and its concerns about the impact of guidelines on the quality and costs of health care, the committee focused on six methodological issues where further research and development is especially desirable:

1. means for setting priorities among topics for guidelines development

2. procedures for securing thoughtful and useful statements of expert judgments

3. methods for analyzing and rating scientific evidence

4. techniques for improving knowledge of health outcomes and giving due importance to patient preferences

5. methods for identifying and projecting the costs of alternative courses of care and comparing their cost-effectiveness

6. mechanisms for identifying and evaluating inconsistent or conflicting guidelines.

Each of the above areas now suffers a variety of minor and major weaknesses in either general procedures or technical methods. The fourth area is (and probably should be) receiving the most attention from the health services research community, but the other topics also warrant more study.

In addition, the committee examined these persistent questions: Who should participate in the process and at what point, in what manner, and for what purpose? Selecting members of guidelines panels and selecting experts to review draft guidelines were underscored as especially critical steps in anticipating the challenges of implementation and in devising guidelines that are credible and useful to those involved in implementation.

A further significant issue is the updating of guidelines, an essential activity, given advances in clinical research and the potential for confusion if guidelines were to include "sunset provisions" (i.e., to be authoritative one day and not the next). Yet updating places an extra burden on existing guidelines panels and organizations. Orderly processes for revising guidelines have yet to be implemented and may require some degree of assistance and coordination from AHCPR and such broad-based professional organizations as the American Medical Association.

At the Interface Between Development and Use

The committee also considered three subjects that arise at the interface between guidelines development and guidelines implementation: local adaptation of guidelines, inconsistent guidelines, and formatting and dissemination. In this context, the term *local* is used broadly to include multihospital systems, nationwide networks of HMOs, or other similar groups that may develop their own guidelines and modify those developed by others.

Local Adaptation of Guidelines

Some local adaptation of national guidelines is probably inevitable and may be useful, because even well-developed guidelines may have gaps and may not foresee significant local objectives or constraints. The process of adapting guidelines can also educate practitioners and serve as a ratifying mechanism that helps win acceptance.

Moreover, within a framework such as is offered by continuous quality improvement, empirical and incremental testing and modification of guidelines may well be appropriate (indeed, even necessary). This kind of testing may not conform to the highest standards of experimental research design, but it can provide a systematic, practical, and direct means of identifying where guidelines—as well as clinical practice—may need revision. Ideally, this kind of local but systematic information will become part of the broader evolutionary framework for guidelines development, revision, and improvement. To this end, the committee urges organizations that adapt guidelines to notify the originating group and explain the circumstances that led to their modifications.

Adaptation may also serve less benign purposes—for example, protecting professional habits and local customs for their own sake or guarding economic self-interest by endorsing unnecessary care or care that others could provide as well or more economically. Casual, "back-of-the-envelope" approaches to adaptation offer particular temptations and opportunities for such unacceptable behavior. Where carefully developed and documented "national" guidelines exist, local adaptation processes should provide explicit rationales that relate to specific, well-defined local conditions or objectives and that take notice of the strength of the case for the original guidelines.

Inconsistent Guidelines

Inconsistent guidelines appear to be unavoidable, even for groups looking at the same scientific evidence and using defensible expert-judgment procedures. As suggested above, inconsistent guidelines provide an opportunity as well as a problem. The opportunity resides in the process of identifying inconsistencies and determining whether they should be tolerated, rejected, or reconciled. A form of disciplined accommodation is suggested to (1) strenuously seek areas of agreement, (2) make rationales for differences explicit and susceptible to comparison with available evidence, (3) reject recommendations or options that conflict with available evidence, and (4) allow options to remain where a case can be made that evidence is inconclusive, professional consensus is split, and variation is unlikely to harm quality of care. In any event, the areas of disagreement point strongly to topics warranting further clinical research.

Formatting and Disseminating Guidelines

The committee had concrete views about steps beyond development. First is effective formatting, which the committee sees as the presentation of guidelines in physical arrangements or media that can be readily understood and applied by practitioners, patients, or other intended groups. Second is effective dissemination—delivering guidelines to the intended audiences in ways that promote the reception, understanding, acceptance, application, and positive impact of the guidelines. Effective dissemination presupposes effective formatting.

The issues relating to dissemination are many, and the committee did not explore them in depth. Certainly, dissemination alone will neither induce use of the information being disseminated nor change behavior, and excessive distribution of information simply contributes to information overload. The committee concluded that a recognition of these complexities and appropriate planning for dissemination are important components of what guideline *developers* should do in the future.

Going Further? Defining Cost-Effective and Minimum Levels of Care

This report recommends that every set of clinical practice guidelines include information on the health and cost implications of alternative preventive, diagnostic, and management strategies for the clinical situation in question. The rationale is that this information can help potential users, who must take financial and other resources into account, to evaluate better the potential consequences of different practices. Should guidelines developers go further?

Specifically, should every set of guidelines include cost-effectiveness as an explicit criterion for judging or recommending what constitutes appropriate care? Should guideline developers necessarily distinguish minimum, essential, or required levels of care in their products? After much debate, the committee concluded that every set of guidelines need not be based on formal judgments of cost-effectiveness; sound guidelines for clinical practice can stand on rigorous assessments of clinical evidence and carefully derived expert judgment. In addition, the committee declined—with some dissent—to recommend that guidelines must include statements of what constitutes minimum or required care for particular clinical problems.

Both these responsibilities may be too expansive for individual guidelines panels or for organizations that face major challenges in following the path for guidelines development set forth in this report. Further, and perhaps more important, committee members could not agree that guidelines developers were, from a policy perspective, the right source of judgments about cost-effectiveness and minimum care; indeed, several members feared that such judgments would complicate the decisions of managers, payers, and policymakers who are actually in a position to make decisions about resources. The committee recognizes, however, that some developers of guidelines may be technically, ethically, and politically positioned to make judgments about cost-effectiveness, particularly when those who are developing guidelines are also the intended users. This report is not meant to forestall such judgments.

Doing More? Guidelines for Informed Patient Decisionmaking

With respect to informed patient decisionmaking, the committee concluded that guideline developers should do more. Good medical care requires shared decisionmaking by practitioners and patients. A commitment to shared decisionmaking, however, does not in itself define what information should be provided to patients under different circumstances. Various organizational and public policies exist that, on the one hand, encourage or dictate the provision of certain information and, on the other hand, discourage or even preclude the provision of other information. Similarly, respect for patient preferences does not in itself answer the technical and policy questions about how to incorporate such preferences into the development or use of practice guidelines.

Two separate paths are suggested here to deal with the difficult practical and ethical questions related to patient decisionmaking and informed consent. One path is the development of treatment- and condition-specific practice guidelines that identify the strength of the evidence and of professional agreement behind statements about appropriate care and that estimate and assess outcomes in terms that patients can perceive as relevant. Strong evidence and consensus regarding a care option should imply strong duties to provide information to patients about that option. Weak evidence and consensus would permit more leeway for other factors to be weighed against these duties.

A second path for improving the conditions for informed patient decisionmaking is the development of a set of general guidelines for patient information and consent. These guidelines would supplement condition- or treatment-specific guidelines, on the one hand, and legally oriented patient consent forms, on the other. Such "patient information guidelines" should be developed by a systematic process similar but not identical to that described for clinical practice guidelines. Once formulated, these guidelines would apply, unless specifically modified by condition-specific guidelines, to broad categories of patient care. The objective in creating such patient information guidelines would be to anticipate and specifically address how information and consent guidelines should cover (a) different kinds of care for (b) different kinds of patients in (c) different delivery systems and settings, given (d) different levels of certainty about the benefits, risks, and costs of care.

ENSURING THE USE OF GOOD GUIDELINES

Even when specific, well-founded guidelines exist, their effective use by patients and practitioners will require a broad range of supportive conditions and organizations. As those involved in programs to manage quality, costs, and liability begin to rely on guidelines, these common uses will provide powerful support for their consistent application in actual clinical practice. In particular, the force of peer influence should not be underestimated.

Practitioner knowledge of guidelines and acceptance of their validity are key conditions for their successful application, but acceptance is not equivalent to behavioral change. Thus, as a practical matter, it may be better strategically or tactically to focus less on knowledge and acceptance and more on what changes behavior in desired directions. More than simple acceptance that a guideline is correct may be required to overcome countervailing forces, in particular, information overload, habitual practice patterns, malpractice fears, and economic disincentives.

Quality Assurance and Improvement

Well-developed, scientifically based practice guidelines have an important role to play in assessing, assuring, and improving the quality of health services provided in this country. Clear, specific guidelines and associated review criteria should help prevent or, alternatively, identify and remedy problems of overuse of care, underuse of care, and poor technical and interpersonal provision of care. Guidelines that have been accepted by those responsible for providing care, those responsible for financing it, and those responsible for monitoring care in the public interest are one means of bridging the chasm between internal and external quality assurance strategies.

With respect to models of continuous quality improvement, the committee urges that their focus on systems problems, improvement of average performance, and reduction of variation be more systematically and explicitly joined with an effort to apply and improve sound guidelines for clinical practice. Specifically:

• Guidelines, medical review criteria, and other evaluative tools should be used both to improve average performance and—as is still important—identify substandard performance;

• Inquiries into how individual practice patterns differ from average patterns should go beyond statistical analysis to consider relevant practice guidelines as benchmarks for performance;

• Both the statistical information from such analyses and the pertinent guidelines should be part of educational feedback on practice patterns;

• Evaluations of performance and outcome data should seek to determine the sources of poor outcomes and deviations from guidelines so that systems problems can be corrected and, if necessary, impaired individuals dealt with through training, counseling, limiting of privileges, or other appropriate mechanisms;[1]

• Evaluations of performance and outcomes data should be used to indicate or determine whether practice guidelines ought to be updated or revised;

• Developers of guidelines and health care institutions should convene educational conferences to acquaint practitioners with specific guidelines and provide an opportunity for them to discuss and plan setting-specific applications;

• Institutional activities to develop or adapt guidelines or review criteria should aspire to incorporate the attributes for guidelines and for review criteria described elsewhere in this report.

Cost Management

On both philosophical and strategic grounds, this committee believes that thoughtfully designed and applied programs to encourage cost-effective use of health care have an important role to play in supporting the wider application of guidelines for clinical practice. Such programs need guidelines and related materials that provide information on the cost-effectiveness of alternative ways of managing particular clinical problems. They also need to be supplemented by explicit programs that employ guidelines and review criteria to monitor the quality and appropriateness of care.

Those who develop review criteria should be guided by the attributes discussed earlier in this report. This recommendation applies to organizations that develop retrospective quality-of-care criteria, that generate prospective preprocedure or preadmission criteria, and that engage in all manner of "review" between these two extremes. Review organizations of all sorts, if they follow these attributes, will perforce do certain things. They will make their review activities as manageable and nonintrusive as possible for both patients and practitioners. They will make their review criteria available to practitioners and others. They will provide an explicit process for appealing negative decisions that is free from unreasonable complexity, delay, or other barriers. In addition, if such an organization identifies quality-of-care problems, it will have procedures for, at a minimum, discussing these problems with the involved practitioner or provider

---

[1] The committee explicitly recognizes the need for protection of privacy and confidentiality as those concepts are understood in usual quality assurance terms (e.g., in actions of Medicare peer review organizations, state medical licensure boards, hospital quality assurance committees, and the like).

and, perhaps, raising the matter with the relevant institutional or professional body or state or federal agent (e.g., the Medicare peer review organization [PRO]).

It is the committee's hope that economic incentives and quality review mechanisms will, in the future, reduce the need for so-called micromanagement of professional and institutional behavior. External utilization review still may have a role in monitoring practice and targeting problem practices, but many payers will admit that they would prefer to rely more on effective self-regulation by practitioners and providers. Consistent with quality improvement principles, they can stress education and feedback to physicians aimed at improving practice rather than punishing errors.

Risk Management and Medical Liability

Guidelines that are based on available scientific evidence and that are clear, specific, and developed by a reputable process should carry greater weight in malpractice decisionmaking than vague, nonspecific guidelines that lack documentation and careful reasoning. Guidelines that can underscore their recommendations with reference to a strong foundation of scientific evidence should be particularly helpful.

Specific statutory recognition of guidelines, which is intended to provide legal protection to conforming clinicians, is desirable but premature. Acceptable legislation that provides immunity from liability would need to specify operational criteria for the organizations developing guidelines or particular criteria for guidelines themselves, or both. The criticisms directed at the variability and weaknesses of review criteria developed or adopted by Medicare PROs and carriers (and the fact that the criteria of the latter groups are often kept secret as well) made the committee reluctant to accept organizational imprimatur alone as a sufficient basis for a grant of immunity. Absent some explicit procedures and standards for assessing the soundness of practice guidelines (as recommended earlier), the committee believes that giving formal legal stature to any guideline at this early stage may create more problems than it solves.

Information and Decision Support Systems

No existing information infrastructure can support the kind of effective, unobtrusive, easy application of guidelines envisioned by continuous quality improvement models, future-oriented utilization management and cost-containment systems, and patient-centered care proposals. Clearly, however, information technologies are being developed that will make the application of guidelines much easier, particularly if other conditions support their use. For clinicians, creating user-friendly decision aids that relate information about specific patients to guidelines that cover similar patients deserves greater emphasis and more effort.

The work of the National Library of Medicine and others to establish some capability of responding to user inquiries and dissemination needs related to guidelines should be encouraged. (The committee also supports efforts by the library to expand its capacity to assist in guideline development through expansion of its Office for Health Services Research Information.) In addition, the committee favors the translation and movement of guidelines into computerized decision aids of various sorts. It recommends, however, that those efforts conform to emerging computer industry standards to enable guidelines (however transformed) to be used on different types of computer-based equipment and systems.

The clinical and health services research communities also have a role to play in smoothing the path from clinical research to better clinical practice and improved health outcomes. If more attention is paid to testing the effectiveness of procedures and patient management strategies in real-life settings rather than only assessing efficacy in highly controlled clinical trials, developers of guidelines will be more likely to have a knowledge base with greater practical relevance. In turn, the more that practitioners and institutions adopt the tools of outcomes management, the more information there will be to evaluate and revise guidelines.

A CRITICAL NEED: MEANS TO ASSESS
THE SOUNDNESS OF GUIDELINES

This committee has strongly urged that processes for developing and revising guidelines be firmly based on scientific evidence and expert clinical judgment *and* that guidelines anticipate the needs of practitioners, patients, and others. How can clinicians, policymakers, and other interested parties determine whether and how different guidelines measure up to these expectations? In the course of this study, many individuals and organizations expressed a strong desire for some kind of independent assessment of practice guidelines. In this context, *assessment* means prospective consideration of the strengths and weaknesses of a set of guidelines based on the attributes of good guidelines identified in Chapter 1. Such advance assessment is distinct from any subsequent evaluation of the impact of guidelines on costs, quality, and other factors.

Greater confidence in the quality of practice guidelines and better understanding of their strengths and limitations would yield several benefits to practitioners, patients and consumers, payers, policymakers, and others with an interest in health care and health care reform. These benefits include (1) firmer judgments about what care should be covered under public and private health benefit programs, (2) better decisions about what information is necessary for informed patient decisionmaking, and (3) stronger assurance for practitioners that compliance with guidelines will reduce their exposure to medical liability.

The design and application of any assessment process will depend on many factors—ethical, political, economic, and organizational. Furthermore, such a process requires at least two basic program components. One is a practical and valid assessment instrument; the other is a feasible administrative structure and process for applying the instrument.

Assessment Instrument

How might one construct an assessment instrument? The approach taken by the committee is presented in Appendix B, which contains the full text of the instrument along with an introduction that allows the appendix to be used as a freestanding document. The instrument is presented as provisional because more practical experience with it is essential. Volunteers from a large number of specialty societies and other experts reviewed a draft document; some also applied it to existing or draft guidelines. The resulting comments and suggestions, which were both extensive and candid, reinforced the committee's initial assumption that the instrument required more practical testing of its utility.[2]

The assessment instrument covers both the process used to develop a specific guidelines document and the substantive content of the document and its recommendations. (The committee did not want an assessment instrument that could allow a set of scientifically invalid or questionable guidelines to receive a "good" rating based on process criteria alone.) In essence, it attempts to operationalize both the substance and process attributes presented in Chapter 1. The committee believes the instrument will be useful as

• an educational tool for those beginning to develop guidelines;
• a self-assessment tool that developers of guidelines can use to check their work; and
• a tool for external groups to use in judging whether a set of guidelines should or should not be recommended or adopted.

Successful application of the assessment instrument for this last purpose depends on several conditions. First, those assessing a set of guidelines must have access to the primary and secondary documentation of the evidence, rationales, and process involved. A summary statement of the

---

[2] In accordance with the IOM'S contract with AHCPR, the provisional instrument was delivered in August 1991 after it had successfully completed the process of report review required by the National Research Council.

recommendations is not sufficient. Second, those undertaking an assessment must individually or collectively possess the methodological and clinical knowledge required to apply the instrument to a particular set of guidelines. Relatively junior or inexperienced individuals can assemble relevant materials and check simple items, but experienced clinicians and methodologists must play key roles. Third, those using the instrument must be prepared to complete a task that will be both complex and tedious.

Assessment Organization

Given a reliable, valid assessment instrument, how might one apply it in a broader evaluative program? The above discussion of the instrument implies little about the characteristics of a specific institutional arrangement for assessing guidelines except that it would require more than trivial resources and stature. In considering recommendations about an assessment organization, the committee raised several questions. Is such an entity needed? What are the minimum conditions for its successful operation? Is there a reasonable probability that these conditions can be achieved?

Is an Assessment Organization Needed?

The committee believes the answer to this question is clearly yes. Existing guidelines vary enormously in quality, and the commitment and ability of developers to improve methods and content will also vary. Similarly, potential users of guidelines differ in their ability to identify the strengths and weaknesses of different guidelines. As the uses of guidelines become more clearly defined and significant, some way to distinguish good, bad, and mediocre guidelines becomes more important. The committee heard repeatedly from practitioners, providers, and others that they wanted guidance about the credibility and soundness of guidelines developed by different organizations. Existing private and public organizations may try to give such help, but acceptance of these efforts may not extend beyond limited constituencies of the involved groups.

An assessment entity could stimulate more demand for credible guidelines; that demand, in turn, could stimulate the commitment of more resources to develop such guidelines. What currently exists is more like a chaotic "market" operating in an environment that has no effective means of distinguishing good products from bad. This was essentially the committee's rationale for stating (see Chapter 5) that it is premature to recommend that federal or state legislatures grant malpractice immunity to practitioners who act in conformance with practice guidelines. An effectively functioning assessment entity would go far to ameliorate the committee's concerns in this area. Such an organizational structure could also help realize the recommendation that utilization management firms and similar organizations improve and make public their review criteria. The incentive provided by the assessment entity for such a move would be that favorable assessments might offer a competitive advantage.

Is an Assessment Organization Feasible?

That a need exists does not mean that a feasible means of meeting it can be devised. The conditions that must prevail for an assessment entity to be practical and viable are numerous. Four such conditions present particular challenges.

• **Effective demand for the product** (i.e., the assessments of guidelines). The product has a clear potential market: providers, public and private payers, government generally, malpractice insurers, and consumer groups. That this potential demand would translate into actual financial and political support, however, is not inevitable. The survival rate of somewhat analogous organizations, such as the Council on Health Care Technology and the National Center for Health Care Technology,[3] is not encouraging, although the entity envisioned by the committee would not undertake the highly controversial task of advising public or private payers on coverage matters.

• **Integrity of the process, participants, and assessments.** Both the actual integrity of the entity and a widespread perception of its integrity must be created and maintained. To this end, considerable attention and sensitivity must be directed toward the choice of sponsors (financial as well as political), selection of managers (members of any board of directors, the executive director and other officers, consultants, and members of assessment panels or teams), and choice of topics and actual guidelines to be assessed. As to the last, explicit criteria and an open priority-setting process would be important.

---

[3] The Council on Health Care Technology was established at the Institute of Medicine through the Health Promotion and Disease Prevention Amendments of 1984, partly in response to a recommendation in the 1983 IOM report, *A Consortium for Assessing Medical Technologies;* it was reauthorized in 1987. A complex system of public and private funding, which essentially called for private-sector financing to be acquired and spent before certain public matching monies (through the National Center for Health Services Research, or NCHSR) became available, proved to be an insufficient base of sustained support. The Council was disbanded at the same time that AHCPR was created (from NCHSR) in the Omnibus Budget Reconciliation Act of 1989. Earlier (1978), Congress created the National Center for Health Care Technology, which withered from lack of political support in the Executive Branch (Rettig, 1991b). A new effort to channel private funds to increase federal technology assessment activities is running into opposition from affected industries (Kent, 1991).

• **Sufficiency of effort**. The necessary participants, methodologies, and other resources must be secured to undertake a reasonable volume of credible, usable assessments on a timely basis. This might be done, for example, by direct employment, subcontracting, creation of resource centers, or other mechanisms. Those involved in the assessments should have (collectively) an excellent understanding of actual clinical practice as well as a thorough grounding in clinical research, research methodologies, outcomes measurement, and cost-effectiveness analysis.

• **Stability of effort**. There is little reason to embark on an enterprise of this sort if one cannot project a reasonable period of existence to attract qualified participants and to support dissemination of results. For such stability, a sufficient, predictable, and visible commitment of political, financial, and other resources is essential.

Is There a Reasonable Probability That These Conditions Will Prevail?

The committee believes that such a reasonable probability exists. Therefore, it recommends the creation of an assessment organization. The following discussion describes an approach that the committee considers plausible and realistic. It highlights four key aspects of such an approach: governance, products, funding, and credibility.

• **Governance.** Entities sponsored, governed, and funded by interested parties may enjoy a higher level and greater predictability of financial and other resources, but such sponsorship or funding can create threats to the real or perceived integrity of the undertaking. The perceived threats can turn on a distinction between public and private sectors per se, or on a distinction between interested and (presumably) not-so-interested parties, regardless of their private- or public-sector status. Even those generally favorable to the concept of an assessment entity—within the committee and outside—have directly conflicting views on the credibility of a public versus a private assessment entity.

AHCPR already has legislative authority to perform the assessment function. Private funds could be added to appropriations for the work of the Forum for Quality and Effectiveness in Health Care to support the assessment function envisioned here.[4] The agency might be viewed, however, as having a conflict of interest in assessing guidelines sponsored by its Forum or guidelines developed by outside contractors on its behalf. Furthermore,

---

[4] In a related context, some private groups, in particular, major insurers, suggested in late 1991 that they would be interested in contributing significant funds to supplement government monies that have been appropriated to AHCPR's Office of Health Technology Assessment for assessing new technologies.

its work would be subject to the usual vagaries of the federal appropriations process, and it would be politically vulnerable to hostile actions from organizations whose guidelines, once assessed, do not pass muster.

Other groups, such as the American Medical Association (AMA), have also offered themselves in the role of "certifier" of guidelines. The AMA, in fact, has drafted its own assessment instrument and developed a process for applying it. Nevertheless, a powerful medical organization could have its own problems of credibility in this role, no matter how well it performs. Clearly, assessment would be a sensitive undertaking when guidelines from one group in the larger association clearly conflicted with or were "prejudicial" to those of another group.

Weighing the various pluses and minuses, the committee finally concluded that an assessment entity would best be organized as a private, not-for-profit organization and that it should have a governing board drawn from a wide range of interested parties, both public and private. The entity must be apart from, but able to work with, the parties that have a stake in guideline development. To forestall criticisms about objectivity and integrity, the board of any such organization would develop clear procedures regarding bias, conflicts of interest, and other issues of accountability.[5]

• **Products and focus.** The proposed assessment entity would have one primary product: periodic publication of assessments of the guidelines issued by public and private organizations. Overseeing publication of the assessments and other dissemination activities would be the responsibility of the governing board.

In terms of publications, the committee believes that a journal is an attractive option. Its articles or reports should combine the academic rigor of top professional journals with the user-oriented style of a publication like *Consumer Reports*. The latter journal has several attractive features.[6] It compares products with a similar purpose rather than reporting on products in isolation. It uses graphics and other devices to great advantage to provide easy-to-assimilate information on the strengths, weaknesses, and characteristics of products. Further, it explicitly recognizes that consumers have different preferences and circumstances that may lead them to different choices based on individual weighing of this information.

An annual review issue might provide summary compilations of the

---

[5] Such procedures would include peer review of the assessments. In addition, the entity might publish both its assessment methodology and its assessments in draft form for public review and comment. The latter would be analogous to the process by which federal regulations are published in the *Federal Register* for comment before final promulgation occurs. AHCPR's Patient Outcomes Research Teams, the committees of the National Academy of Sciences, and similar organizations offer other model procedures.

[6] The committee is not recommending, however, that the assessment entity be modeled directly on Consumers Union.

assessments. Both the quarterly issues and the annual collection would, ideally, be indexed by the National Library of Medicine in a manner similar to its plans for AHCPR guidelines; short synopses of the assessments might even be available through NLM on-line services. Teleconferences or workshops organized around particularly controversial or important assessments might also be considered as dissemination strategies. The assessment methodology or methodologies could be made available to interested parties as a freestanding publication, which might be similar to the provisional instrument presented in Appendix B.

The assessment organization might eventually move into other dissemination, educational, and clearinghouse activities if its initial efforts proved to be successful. For example, it might provide training sessions for organizations interested in learning how guidelines would be assessed. It might also produce assessments or commentaries on related items such as medical review criteria, commercial software products, software standards such as those promulgated by the American Society for Testing and Materials, and new graphic display techniques. Another information dissemination effort might be the production of occasional special publications or the sponsorship of conferences (with published proceedings) or workshops for the exchange of ideas and new developments. The organization might even publish—but not develop—guidelines that met its assessment standards or, in some cases, publish economic analyses for guidelines that did not include them.

The committee emphasizes, however, that it sees the organization's central mission as assessing guidelines. In keeping with the proposed user orientation, the assessment entity should *seek out* guidelines to assess as well as accept submissions. For example, it could focus on clinical topics of particular interest for which multiple sets of guidelines exist. This appears, from anecdotal evidence, to be a critical need—one the AHCPR Forum is being asked to address by developing definitive guidelines in certain areas. An organization that can sort out good from not-so-good guidelines might help to conserve the funds of guideline developers for work on clinical problems that are not so widely endowed with conflicting (or any) contemporary guidelines.

A proactive search strategy is likely to uncover second-rate guidelines that the sponsors would not submit on their own. Other kinds of user-oriented assessments of such guidelines would seek to be constructive rather than merely critical and to provide encouragement to developers of guidelines to improve their processes and products. One measure of the assessment entity's success will be the extent to which, over time, developers of guidelines seek its assessments.

• **Funding.** Funding from both public and private sources is desirable, and it could be in the form of start-up monies, long-term core support, special project grants, and purchase of products and services. Of these, long-term core financing is the most important, and uncertainty about public or private willingness to move from general expressions of interest to actual financial support constitutes the major short-term challenge to the creation of an assessment entity.

Once core funding is secured, additional financing could be obtained in several ways. One would be to charge a substantial subscription for the products of the organization. The subscription response would provide an early test of market appeal and feasibility. Another source of revenue could come from training or other activities, for which fees would be at least sufficient to recoup costs.

• **Credibility.** All the features described above are intended to provide the assessment organization with initial and continuing credibility. To further the entity's credibility, a key objective should be the creation of a virtual "fail-safe" mechanism to prevent clinically flawed guidelines from receiving a generally favorable assessment. Achieving this objective may require a pretesting process. An important first step is for AHCPR to test the IOM's provisional assessment instrument and to compare the results with pretests of its guidelines. Another key to credibility is for the procedures used by the assessment organization, as well as the assessment instrument and other tools, to be open and in the public domain.

The assessment organization should have a user orientation that extends to a range of interested parties. Still, its assessments should be *particularly* attuned to everyday clinical practice and sensitive to the reliance of practitioners on their professional societies for guidance and support. For long-lasting credibility, establishing a constructive relationship with these professional societies must be a priority.

The committee was acutely interested in the potential for legislation to grant legal immunity to practitioners who practiced in accord with guidelines that received positive assessments. It concluded, however, that a specific recommendation must await the specific policy decisions and operating strategies that will emerge only as the assessment entity shifts from concept to reality. As that happens, the future legal use of assessments should be an explicit interest.

RESEARCH AGENDA

In addition to developing its proposal regarding the assessment entity described earlier, the committee drew some conclusions about research to help answer certain questions about practice guidelines. The points noted below are narrowly aimed at guidelines development, implementation, and evaluation. Most generally, the committee urges continued investment in research on effectiveness and outcomes of health care and in programs for technology assessment. These activities are a necessary part of the scientific and analytic support for clinical decisionmaking and guidelines development. They also support management and policy decisionmaking about how to allocate limited resources among alternative uses.

Yet another priority is the testing and improvement of methods for guideline and criteria development, dissemination, application, and evaluation. Chapters 6 and 7 noted a number of outstanding technical and methodologic issues relating to cost-effectiveness analysis, weighing and combining evidence, consensus development and expert judgment. Clarifying the statistical aspects of, say, meta-analysis or effect sizes as they relate to amassing and interpreting scientific evidence is another. Other questions warranting attention include the effects of different ways of phrasing recommendations on the understanding or behavior (or both) of clinicians and patients and, perhaps, whether translation into languages other than English changes the meaning or import of those recommendations in unanticipated ways.

One early, specific research activity should be the testing and perhaps refining of the provisional assessment instrument. Here, the questions include reliability, in its application by different users; validity, in the sense that it will discriminate well between good and not-so-good guidelines (or development processes); and practicality. Formal investigation of the feasibility and utility of the instrument for the entire guidelines enterprise—and its revamping as necessary—strikes the committee as a likely prerequisite for the success of any assessment entity.

A middle step in understanding the impact of guidelines is an understanding of adoption and diffusion patterns. In this instance, one important question involves the role of opinion leaders and so-called pacesetter physicians; related issues concern graduate medical education (or graduate training in all the health professions now engaged in guidelines development). Of particular interest may be the extent to which physicians in residency training are an appropriate target audience; both guidelines and materials about the importance of being involved in guidelines development and implementation throughout their careers would be appropriate matters to emphasize.

A clear priority is research on the actual impact of clinical practice guidelines on what clinicians and patients do and on the health status of patients and populations. This research focus is of a piece with studying how to change practitioner and patient behavior—a significant question for the quality assurance field in particular. Although impact can be addressed in part through proxy measures (e.g., measures relating to dissemination), an appreciation of whether given guidelines *really make a difference* in practice patterns, lifestyles, and the like will require complex, longitudinal studies. Ideally, these might be planned as randomized clinical trials; short of that, various types of demonstration projects and efforts similar to those of the AHCPR Patient Outcomes Research Team (PORT) program might be considered.

A related objective should be to determine how traditional clinical trials might be redesigned and extended so that the dissemination, application, and impact of practice guidelines could be studied in actual health care delivery settings. In this formulation, the findings from such studies, for instance, in groups of academic medical centers together with participating practices in the community, might later be used to improve and update the guidelines under study.

Finally, in much the same manner that "no-difference" results in clinical trials and health services research can be illuminating, understanding why seemingly good guidelines have had no impact (or why seemingly poor ones did have an effect) may be a fruitful avenue of investigation. Such research could identify facilitating or complicating factors, either intrinsic to the guideline topic or extrinsic to it but prevalent in the broader health care environment, that might be taken into account as the guidelines enterprise moves into higher gear during the 1990s. Work along these lines (e.g., as case studies) might be a profitable interim step while more complex longitudinal investigations are being planned and conducted.

FINAL NOTE: GUIDELINES AND HEALTH CARE REFORM

During its deliberations, the committee was quite conscious of the intense debate occurring about broad health care reform in this country and about the contributions that practice guidelines might make to workable reform. In the committee's view, reform concerns two issues: access and cost. Politically, expansion of access is contingent on some sense that the rate of escalation in health care costs can be reduced.

The committee's discussions of cost-effectiveness and minimum care have already touched on these concerns. As noted earlier, the committee has expressed reservations about assigning guideline developers the task of recommending what care is worth paying for. Consequently, it recommended that guideline developers concentrate instead on providing the clinical information, judgments, and rationales on which policymakers, payers, managers, and others might base such decisions.

Some proposals for reform include provisions for clinical practice guidelines that would seem generally consistent with the committee's views on who should make judgments about what is worth covering under public or private health benefits plans. For example, one proposal would create a Health Standards Board to design a set of "uniform effective health benefits" that would be "responsive to public values about the appropriateness of various treatments,[7] incorporate scientifically based information on treatment effectiveness, and be sensitive to considerations of cost in terms of the net benefits of services" (Ellwood, 1991, p. 1). A similar proposal (Brook, 1991) would establish a public governing body to oversee work by interdisciplinary teams based at academic medical centers to develop necessary-care guidelines;[8] federal legislation would require all health plans to cover this care. Chapter 6 raised several questions about the technical and ethical challenges involved in making such judgments, whether the decisionmakers be developers of guidelines, insurers, or public officials.

A contrasting approach relies not on guidelines that define uniform coverage policies but on guidelines that provide for varying standards of care (Havighurst, 1990a). Health plans would adopt different guidelines (perhaps those certified as meeting a minimum standard of acceptability), and consumers could choose what level of care they were willing and able to purchase. In theory, both health plans and consumers would make judgments about what care is worth covering. Chapter 5 raised some questions about this proposal, but the discussion of inconsistent guidelines in Chapter 7 made clear that inconsistencies were not necessarily unacceptable, for example, when the guidelines reflected different value judgments about what was an important benefit (and documented this as part of the rationale for their recommendations).

These and other proposals for health care reform raise many questions that are beyond the scope of this committee's charge. Some of the health care reform proposals that are described above and that are being widely discussed in the health policy literature and lay media envision sweeping changes in the nation's health care delivery and financing systems. These changes would certainly place guidelines in a framework of incentives for cost containment that is different from what currently exists. The specifics vary, but the basic ideas are that the reforms would override state benefit

---

[7] In Ellwood's terms (1991), these values would relate to "the value of a service to society (e.g., public health impact, social costs, community compassion), the value of a service to the individual at risk, and the extent to which a service is considered an essential component of a basic level of health care below which no person should fall. Public values can be periodically assessed through surveys, focus groups, public hearings, and other community meeting formats" (p. 1). This is roughly similar to the process used in Oregon (see Chapter 6). Presumably, the Health Standards Board would limit the extent to which public distaste for some kinds of health problems (e.g., sexually transmitted diseases, smoking-related illness) could dictate coverage.

[8] Necessary care "(1) is appropriate (medical benefit exceeds medical risk); (2) produces important benefits to the patients receiving it; and (3) would be considered improper for physicians not to recommend to the patient. It would disturb both primary care physicians and specialists if it were not provided" (Brook, 1991, p. 3000).

mandates, circumvent court-ordered coverage in individual cases, rewrite malpractice laws, reduce administrative costs through single-payer arrangements, and limit the coverage eligible for tax deductibility.

Some reforms—for example, those that envision practice guidelines as the basis for defining a basic benefits package for all health insurance plans— would put a premium on the kinds of credible, accountable processes for developing and applying guidelines that are described in this report. The danger in such proposals is that the potential contributions guidelines have to make in improving the quality of health care and health outcomes may be lost in a perception that guidelines serve only cost-containment purposes. The committee sees, therefore, both unprecedented opportunities for the clinical practice guidelines movement as well as exceptional challenges in the years ahead.

References

AAP (American Academy of Pediatrics). *Report of the Committee on Infectious Diseases* (22nd ed.). Elk Grove Village, Ill.: American Academy of Pediatrics, 1991.

Aaron, H. *Serious and Unstable Condition: Financing America's Health Care.* Washington, D.C.: Brookings Institution, 1991.

ACC (American College of Cardiology). Symposium on Quality and Cost-Conscious Cardiovascular Care: Role of Decision Modeling. *Journal of the American College of Cardiology* 14(3 Suppl. A):1A-76A, September 1989.

Ackerman, F., and Nash, D. Teaching the Tenets of Quality: A Survey of Medical Schools and Programs in Health Administration. *Quality Review Bulletin* 17:200-203, 1991.

ACP (American College of Physicians). *Clinical Efficacy Assessment Project: Procedural Manual.* Philadelphia, Pa.: The College, 1986.

ACP. *Common Diagnostic Tests: Use and Interpretation.* H. Sox, ed. Philadelphia, Pa.: The College, 1987.

ACPM (American College of Preventive Medicine). The American College of Preventive Medicine: Long-Range Plans. *American Journal of Preventive Medicine* 5:56-58, 1989.

ACS (American Cancer Society). Who We Are. What We Do. Where We're Going. Atlanta, Ga.: American Cancer Society, Inc., March 1990.

Adams, J. Three Surveillance and Query Languages for Medical Care. *M.D. Computing* 3:11-19, 1986.

AHCPR (Agency for Health Care Policy and Research). *Program Note. Medical Treatment Effectiveness Research.* Rockville, Md.: U.S. Department of Health and Human Services, Agency for Health Care Policy and Research, March 1990.

AHCPR. Effective Dissemination of Health Services Research Findings and Medical Practice Guidelines. RFA AHCPR-91-01. *NIH Guide for Grants and Contracts*, February 15, 1991.

AMA (American Medical Association). *Attributes to Guide the Development of Practice Parameters*. Chicago, Ill.: The Association, April 1990a.

AMA. *Legal Implications of Practice Parameters*. Chicago, Ill.: The Association, 1990b.

AMA. *Practice Parameters Update*. 1(1):16, August 1990c.

AMA. *Directory of Practice Parameters*. Chicago, Ill.: The Association, October 1991a.

AMA, Council on Ethical and Judicial Affairs. Guidelines for the Appropriate Use of Do-Not-Resuscitate Orders. *Journal of the American Medical Association* 265:1868-1871, 1991b.

AMRA (American Medical Record Association). Continuous Quality Improvement References. Supplemental Material in *QA Section Connection* 11(6), 1991.

ANA (American Nurses Association). Testimony before the Institute of Medicine Committee on Clinical Practice Guidelines, Washington, D.C., December 3, 1990.

Annas, G. Restricting Doctor-Patient Conversations in Federally Funded Clinics. *New England Journal of Medicine* 325:362-364, 1991.

ASIM (American Society of Internal Medicine). 1989 House of Delegates: Guidelines for the Development of Practice Guidelines. Report of the Board of Trustees, Report K. Philadelphia, Pa., 1989, p. 8.

ASIM. Testimony on Practice Guidelines and Volume of Services before the U.S. House of Representatives, Committee on Ways and Means. Washington, D.C., May 3, 1990.

ASTM (American Society for Testing and Materials). Draft Standard Specification for Transferring Modular Medical Knowledge Bases. Committee on Computerized Systems and Subcommittee on Health Knowledge Representation. Philadelphia, Pa.: May 29, 1991.

Audet, A., Greenberg, S., and Field, M. Medical Practice Guidelines: Current Activities and Future Directions. *Annals of Internal Medicine* 113:709-714, 1990.

Avorn, J., and Soumerai, S. Improving Drug-Therapy Decisions through Educational Outreach: A Randomized Controlled Trial of Academically Based "Detailing." *New England Journal of Medicine* 308:1447-1463, 1983.

Ball, J. Professional Society Perspectives. In: *Proceedings of a Medical Practice Guidelines Workshop—Issues for Internal Medicine*, sponsored by the Agency for Health Care Policy and Research and the Internal Medicine Center to Advance Research and Education, Washington, D.C., June 8-9, 1990, pp. 69-75.

Barnett, G.O., Winickoff, R., Dorsey, J., et al. Quality Assurance through Automated Monitoring Systems and Concurrent Feedback Using a Computer Based Medical Information System. *Medical Care* 16:962-970, 1978.

Barry, M.J., Mulley, A.G., Fowler, F.J., et al. Watchful Waiting vs. Immediate Transurethral Resection for Symptomatic Prostatism: The Importance of Patients' Preferences. *Journal of the American Medical Association* 259:3010-3017, 1988.

Batalden, P., and Buchanan, E.D. Industrial Models of Quality Improvement. In: *Providing Quality Care: The Challenge to Clinicians*, N. Goldfield and D. Nash, eds. Philadelphia, Pa.: American College of Physicians, 1989.

Beauchamp, T., and Childress, J. *Principles of Biomedical Ethics.* New York, N.Y.: Oxford University Press, 1983.

Becker, M. In Hot Pursuit of Health Promotion: Some Admonitions. In: *Health at Work.* S. Weiss, J. Fielding, and A. Baum, eds. Hillsdale, N.J.: Lawrence Erlbaum Associates, 1991.

Bergner, M. Measurement of Health Status. *Medical Care* 23:696-704, 1985.

Berkow, R., ed. *The Merck Manual,* 14th ed. Rahway, N.J.: Merck Sharp & Dohme Research Laboratories (Division of Merck and Co., Inc.), 1982.

Berlin, J.A., Laird, N.M., Sacks, H.S., and Chalmers, T.C. A Comparison of Statistical Methods for Combining Event Rates from Clinical Trials. *Statistics in Medicine* 8:141-151, 1989.

Berwick, D. Continuous Improvement as an Ideal in Health Care. Sounding Board. *New England Journal of Medicine* 320:53-56, 1989.

Berwick, D.M., Godfrey, A.B., and Roessner, J. *Curing Health Care: New Strategies for Quality Improvement.* San Francisco, Calif.: Jossey-Bass Publishers, 1990.

Billings, J. The Emergence of Quality as a Major Health Policy Issue. In: *Medical Quality and the Law. Report of the 1989 Chief Justice Earl Warren Conference on Advocacy in the United States.* J. Billings, N. Goldfield, C. Havighurst, et al., eds. Washington, D.C.: Roscoe Pound Foundation, 1990, pp. 21-35.

Blumstein, J. Presentation at RAND Conference on Changing the Health Care Delivery System and Its Implications for Liability Law, Dallas, Texas, June 10-11, 1991.

Borbas, C., Stump, M., Dedeker, K., et al. The Minnesota Clinical Comparison and Assessment Project. *Quality Review Bulletin* 16:87-92, 1990.

Bouxsein, P. Commentary. Standards of Care in Medicine. *Inquiry* 25: 450-451, 1988.

Bovbjerg, R. Legislation on Medical Malpractice: Further Developments and a Report Card. *University of California at Davis Law Review* 22:499-560, 1989.

Brassard, M. *The Memory Jogger. A Pocket Guide of Tools for Continuous Improvement.* Methuen, Mass.: GOAL/QPC, 1985; 2d ed., 1988.

Brennan, T. Review of the American Medical Association's General Counsel's Office Report on the Impact of Parameters of Care or Practice Guidelines on the Potential Liability of Physicians, Medical Societies and Payers. Unpublished paper prepared at the request of the Physician Payment Review Commission (PPRC), 1990.

Brennan, T. *Just Doctoring: Medical Ethics in the Liberal State.* Berkeley, Calif.: University of California Press, 1991a. (See especially Chapter 5, "Informed Consent," pp. 97-120.)

Brennan, T. Practice Guidelines and Malpractice Litigation: Collision or Cohesion. *Journal of Health Politics, Policy and Law* 16:67-85, 1991b.

Brennan, T., Leape, L., Laird, N., et al. Incidence of Adverse Events and Negligence in Hospitalized Patients: Results of the Harvard Medical Practice Study I. *New England Journal of Medicine* 324:370-376, 1991.

Brett, A., and McCullough, L. When Patients Request Specific Interventions. *New England Journal of Medicine* 315:1347-1351, 1986.

Brightbill, T. Medical Databases: Amazing Potential Hidden in a Maze of Complex Commands. *Healthweek*, August 27, 1990, pp. 27-35.

Brinkley, J. U.S. Releasing Lists of Hospitals with Abnormal Mortality Rates. *New York Times*, March 12, 1986, p. 1.

Brock, D., and Wartman, S. When Competent Patients Make Irrational Choices. *New England Journal of Medicine* 322:1595-1599, 1990.

Brodnik, M., and Johns, M., eds. Standards for Clinical Information Processing. *Topics in Health Record Management* 11(4):1991.

Brook, R. Practice Guidelines and Practicing Medicine: Are They Compatible? *Journal of the American Medical Association* 262:3027-3030, 1989.

Brook, R. Practice Guidelines (In Reply). *Journal of the American Medical Association* 263:3022, 1990.

Brook, R. Health, Health Insurance, and the Uninsured. *Journal of the American Medical Association* 265:2998-3002, 1991.

Brook, R., and Williams, K. Evaluation of the New Mexico Peer Review System, 1971-1973. *Medical Care* 14(12, Suppl.):1-122, 1976.

Brook, R., Williams, K., and Rolph, J., with the assistance of Mori, B.M. Controlling the Use and Cost of Medical Services: The New Mexico Experimental Medical Care Review Organization—A Four-Year Case Study. *Medical Care* 16(9, Suppl.): 1-76, 1978.

Brook, R., Chassin, M., Park, R., et al. A Method for Detailed Assessment of the Appropriateness of Medical Technologies. *International Journal of Technology Assessment in Health Care* 2:53-63, 1986.

Brown, L. The National Politics of Oregon's Rationing Plan. *Health Affairs* 10:28-51, 1991.

Brown, R.E., Sheingold, S.H., and Luce, B.R. *Options of Using Practice Guidelines in Reducing the Volume of Medically Unnecessary Services.* BHARC-013/89/027. Washington, D.C.: Battelle Human Affairs Research Center, 1989.

Burda, D. Total Quality Management Becomes Big Business. *Modern Healthcare* 21:25-29, 1991a.

Burda, D. The Two (Quality) Faces of HCHP. *Modern Healthcare* 21:28-32, 1991b.

Callahan, D. *Setting Limits: Medical Goals in an Aging Society.* New York, N.Y.: Simon and Schuster, 1987.

Canadian Task Force on the Periodic Health Examination. The Periodic Health Examination. *Canadian Medical Association Journal* 121:1194-1254, 1979.

Causey, W. Improve Quality and the Bottom Line Will Follow. *QI/TQM* [Quality Improvement/Total Quality Management] 1:1-3, 1991.

Chassin, M. Standards of Care in Medicine. *Inquiry* 25:437-450, 1988.

Chassin, M.R., Kosecoff, J., Park, R.E., et al. *Indications for Selected Medical and Surgical Procedures—A Literature Review and Ratings of Appropriateness: Coronary Angiography.* R-3201/1-CWF/HF/HCFA/PMT/RWJ. Santa Monica, Calif.: The RAND Corporation, 1986a.

Chassin, M.R., Brook, R.H., Park, R.E., et al. Variations in the Use of Medical and Surgical Services by the Medicare Population. *New England Journal of Medicine* 14:285-290, 1986b.

Chassin, M.R., Kosecoff, J., Park, R.E., et al. Does Inappropriate Use Explain Geographic Variations in the Use of Health Care Services? A Study of Three Procedures. *Journal of the American Medical Association* 258:2533-2537, 1987.

Chassin, M.R., Park, R.E., Lohr, K.N., Keesey, J., and Brook, R.H. Differences among Hospitals in Medicare Patient Mortality. *Health Services Research* 24:1-31, 1989.

CMSS (Council of Medical Specialty Societies). Standards of Quality in Patient Care: The Importance and Risks of Standard Setting. In: *Proceedings of an Invitational Conference.* Washington, D.C., September 25-26, 1987.

Coombs, J. Implementing Practice Guidelines. Presentation at the American Hospital Association Hospital-Medical Staff Leadership Forum. Hilton Head, S.C., November 7, 1991.

Costich, J.F. Denial of Coverage for "Experimental" Medical Procedures: The Problem of De Novo Review under ERISA. *Kentucky Law Journal* 79(4):801-827, 1990-1991.

Darby, M. HCFA Pilot Test Lays Ground for Physician Office Review. *Report on Medical Guidelines & Outcomes Research* 2:6-7, October 1, 1991a.

Darby, M. US Medical Schools Have Not Embraced Guidelines. *Report on Medical Guidelines & Outcomes Research* 2:5-6, July 1, 1991b.

Deming, W.E. *Out of the Crisis.* Cambridge, Mass.: Massachusetts Institute of Technology Press, 1986.

Dersimonian, R., Charette, L., and McPeek, B. Reporting on Methods in Clinical Trials. *New England Journal of Medicine* 306:1332, 1982.

Detsky, A., and Naglie, I. A Clinician's Guide to Cost-Effectiveness Analysis. *Annals of Internal Medicine* 113:147-154, 1990.

Donabedian, A. Evaluating the Quality of Medical Care. *Milbank Memorial Fund Quarterly* 44:166-203, July (part 2) 1966.

Donabedian, A. *Explorations in Quality Assessment and Monitoring*; Vol. 1. *The Definition of Quality and Approaches to Its Assessment*; Vol. 2. *The Criteria and Standards of Monitoring*; Vol. 3. *The Methods and Findings of Quality Assessment and Monitoring: An Illustrated Analysis.* Ann Arbor, Mich.: Health Administration Press, 1980, 1982, 1985.

Donabedian, A. Reflections on the Effectiveness of Quality Assurance. In: R.H. Palmer, A. Donabedian, and G.J. Povar. *Striving for Quality in Health Care: An Inquiry into Policy and Practice.* Ann Arbor, Mich.: Health Administration Press, 1991.

Donaldson, M.S., and Lohr, K. N. A Quality Assurance Sampler: Methods, Data, and Resources. In Institute of Medicine. *Medicare: A Strategy for Quality Assurance. Vol. 2: Sources and Methods.* K.N. Lohr, ed. Washington, D.C.: National Academy Press, 1990.

Dreifus, L.S. A Case History: Developing Guidelines for Cardiac Pacemakers. *The Internist* 31(5):12-16, 1990.

Eckman, M., Wong, J., and Pauker, S. The Role of Clinical Decision Analysis in Medical Quality Management. In: *Health Care Quality Management for the 21st Century.* J. Couch, ed. Tampa, Fla.: American College of Physicians, 1991.

Eddy, D. Variations in Physician Practice: The Role of Uncertainty. *Health Affairs* 3:74-89, 1984.

Eddy, D. Selecting Technologies for Assessment. *International Journal of Technology Assessment in Health Care* 5:485-501, 1989.

Eddy, D. Anatomy of a Decision. *Journal of the American Medical Association* 263:441-443, 1990a.

Eddy, D. The Challenge. *Journal of the American Medical Association* 263:287-290, 1990b.

Eddy, D. Comparing Benefits and Harms: The Balance Sheet. *Journal of the American Medical Association* 263:2493-2505, 1990c.

Eddy, D. Connecting Value and Costs: Whom Do We Ask, and What Do We Ask Them? *Journal of the American Medical Association* 264:1737-1739, 1990d.

Eddy, D. Designing a Practice Policy—Standards, Guidelines, and Options. *Journal of the American Medical Association* 263:3077-3084, 1990e.

Eddy, D. Guidelines for Policy Statements: The Explicit Approach. *Journal of the American Medical Association* 263:2239-2243, 1990f.

Eddy, D. Practice Policies—Guidelines for Methods. *Journal of the American Medical Association* 263:1839-1841, 1990g.

Eddy, D. Practice Policies—What Are They? *Journal of the American Medical Association* 263:877-880, 1990h.

Eddy, D. Practice Policies: Where Do They Come From? *Journal of the American Medical Association* 263:1265-1275, 1990i.

Eddy, D. Resolving Conflicts in Practice Policies. *Journal of the American Medical Association* 264:389-391, 1990j.

Eddy, D. Should We Change the Rules for Evaluating Medical Technologies? In: Institute of Medicine, *Modern Methods of Clinical Investigation.* Annetine C. Gelijns, ed. Washington, D.C.: National Academy Press, 1990k.

Eddy, D. What Do We Do About Costs? *Journal of the American Medical Association* 264:1161-1170, 1990l.

Eddy, D., ed. *Common Screening Tests.* Philadelphia, Pa.: American College of Physicians, 1991a.

Eddy, D. How to Think About Screening. In: *Common Screening Tests.* D. Eddy, ed. Philadelphia, Pa.: American College of Physicians, 1991b.

Eddy, D. (in collaboration with the Council of Medical Specialty Societies). *A Manual for Assessing Health Practices and Designing Practice Policies: The Explicit Approach.* Philadelphia, Pa.: American College of Physicians, 1991c.

Eddy, D. Oregon's Methods: Did Cost-effectiveness Analysis Fail? *Journal of the American Medical Association* 266:2135-2141, 1991d.

Eddy, D. Rationing by Patient Choice. *Journal of the American Medical Association* 265:105-108, 1991e.

Eddy, D., and Billings, J. The Quality of Medical Evidence: Implications for Quality of Care. *Health Affairs* 7:19-32, 1988.

Edwards, D. The Maine 5-Year Medical Demonstration Project. Presentation at the Agency for Health Care Policy and Research Conference on Medical Liability Issues, Washington, D.C., February 28, 1991.

Egan, T. Oregon Shakes Up Pioneering Health Plan for the Poor. *New York Times,* February 22, 1991, p. A11.

Eichorn, J., Cooper, R., and Cullen, M. Standards for Patient Monitoring during

Anesthesia at Harvard Medical School. *Journal of the American Medical Association* 246:1017-1020, 1986.

Eisenberg, J. Physician Utilization: The State of Research About Physicians' Practice Patterns. *Medical Care* 23:461-483, 1985.

Eisenberg, J. *Doctors' Decisions and the Cost of Medical Care: The Reasons for Doctors' Practice Patterns and the Ways to Change Them.* Ann Arbor, Mich.: Health Administration Press Perspectives, 1986.

Elliott, C. Computer-Assisted Quality Assurance: Development and Performance of a Respiratory Care Program. *Quality Review Bulletin* 17:85-90, 1991.

Ellwood, P. Shattuck Lecture. Outcomes Management: A Technology of Patient Experience. *New England Journal of Medicine* 318:1549-1556, 1988.

Ellwood, P. Uniform Effective Health Benefits. Policy Document No. 3 (of four). Unpublished paper prepared for the Jackson Hole Group, August 30, 1991.

Faden, R., and Beauchamp, T. *A History and Theory of Informed Consent.* New York, N.Y.: Oxford University Press, 1986.

Fink, A., Kosecoff, J., Chassin, M., and Brook, R. Consensus Methods: Characteristics and Guidelines for Use. *American Journal of Public Health* 74:979-983, 1984.

Fitzpatrick, T. Utilization Review and Control Mechanisms: From the Blue Cross Perspective. *Inquiry* 2:16-29, 1965.

Fliegel, T. Knowledge-Based Systems: Trying to Define a Role That's Wise. *Healthweek*, June 11, 1990, pp. 61-63.

Fowler, F.J. *Prostatism Form 4.1: TyPE Specification.* Minneapolis, Minn.: InterStudy, 1991.

Fowler, F.J., Wennberg, J.E., Timothy, R.P., et al. Symptom Status and Quality of Life Following Prostatectomy. *Journal of the American Medical Association* 259:3018-3022, 1988.

Fox, D., and Leichter, H. Rationing Care in Oregon: The New Accountability. *Health Affairs* 10:7-27, 1991.

Foxman, B., Valdez, R.B., Lohr, K.N., et al. The Effect of Cost Sharing on the Use of Antibiotics in Ambulatory Care: Results from a Population-Based Randomized Controlled Trial. *Journal of Chronic Diseases* 40:429-437, 1987.

Frame, P.S., and Carlson, S.J. A Critical Review of Periodic Health Screening Using Specific Screening Criteria. *Journal of Family Practice* 2:283-289, 1975.

Frisch, S. The Case of the Numb Chin: Benefits of Searching Electronic Literature. *ACP [American College of Physicians] Observer* 11(4):6-7, 1991.

Gabrieli, E. Need for Standards in Medical Communication. *Topics in Health Record Management: Standards for Clinical Information Processing* 11(4):27-36, 1991.

GAO (General Accounting Office). *Medical Malpractice: A Framework for Action.* GAO/HRD-87-73. Washington, D.C.: General Accounting Office, 1987.

GAO. *Medical ADP Systems: Automated Medical Records Hold Promise to Improve Patient Care.* GAO/IMTEC-91-C. Washington, D.C.: General Accounting Office, 1991a.

GAO. *Practice Guidelines: The Experience of Medical Specialty Societies.* GAO/PEMD-91-11. Washington, D.C.: General Accounting Office, 1991b.

Gardner, E. The Coming Evolution in Computer Systems. *Modern Healthcare* 20(6):29-44, 1990a.

Gardner, E. Hospitals Not in a Hurry to Plug in Computers by the Bedside. *Modern Healthcare* 20(28):31-55, 1990b.

Gardner, E. Going on Line with Outsiders. *Modern Healthcare* 21(28):35-48, 1991.

Gardner, E., and Perry, L. Assessing Computer Links' Risks and Rewards. *Modern Healthcare* 19(47):20-31, 1989.

Garnick, D.W., Hendricks, A.M., and Brennan, T.A. Can Practice Guidelines Reduce the Number and Costs of Malpractice Claims? *Journal of the American Medical Association* 266:2856-2860, 1991.

Garvin, D.A. *Managing Quality: The Strategic and Competitive Edge.* New York, N.Y.: The Free Press, A Division of Macmillan, 1988.

Gertman, P.M., and Restuccia, J.D. The Appropriateness Evaluation Protocol. *Medical Care* 19:855-871, 1981.

Glass, G.V. Primary, Secondary, and Meta-Analysis of Research. *Educational Researcher* 5:3-8, 1976.

Goldman, L., Cook, E.F., Brand, D.A., et al. A Computer Protocol to Predict Myocardial Infarction in Emergency Department Patients with Chest Pain. *New England Journal of Medicine* 318:797-803, 1988.

Goldstein, A. Poor Required to Have Own Doctor Under Md.'s New Medicaid Program. *Washington Post*, December 10, 1991, p. A1, A10.

Gosfield, A. *PSROs: The Law and the Health Consumer.* Cambridge, Mass.: Ballinger Publishing Co., 1975.

Gosfield, A. PROs: A Case Study in Utilization Management and Quality Assurance. In: *1989 Health Law Handbook.* New York, N.Y.: Clark Boardman Company, Ltd., 1989, pp. 361-398.

Gosfield, A. Presentation at the RAND Conference on the Changing Health Care Delivery System and Its Implications for Liability Law, Dallas, Texas, June 10-11, 1991a.

Gosfield, A. Value Purchasing and Effectiveness: Legal Implications. In: *1991 Health Law Handbook.* New York, N.Y.: Clark Boardman Company, Ltd., 1991b.

Gottlieb, L., Margolis, C., and Schoenbaum, S. Clinical Practice Guidelines at an HMO: Development and Implementation in a Quality Improvement Model. *Quality Review Bulletin* 16:80-86, 1990.

Granneman, T. Priority Setting: A Sensible Approach to Medicaid Policy? *Inquiry* 28:300-305, 1991.

Green, L. Dissemination Strategies for Consumers. Paper prepared for the Conference to Develop a Research Agenda for Outcomes and Effectiveness Research, conducted by the Foundation for Health Services Research and the Alpha Center, Arlington, Va., April 14-16, 1991.

Greenfield, S. The State of Outcomes Research: Are We on Target? *New England Journal of Medicine* 320:1142-1143, 1989.

Greenfield, S. The Effect of Local Physician Participation in Guideline Development on Patient Outcome and Adherence to the Guidelines: A Controlled Prospective Trial. Unpublished paper, New England Medical Center, Boston, Mass., December 1991.

Grossman, J. Emerging Medical Quality Management Support Systems for Hospitals. In: *Health Care Quality Management for the 21st Century*. J. Couch, ed. Tampa, Fla.: American College of Physician Executives, 1991.

Gschwend, R. Commentary: Medical Specialty Societies and the Development of Practice Policies. *Quality Review Bulletin* 16:58-59, 1990.

Gunnar, R., Passamani, E., Bourdillon, P., et al. Guidelines for the Early Management of Patients with Acute Myocardial Infarction. ACC/AHA Task Force Report. *Journal of the American College of Cardiology* 16:249-292, 1990.

Hadorn, D. Defining Basic Health Benefits Using Clinical Guidelines: A Model Proposal for Discussion. Paper prepared for the conference on "Creating a Fair and Reasonable Basic Benefit Plan Using Clinical Guidelines," sponsored by the California Public Employees' Retirement System's Health Benefits Advisory Council, Sacramento, Calif., April 24-26, 1991a.

Hadorn, D. Necessary-Care Guidelines: Using an Explicit Standard of Proof to Define Health Care Needs. Paper prepared for the conference on "Creating a Fair and Reasonable Basic Benefit Plan Using Clinical Guidelines," sponsored by the California Public Employees' Retirement System's Health Benefits Advisory Council, Sacramento, Calif., April 24-26, 1991b.

Hadorn, D.C. Setting Health Care Priorities in Oregon: Cost-Effectiveness Meets the Rule of Rescue. *Journal of the American Medical Association* 265:2218-2225, 1991c.

Hadorn, D., and Brook, R. The Health Care Resource Allocation Debate. *Journal of the American Medical Association* 266:3328-3331, 1991.

Hall, M. The Malpractice Standard under Health Care Cost Containment. *Law, Medicine and Health Care* 17(4):347-355, 1989.

Hall, M. The Legal Implications of Medical Practice Guidelines: An Evaluation of the AMA Report [American Medical Association's General Counsel's Office Report on the Impact of Parameters of Care or Practice Guidelines on the Potential Liability of Physicians, Medical Societies and Payers]. Unpublished paper prepared at the request of the Physician Payment Review Commission (PPRC), January 1990.

Hall, M. The Defensive Effect of Medical Practice Policies in Malpractice Litigation. *Law and Contemporary Problems* 54:199-245, 1991.

Hammond, W. Health Level 7: An Application Standard for Electronic Medical Data Exchange. *Topics in Health Record Management: Standards for Clinical Information Processing* 11(4):59-66, 1991.

Hammons, T. The Use and Contribution of Practice Guidelines. Background paper prepared for the Conference to Develop a Research Agenda for Outcomes and Effectiveness Research, conducted by the Foundation for Health Services Research and the Alpha Center, Arlington, Va., April 14-16, 1991.

Harvard Medical Practice Study. *Patients, Lawyers and Doctors*. Cambridge, Mass.: Harvard Medical School, 1990.

Hattwick, M.A., Hart, R.J., and Weiss, S. Using the Information Tool to Improve Preventive Medical Care. In: *Proceedings of the Fifth Annual Symposium on Computer Applications in Medical Care*. New York: Institute of Electrical and Electronic Engineers, November 1981, pp. 182-186.

Havighurst, C. Practice Guidelines and the Law. Unpublished memorandum to G.T. Hammons, Physician Payment Review Commission, January 16, 1990a.

Havighurst, C. Practice Guidelines for Medical Care: The Policy Rationale. *St. Louis University Law Journal* 34:777-819, 1990b.

Havighurst, C. Practice Guidelines as Legal Standards Governing Physician Practice. *Law and Contemporary Problems* 54:87-117, Spring 1991a.

Havighurst, C. Why Preserve Private Health Care Financing? Paper prepared for conference on American Health Policy: Critical Issues for Reform, sponsored by American Enterprise Institute for Public Policy Research in Washington, D.C., October 3-4, 1991b.

Havighurst, C., and Metzloff, T.S. 1232—A Late Entry into the Race for Malpractice Reform. *Law and Contemporary Problems* 54:179-197, 1991.

Hayward, R.S., Steinberg, E.P., Ford, D.E., et al. Preventive Care Guidelines: 1991. In: *Common Screening Tests.* D.M. Eddy, ed. Philadelphia, Pa.: American College of Physicians, 1991.

HCFA (Health Care Financing Administration). *Medicare Hospital Mortality Information: 1986 and Annually Thereafter.* Washington, D.C.: Government Printing Office, 1987-1991.

Hedges, L.V., and Olkin, I. *Statistical Methods for Meta-Analysis.* New York, N.Y.: Academic Press, 1985.

Helvestine, W. Legal Implications of Utilization Review. In: Institute of Medicine. *Controlling Costs and Changing Patient Care? The Role of Utilization Management.* B.H. Gray and M.J. Field, eds. Washington, D.C.: National Academy Press, 1989, pp. 169-204.

Hillman, A. Disclosing Information and Treating Patients as Customers: A Review of Selected Issues. *HMO Practice* 5:37-41, 1991.

Hinterbuchner, L. Letter to the Editor. *ACP Observer* 11:5 November 1991.

Hirshfield, E. Economic Considerations in Treatment Decisions and the Standard of Care in Medical Malpractice Litigation. *Journal of the American Medical Association* 264:2004-2012, 1990a.

Hirshfield, E. Practice Parameters and the Malpractice Liability of Physicians. *Journal of the American Medical Association* 263:1556-1562, 1990b.

Holzer, J. The Advent of Clinical Standards for Professional Liability. *Quality Review Bulletin* 16:71-79, 1990.

Hoogwerf, B. *Diabetes Form 2.1: TyPE Specification.* Minneapolis, Minn.: InterStudy, 1989.

Hripcsak, G., Clayton, T., Pryor, T., et al. The Arden Syntax for Medical Logic Modules. In: *Proceedings of the Fourteenth Annual Symposium on Computer Applications in Medical Care.* R. Miller, ed. Washington, D.C.: IEEE Computer Society Press, 1990, pp. 200-204.

IMCARE (Internal Medicine Center to Advance Research and Education). *Medical Practice Guidelines Workshop: Issues for Internal Medicine.* Washington, D.C.: IMCARE, 1990.

IMCARE. IMCARE News & Reviews. *The Internist* 32:43, 1991.

InterQual, Inc. *The ISD-A Review System.* Chicago, Ill.: InterQual, Inc., 1987.

InterStudy. *An Introduction to InterStudy's Outcomes Management System.* Minneapolis, Minn.: InterStudy, 1991.

IOM (Institute of Medicine). *Assessing Medical Technologies.* Council on Health Care Technology. Washington, D.C.: National Academy Press, 1985.

IOM. *Medical Technology Assessment Directory.* Washington, D.C.: National Academy Press, 1988.

IOM. *Controlling Costs and Changing Patient Care? The Role of Utilization Management.* B. Gray and M. Field, eds. Washington, D.C.: National Academy Press, 1989a.

IOM. *Effectiveness Initiative: Setting Priorities for Clinical Conditions.* K. Lohr and R. Rettig, eds. Washington, D.C.: National Academy Press, 1989b.

IOM. *Acute Myocardial Infarction: Setting Priorities for Effectiveness Research.* P. Mattingly and K. Lohr, eds. Washington, D.C.: National Academy Press, 1990a.

IOM. *Breast Cancer: Setting Priorities for Effectiveness Research.* K.N. Lohr, ed. Washington, D.C.: National Academy Press, 1990b.

IOM. *Clinical Practice Guidelines: Directions for a New Program.* M.J. Field and K.N. Lohr, eds. Washington, D.C.: National Academy Press, 1990c.

IOM. *Consensus Development at the NIH: Improving the Program.* Washington, D.C.: National Academy Press, 1990d.

IOM. *Effectiveness and Outcomes in Health Care: Proceedings of an Invitational Conference.* K.A. Heithoff and K.N. Lohr, eds. Washington, D.C.: National Academy Press, 1990e.

IOM. *Hip Fracture: Setting Priorities for Effectiveness Research.* K.A. Heithoff and K.N. Lohr, eds. Washington, D.C.: National Academy Press, 1990f.

IOM. *Improving Consensus Development for Health Technology Assessment: An International Perspective.* C. Goodman and S.R. Baratz, eds. Washington, D.C.: National Academy Press, 1990g.

IOM. *Medical Innovation at the Crossroads.* Vol. 1. *Modern Methods of Clinical Investigation.* A. Gelijns, ed. Washington, D.C.: National Academy Press, 1990h.

IOM. *Medicare: A Strategy for Quality Assurance,* 2 vols. K.N. Lohr, ed. Washington, D.C.: National Academy Press, 1990i.

IOM. *National Priorities for the Assessment of Clinical Conditions and Medical Technologies: Report of a Pilot Study.* M.E. Lara and C. Goodman, eds. Washington, D.C.: National Academy Press, 1990j.

IOM. *The Artificial Heart: Prototypes, Policies, and Patients.* J.R. Hogness and M. VanAntwerp, eds. Washington, D.C.: National Academy Press, 1991a.

IOM. *The Computer-based Patient Record: An Essential Technology for Health Care.* R. Dick and E.B. Steen, eds. Washington, D.C.: National Academy Press, 1991b.

IOM. *Information Services for Health Services Researchers: A Report to the National Library of Medicine.* J. Harris-Wehling and L. Morris, eds. Washington, D.C.: National Academy Press, 1991c.

IOM. *Kidney Failure and the Federal Government.* R.A. Rettig and N.G. Levinsky, eds. Washington, D.C.: National Academy Press, 1991d.

IOM. *Setting Priorities for Health Technology Assessment: A Model Process.* M.S. Donaldson and H.C. Sox, Jr., eds. Washington, D.C.: National Academy Press, 1992.

Jacoby, I. Biomedical Technology Information Dissemination and the NIH Consensus Development Process. *Knowledge: Creation, Diffusion, Utilization* 5(2):245-261, 1983.

Jacoby, I. The Consensus Development Program of the National Institutes of Health: Current Practices and Historical Perspectives. *International Journal of Technology Assessment in Health Care* 1:420-432, 1985.

Javitt, C., and Ware, J. *Cataract Form 1.1: TyPE Specification.* Minneapolis, Minn.: InterStudy, 1990.

Jencks, S.F., Williams, D.K., and Kay, T.L. Assessing Hospital Associated Deaths from Discharge Data. The Role of Length of Stay and Comorbidities. *Journal of the American Medical Association* 260:2240-2246, 1988a.

Jencks, S.F., Daley, J., Draper, D., et al. Interpreting Hospital Mortality Data. The Role of Clinical Risk Adjustment. *Journal of the American Medical Association* 260:3159-3163, 1988b.

Jennison, K. Total Quality Management—Fad or Paradigmatic Shift? In: *Health Care Quality Management for the 21st Century.* J. Couch, ed. Tampa, Fla.: American College of Physician Executives, 1991.

Jonsen, A., and Toulmin, S. *The Abuse of Casuistry: A History of Moral Reasoning.* Berkeley, Calif.: University of California Press, 1988.

Kahan, J., Kanouse, D., and Winkler, J. Stylistic Variations in National Institutes of Health Consensus Statements, 1979-1983. *International Journal of Technology Assessment in Health Care* 4:289-304, 1988.

Kahn, K.L., Roth, C.P., Fink, A., et al. *Indications for Selected Medical and Surgical Procedures: A Literature Review and Ratings of Appropriateness. Colonoscopy.* R-3204/5-CWF/HF/HCFA/PT/RWJ. Santa Monica, Calif.: The RAND Corporation, 1986.

Kanouse, D., and Jacoby, I. When Does Information Change Practitioners' Behavior? *International Journal of Technology Assessment in Health Care* 4:27-33, 1988.

Kanouse, D., Brook, R., Winkler, J., et al. *Changing Medical Practice Through Technology Assessment: An Evaluation of the National Institutes of Health Consensus Development Program.* R-3452-NIH. Santa Monica, Calif.: The RAND Corporation, 1989.

Kaplan, S., and Ware, J. The Patient's Role in Health Care and Quality Assessment. In: *Providing Quality Care: The Challenge to Clinicians.* N. Goldfield and D. Nash, eds. Philadelphia, Pa.: American College of Physicians, 1989, pp. 25-68.

Kapp, M. Enforcing Patient Preferences. *Journal of the American Medical Association* 261:1935-1938, 1989.

Kapp, M. Health Care Risk Management: The Challenge of Measuring Costs and Benefits. Quality Review Bulletin 16:166-169, 1990.

Kassirer, J.P. Our Stubborn Quest for Diagnostic Certainty. *New England Journal of Medicine* 320:1489-1491, 1989.

Kellie, S., and Kelly, J. Medicare Peer Review Organization Preprocedure Review Criteria: An Analysis of Criteria for Three Procedures. *Journal of the American Medical Association* 265:1265-1270, 1991.

Kelly, J., and Swartwout, J. Commentary: Development of Practice Parameters by Physician Organizations. *Quality Review Bulletin* 16:54-57, 1990.

Kent, C. Technology Assessment: A Stronger Federal Role? *Medicine and Health Perspectives* December 16, 1991 (n.p.).

Kinney, E., and Wilder, M. Medical Standard Setting in the Current Malpractice

Environment: Problems and Possibilities. *University of California Davis Law Review* 22:421-450, 1989.

Kirklin, J.W., Akins, C.W., Blackstone, E.H., et al. Guidelines and Indications for Coronary Artery Bypass Graft Surgery. A Report of the American College of Cardiology/American Heart Association. *Journal of the American College of Cardiology* 17:543-589, 1991.

Kosecoff, J., Kanouse, D., Rogers, W., et al. Effects of the National Institutes of Health Consensus Development Program on Physician Practice. *Journal of the American Medical Association* 258:2708-2713, 1987.

Kosterlitz, J. Cookbook Medicine. *National Journal*, March 9, 1991, pp. 574-577.

Krakauer, H. The Uniform Clinical Data Set. In: *Effectiveness and Outcomes in Health Care.* K.A. Heithoff and K.N. Lohr, eds. Washington, D.C.: National Academy Press, 1990.

Krakauer, H., and Bailey, R.C. Epidemiologic Oversight of the Medical Care Provided to Medicare Beneficiaries. *Statistics in Medicine* 10:521-540, 1991.

Kritchevsky, S.B., and Simmons, B.P. Continuous Quality Improvement: Concepts and Applications for Physician Care. *Journal of the American Medical Association* 266:1817-1823, 1991.

L'Abbe, K.A., Detsky, A.S., and O'Rourke, K. Meta-Analysis in Clinical Research. *Annals of Internal Medicine* 107:224-233, 1987.

Langsley, D. Medical Competence and Performance Assessment: A New Era. *Journal of the American Medical Association* 266:977-980, 1991.

Leape, L. Practice Guidelines and Standards: An Overview. *Quality Review Bulletin* 16:42-49, 1990.

Littenberg, B., Garber, A.M., and Sox, Jr., H.C. The Resting Electrocardiogram as a Screening Test: A Clinical Analysis. *Common Screening Tests.* D.M. Eddy, ed. Philadelphia, Pa.: American College of Physicians, 1991.

Little, L. Swedish Practice Guidelines Failed, Group Told. *American Medical News* June 8, 1990, p. 4.

Lo, B. Unanswered Questions About DNR Orders. *Journal of the American Medical Association* 265:1874-1875, 1991.

Localio, A., Lawthers, A., Brennan, T., et al. Relation Between Malpractice Claims and Adverse Events Due to Negligence: Results of the Harvard Medical Practice Study III. *New England Journal of Medicine* 325:245-251, 1991.

Lohr, K.N. Outcome Measurement: Concepts and Questions. *Inquiry* 25:37-50, 1988.

Lohr, K.N. guest ed. Advances in Health Status Assessment. Proceedings of a Conference. *Medical Care* 27(3, Suppl.):S1-S294, 1989.

Lohr, K.N., guest ed. Advances in Health Status Assessment: Fostering the Application of Health Status Measures in Clinical Settings. *Medical Care* 30 (Supplement), 1992 (forthcoming).

Lohr, K.N., and Harris-Wehling, J. Medicare: A Strategy for Quality Assurance. I. A Recapitulation of the Study and a Definition of Quality of Care. *Quality Review Bulletin* 17:6-9, 1991.

Lohr, K.N., and Ware, Jr., J.E., guest eds. Proceedings of the Advances in Health Assessment Conference. *Journal of Chronic Diseases* 40 (Suppl.):S1-S193, 1987.

Lohr, K.N., Brook, R.H., Kamberg, C.J., et al. Use of Medical Care in the Rand Health Insurance Experiment. Diagnosis- and Service-Specific Analyses in a Randomized Controlled Trial. *Medical Care* 24(Sept. Suppl.):S1-S87, 1986.

Lomas, J. Words Without Action: The Production, Dissemination, and Impact of Consensus Recommendations. *Annual Review of Public Health* 12:41-65, 1991.

Lomas, J., and Haynes, R.B. A Taxonomy and Critical Review of Tested Strategies for the Application of Clinical Practice Recommendations: From "Official" to "Individual" Clinical Policy. *American Journal of Preventive Medicine* 4(4 Suppl.):77-94, 1988.

Lomas, J., Anderson, K., Dominck-Pierre, et al., Do Practice Guidelines Guide Practice? *New England Journal of Medicine* 321:1306-1311, 1989.

Lomas, J., Enkin, M., Anderson, G.M., et al. Opinion Leaders vs Audit and Feedback to Implement Practice Guidelines. Delivery after Previous Cesarean Section. *Journal of the American Medical Association* 265:2202-2207, 1991.

Luce, B.R., Weschler, J.M., and Underwood, C. The Use of Quality-of-Life Measures in the Private Sector. In: *Quality of Life and Technology Assessment.* F. Mosteller and J. Falotico-Taylor, eds. Council on Health Care Technology Monograph. Washington, D.C.: National Academy Press, 1989.

Lundsgaarde, H., Fischer, P., and Steele, D. Human Problems in Computerized Medicine. *Publications in Anthropology, 13*, Lawrence, Kan.: University of Kansas, 1981.

Macchiaroli, J. Medical Malpractice Screening Panels: Proposed Model Legislation to Cure Judicial Ills. *George Washington Law Review* 58(2):181-261, 1990.

Margolis, C., Gottlieb, L., Barak, N., and Pearson, S. Development of Tools for Algorithmic Analysis of Practice Guidelines. Paper prepared for the Institute of Medicine Committee on Clinical Practice Guidelines, Washington, D.C., 1991.

Maryland Hospital Association, Quality Indicator Project. *Guidebook for Quality Indicator Data. A Continuous Improvement Model.* Lutherville, Md.: The Maryland Hospital Association, 1990.

Mazur, D. Why the Goals of Informed Consent Are Not Realized: Treatise on Informed Consent for the Primary Care Physician. *Journal of General Internal Medicine* 3:370-380, 1988.

McCall, N., Rice, T., and Sangl, J. Consumer Knowledge of Medicare and Supplemental Health Insurance Benefits. *Health Services Research* 20:633-657, 1986.

McCormick, B. Defense Lawyers Raise Questions About Maine Parameters Project. *American Medical News*, May 6, 1991, pp. 1, 27-28.

McCullough, L. An Ethical Model for Improving the Patient-Physician Relationship. *Inquiry* 25:454-468, 1988.

McDonald, C.J. Computer Reminders, the Quality of Care and the Nonperfectability of Man. *New England Journal of Medicine* 295:1351-1355, 1976.

McDonald, C.J., Hui, S., Smith, D., et. al. Reminders to Physicians from an Introspective Computer Medical Record. *Annals of Internal Medicine* 100:130-138, 1984.

McDonald, C.J., Blevins, L., Tierney, W.M., et al. The Regenstrief Medical Records. *MD Computing* 5:34-37, 1988.

McDonald, C.J., Martin, D., and Overhage, J. Standards for the Electronic Transfer of Clinical Data: Progress and Promise. *Topics in Health Record Management: Standards for Clinical Information Processing* 11(4):1-14, 1991.

McDowell, I., and Newell, C. *Measuring Health. A Guide to Rating Scales and Questionnaires.* New York: Oxford University Press, 1987.

McGinn, P. Practice Standards Leading to Premium Reductions. *American Medical News*, December 2, 1988, p. 1, 28.

McGuire, L. A Long Run for a Short Jump: Understanding Clinical Guidelines. *Annals of Internal Medicine* 113:705-708, 1990.

McPherson, K., Wennberg, J.E., Hovind, O.B., et al. Small-Area Variation in the Use of Common Surgical Procedures: An International Comparison of New England, England, and Norway. *New England Journal of Medicine* 307:1310-1314, 1982.

Megargle, R. Role of ASTM in Computer Information Standards for Medicine. *Topics in Health Record Management: Standards for Clinical Information Processing* 11(4):17-26, 1991.

Miike, L. Medical Practice Guidelines and Tort Liability: Review and Comment of the Analysis by the Office of General Counsel, American Medical Association [the American Medical Association's General Counsel's Office Report on the Impact of Parameters of Care or Practice Guidelines on the Potential Liability of Physicians, Medical Societies and Payers]. Unpublished paper prepared at the request of the Physician Payment Review Commission (PPRC), December 1989.

Miller, F. Informed Consent for the Man on the Clapham Omnibus: An English Cure for "The American Disease"? *Western New England Law Review* 9(1):169-190, 1987.

Miller, F. Practice Guidelines and Medical Malpractice Liability. Paper commissioned for the Institute of Medicine Study of Clinical Practice Guidelines. April 1991.

Mills, D.H., and Lindgren, O. Impact of Liability Litigation on Quality of Care. In: *Health Care Quality Management for the 21st Century.* J. Couch, ed. Tampa, Fla.: American College of Physician Executives, 1991.

Mor, V. Cancer Patients' Quality of Life over the Disease Course: Lessons from the Real World. *Journal of Chronic Diseases* 40:535-544, 1987.

Morlock, L., Lindgren, O., and Mills, D. Malpractice, Clinical Risk Management, and Quality Assessment. In: *Providing Quality Care: The Challenge to Clinicians.* N. Goldfield and D. Nash, eds. Philadelphia, Pa.: American College of Physicians, 1989.

Morreim, E. Stratified Scarcity: Redefining the Standard of Care. *Law, Medicine and Health Care* 17:356-367, 1989.

Morris, L. Introduction to the Blue Cross and Blue Shield Association Guidelines. In: *Common Diagnostic Tests: Use and Interpretation.* H. Sox, ed. Philadelphia, Pa.: American College of Physicians, 1987, pp. 331-374.

Mosteller, F., and Falotico-Taylor, J., eds. *Quality of Life and Technology Assessment.* Council on Health Care Technology Monograph. Washington, D.C.: National Academy Press, 1989.

Mullan, F., and Jacoby, I. The Town Meeting for Technology: The Maturation of Consensus Conferences. *Journal of the American Medical Association* 254:1068-1072, 1985.

Mulley, Jr., A.G. Assessing Patients' Utilities: Can the Ends Justify the Means? *Medical Care* 27(3, Suppl.):S269-S281, 1989.

Mulley, Jr., A.G. Finding Common Ground. *HMQ [Health Management Quarterly]* 13(2):16-19, 1991.

Mulrow, C.D. The Medical Review Article: State of the Science. *Annals of Internal Medicine* 106:485-488, 1987.

Nash D., ed. *Clinical Outcomes: Managing Patients and the Total Cost of Care.* Doylestown, Pa.: Health Sciences Institute, 1990a.

Nash, D. Overcoming Resistance in Developing a Quality Focus. *Clinical Outcomes* 1(2):2-3, 1990b.

National Association of Private Psychiatric Hospitals. *Benefits Watch Survey.* Washington, D.C.: The Association, May 1991.

National Council on Patient Information and Education. Educational Resources. In: *Talk About Prescriptions Month.* Washington, D.C.: The Council, October 1991, pp. 12-17.

National Research Council. *Improving Risk Communication.* Washington, D.C.: National Academy Press, 1989.

Newman, T.B., Browner, W.S., and Hulley, S.B. The Case Against Childhood Cholesterol Screening. *Journal of the American Medical Association* 264:3039-3043, 1990.

Neugebauer, E., Troidl, H., Wood-Dauphinee, S., Eypasch, E., and Bullinger, M. Quality-of-Life Assessment in Surgery: Results of the Meran Consensus Development Conference. *Journal of Theoretical Surgery* 6:123-137, 1991.

New York Business Group on Health. Risk-Related Health Insurance: Incentives for Healthy Lifestyles. Discussion Paper Series 10 (Supp. 1), May 1990.

NIH (National Institutes of Health) Consensus Conference. Intravenous Immunoglobulin: Prevention and Treatment of Disease. *Journal of the American Medical Association* 264:3189-3193, 1990.

Nuckolls, J. Practicing Physician Considerations. Medical Practice Guidelines Workshop: Issues for Internal Medicine. Sponsored by the Agency for Health Care Policy and Research and the Internal Medicine Center to Advance Research and Education, Washington, D.C., June 8-9, 1990, pp. 58-63.

O'Donnell, M. Battle of the Clotbusters. *British Medical Journal* 302:1259-1261, 1991.

O'Leary, D. Accreditation in the Quality Improvement Mold—A Vision for Tomorrow. *Quality Review Bulletin* 17:72-77, 1991.

OMAR (Office of Medical Applications of Research), National Institutes of Health. *Guidelines for the Selection and Management of Consensus Development Conferences.* Bethesda, Md.: U.S. Government Printing Office, 1988.

OTA (Office of Technology Assessment). *Assessing the Efficacy and Safety of Medical Technologies.* OTA-H-75. Washington, D.C., 1978.

OTA. *Preventive Health Services for Medicare Beneficiaries: Policy and Research Issues.* Special Report. OTA-H-416. Washington, D.C.: U.S. Government Printing Office, 1990.

Oxman, A.D., and Guyatt, G.H. Guidelines for Reading Literature Reviews. *Canadian Medical Association Journal* 138:697-703, 1988.

Park, R.E., Fink, A., Brook, R.H., et al. Physician Ratings of Appropriate Indications for Six Medical and Surgical Procedures. R-3280-/CWF/HF/PMT/RWJ. Santa Monica, Calif.: The RAND Corporation, 1986.

Patrick, D.L., and Erickson, P. What Constitutes Quality of Life? Concepts and Definitions. *Quality of Life and Cardiovascular Care* 4:103-127, 1988.

Payne, S.M. Identifying and Managing Inappropriate Hospital Utilization: A Policy Synthesis. *Health Services Research* 22:710-769, 1987.

Pellegrino, E. Rationing Health Care: The Ethics of Medical Gatekeeping. *Journal of Contemporary Health Law and Policy* 2:23-45, 1986.

Perry, S. The NIH Consensus Development Program: A Decade Later. *New England Journal of Medicine* 317:485-488, 1987.

Perry, S. Consensus Development: An Historical Note. *International Journal of Technology Assessment in Health Care* 4:481-488, 1988.

Pestotnik, S., Evans, R., Burke, J., et al. Therapeutic Antibiotic Monitoring: Surveillance Using a Computerized Expert System. *American Journal of Medicine* 88:43-48, 1990.

Phelps, C., and Parente, S. Priority Setting in Medical Technology and Medical Practice Assessment. *Medical Care* 28:703-723, 1990.

Pierce, Jr., E. The Development of Anesthesia Guidelines and Standards. *Quality Review Bulletin* 16:61-64, 1990.

Povar, G. Clinical Guidelines: Addressing the Ethical Dimensions. Paper commissioned for the Institute of Medicine Study of Clinical Practice Guidelines, Washington, D.C., April 1991.

PPRC (Physician Payment Review Commission). *Annual Report to Congress.* Washington, D.C.: 1988, 1989, 1990.

President's Commission for the Study of Ethical Problems in Medicine and Biomedical and Behavioral Research. *Summing Up: The Ethical and Legal Problems in Medicine and Biomedical and Behavioral Research.* Washington, D.C.: The Commission, pp. 21, 67, 69, 77-78, 1983.

Project Hope. A Study of the Preadmission Review Process. Prepared for the Prospective Payment Assessment Commission, Chevy Chase, Md., November 1987.

QI/TQM [Quality Improvement/Total Quality Management]. Vol. 1, no. 1. Atlanta, Ga.: American Health Consultants, Inc., July 1991.

QRC [Quality Resource Center] Update. Profile. Three Hospital Projects Aim for Quality Improvement. Washington, D.C.: Washington Business Group on Health, Summer 1991, p. 4.

Quality Connection. *News from the National Demonstration Project on Quality Improvement in Health Care.* Brookline, Mass.: National Demonstration Project, c/o Harvard Community Health Plan, 1991-.

Quality Exchange. *A Newsletter on Quality of Care Issues from The Johns Hopkins University.* Baltimore, Md.: The Johns Hopkins University School of Hygiene and Public Health, 1991-.

Redelmeier, D., and Tversky, A. Discrepancy Between Medical Decisions for Individual Patients and for Groups. *New England Journal of Medicine* 322:1162-1164, 1990.

Reiser, R. A Commentary on the Rationale of the Diet-Heart Statement of the American Heart Association. *American Journal of Clinical Nutrition* 40:654-658, 1984.

Resnicow, K., Berenson, G., Shea, S., et al. Commentary: The Case Against "The Case Against Childhood Cholesterol Screening." *Journal of the American Medical Association* 265:3003-3005, 1991.

Rettig, R. Origins of the Medicare Kidney Disease Entitlement. In: *Biomedical Politics.* K. Hanna, ed. Washington, D.C.: National Academy Press, 1991a.

Rettig, R. Technology Assessment: An Update. *Investigative Radiology* 26:165-173, 1991b.

Robb, J. Health Insurance Rating Reform: Who Should Carry the Burden? Presentation at the conference on Incentive Systems and Risk-Rated Health Insurance, sponsored by Park Nicollet Medical Foundation and MedCenters, Minneapolis, Minnesota, October 28, 1991.

Robinson, M. Annotated Directory of Medical Practice Guidelines. *Report on Medical Guidelines and Outcomes Research.* March 1991.

Roper, W., and Hackbarth, G. HCFA's Agenda for Promoting High-Quality Care. *Health Affairs* 7:91-98, 1988.

Roper, W., Winkenwerder, W., Hackbarth, G., and Krakauer, H. Effectiveness in Health Care: An Initiative to Evaluate and Improve Medical Practice. *New England Journal of Medicine* 319:1197-1202, 1988.

Rovner, S. Back to Basics of Baby Care. *Washington Post Health,* December 17/24, 1991, p. 9.

Russell, L. *Is Prevention Better Than Cure?* Washington, D.C.: Brookings Institution, 1986.

Sacks, H.S., Berrier, J., Reitman, O., Ancoma-Berk, V.A., and Chalmers, T.C. Meta-Analysis of Randomized Controlled Trials. *New England Journal of Medicine* 316:450-455, 1987.

Schoenbaum, S. Consensus and the Quality Improvement Cycle. Medical Practice Guidelines Workshop: Issues for Internal Medicine. Sponsored by the Agency for Health Care Policy and Research and the Internal Medicine Center to Advance Research and Education. Washington, D.C., June 8-9, 1990, pp. 100-106.

Schroeder, S. Strategies for Reducing Medical Costs by Changing Physicians' Behavior: Efficacy and Impact on Quality of Care. *International Journal of Technology Assessment in Health Care* 3:39-50, 1987.

Schulman, S. Clinical Practice Guidelines and Malpractice Law: An Evolving Standard of Care. *Food Drug Cosmetic Law Journal* 46:97-106, 1991.

Silberman, C.E. From the Patient's Bed. *HMQ [Health Management Quarterly]* 13(2):12-15, 1991.

Simmons, J. C. Developing Medical Practice Guidelines: IMCARE's Workshop. Special Report. *The Internist* 31(7):14-16, 1990.

Sipress, A. Cigarettes, Other Habits, Can Cost Someone a Job: Concerned About the Price of Health Insurance, Companies Seek to Control Employee Behavior. *Washington Post Health,* April 30, 1991, p. 7.

Siu, A., and Mittman, B. Implementing the Findings from Effectiveness and Outcomes Research. Paper prepared for the Conference to Develop a Research Agenda for Outcomes and Effectiveness Research, conducted by the Foundation for Health Services Research and Alpha Center, Arlington, Virginia, April 14-16, 1991.

Smith, G. Maine's Liability Demonstration Project—Relating Liability to Practice Parameters. In: AMA *State Health Legislation Report,* Winter 1990, pp. 1-5.

Solomon, D.H., Brook, R.H., Fink, A., et al. *Indications for Selected Medical and Surgical Procedures: A Literature Review and Ratings of Appropriateness. Cholecystectomy.* R-3204/3-CWF/HF/HCFA/PMT/RWJ. Santa Monica, Calif.: The RAND Corporation, 1986.

Sommer, A., Weiner, J., and Gamble, L. Developing Specialtywide Standards of Practice: The Experience of Ophthalmology. *Quality Review Bulletin* 16:65-70, 1990.

Soumerai, S.B., and Avorn, J. Principles of Education Outreach ("Academic Detailing") to Improve Clinical Decision Making. *Journal of the American Medical Association* 263:549-556, 1990.

Sox, Jr., H.C., ed. *Common Diagnostic Tests: Use and Interpretation.* Philadelphia, Pa.: American College of Physicians, 1987; 2d ed., 1990.

Spilker, B., ed. *Quality of Life Assessments in Clinical Trials.* New York, N.Y.: Raven Press, 1990.

Stocker, M. Quality Assurance in an IPA. *HMO Practice* 3(5):1883-1887, 1989.

Tarlov, A.R., Ware, Jr., J.E., Greenfield, S., et al. The Medical Outcomes Study. *Journal of the American Medical Association* 262:925-930, 1989.

Terry, P. A Dangerous Innovation. *HealthAction Managers,* February 25, 1991, pp. 1, 8-9.

Thacker, S.B. Meta-Analysis: A Quantitative Approach to Research Integration. *Journal of the American Medical Association* 259:1685-1689, 1988.

Thompson, R.S., Tapling, S., Carter, A.P., et al. A Risk Based Breast Cancer Screening Program. *HMO Practice* 2:177-191, September-October 1988.

Tierney, W., Miller, M., and McDonald, C. Informing Physicians of Test Charges Reduces Outpatient Test Ordering. *New England Journal of Medicine* 322:1499-1504, 1990.

U.S. House of Representatives, Committee on Ways and Means. *Medical Malpractice.* Washington, D.C.: U.S. Government Printing Office, 1990.

USPSTF (U.S. Preventive Services Task Force). *Guide to Clinical Preventive Services: An Assessment of the Effectiveness of 169 Interventions.* Baltimore, Md.: Williams & Wilkins, 1989.

Utilization Review Newsletter. PROs Develop Uniform Surgical Criteria. April 26, 1991a, p. 3.

Utilization Review Newsletter. Quality Management Programs Get Only 1% of Most Hospital Budgets. October 3, 1991b, p. 1.

Veatch, R. Should Basic Care Get Priority? Doubts About Rationing the Oregon Way. *Kennedy Institute of Ethics Journal* 1:188-206, 1991.

Walton, M. *The Deming Management Method.* New York, N.Y.: Dodd, Mead & Company, 1986.

Weinstein, M., and Stason, B. Foundations of Cost-effectiveness Analysis for Health and Medical Practices. *New England Journal of Medicine* 296:716-721, 1977.

Weinstein, M., Read, J., MacKay, D., et al. Cost-Effective Choice of Antimicrobial Therapy for Serious Infections. *Journal of General Internal Medicine* 1:351-363, 1986.

Welch, H.G., Meehan, K., and Goodnough, L. Prudent Strategies for Elective

Red Blood Cell Transfusion. Draft background paper for the American College of Physicians Clinical Efficacy Assessment Project, Philadelphia, Pa., September 1, 1991.

Wenger, N., Mattson, M., Furberg, C., and Elinson, J., eds. *Assessment of Quality of Life in Clinical Trials of Cardiovascular Therapies.* New York: LeJacq Publishing Inc., 1984.

Wennberg, J. Dealing with Medical Practice Variations: A Proposal for Action. *Health Affairs* 3:6-32, 1984.

Wennberg, J. What is Outcomes Research? In: Institute of Medicine, *Medical Innovation at the Crossroads.* Vol. 1, *Modern Methods of Clinical Investigation.* A. Gelijns, ed. Washington, D.C.: National Academy Press, 1990.

Wennberg, J. Unwanted Variations in the Rules of Practice. *Journal of the American Medical Association* 265:1306, 1991.

Wennberg, J., and Gittelsohn, A. Small Area Variations in Health Care Delivery. *Science* 142:1102-1108, 1973.

Wennberg, J., and Gittelsohn, A. Variations in Medical Care Among Small Areas. *Scientific American* 246:120-134, 1982.

Wennberg, J., Mulley, A., Hanley, D., et al. An Assessment of Prostatectomy for Benign Urinary Tract Obstruction. *Journal of the American Medical Association* 259:3027-3030, 1988.

Wennberg, J., Roos, N., Sola, L., et al. Use of Claims Data Systems to Evaluate Health Care Outcomes. Mortality and Reoperation Following Prostatectomy. *Journal of the American Medical Association* 257:933-936, 1987.

White, L., and Ball, J. Special Article: Integrating Practice Guidelines with Financial Incentives. *Quality Review Bulletin* 16:50-53, 1990.

Williamson, J. Medical Quality Management Systems in Perspective. In: *Health Care Quality Management for the 21st Century.* J. Couch, ed. Tampa, Fla.: American College of Physician Executives, 1991.

Winslow, C.M., Solomon, D.H., Chassin M.R., et al. The Appropriateness of Carotid Endarterectomy. *New England Journal of Medicine* 318:721-727, 1988a.

Winslow, C.M., Kosecoff, J., Chassin, M.R., et al. The Appropriateness of Performing Coronary Artery Bypass Surgery. *Journal of the American Medical Association* 260:505-509, 1988b.

Winslow, C.M. The Role of Guidelines in Achieving Rational Health Care Management. *The Internist* 31:14-16, 1990.

Woolf, S. *Interim Manual for Clinical Practice Guideline Development: A Protocol for Expert Panels Convened by the Office of the Forum for Quality and Effectiveness in Health Care.* Internal document, Agency for Health Care Policy and Research, October, 1990a.

Woolf, S. Practice Guidelines: A New Reality in Medicine. *Archives of Internal Medicine* 150:1811-1818, 1990b.

Woolf, S. Practice Guidelines (To the Editor). *Journal of the American Medical Association* 263:3021, 1990c.

Wortman, P., and Vinokur, A. *Evaluation of the National Institutes of Health Consensus Development Process, Phase I: Final Report.* Ann Arbor, Mich.: Institute for Social Research, University of Michigan, 1982.

Wortman, P., Vinokur, A., and Sechrest, L. Do Consensus Conferences Work? A Process Evaluation of the NIH Consensus Development Program. *Journal of Health Politics, Policy and Law* 13:469-498, 1988.

Young, L. Utilization Review and Control Mechanisms: From the Blue Shield Perspective. *Inquiry* 2:5-15, 1965.

APPENDIXES

A

Examples of Clinical Practice Guidelines and Related Materials[1]

This appendix, which is a collection of clinical practice guidelines and related materials,[2] has three main purposes. First, for readers not familiar with guidelines, it presents samples that may make the text of this report more concrete. Second, it illustrates how guidelines can differ. Third, the appendix discusses the topic of formatting, which is in some ways a step between development and implementation.

Apart from the sponsoring agency or organization, guidelines can vary (as noted in Chapter 1) in at least five key ways:

- **Clinical orientation**—whether the chief focus is a clinical condition, a technology (broadly defined), or a process.
- **Clinical purpose**—whether they advise about screening and prevention, evaluation or diagnosis, aspects of treatment, or other dimensions, or more discrete aspects of health care.
- **Complexity**—whether the guidelines are relatively straightforward in presentation and discussion or are marked by considerable detail, complicated logic, or lengthy narrative and documentation. For purposes of the descriptions in this appendix, complexity is indicated simply as high, medium, or low.

---

[1] This appendix was compiled chiefly by Holly Dawkins, the IOM research assistant for this study.

[2] For purposes of simplification, the term guideline is used quite broadly, and it encompasses materials that do not fit neatly into IOM's definition of practice guidelines.

243

• **Format**—whether the guidelines are formatted as free text, tables, if-then statements, critical pathways, decision paths, or algorithms.
• **Intended users**—whether they are intended for practitioners, patients, or others.

The next section of this appendix discusses the ways guidelines may be formatted. The rest of the appendix presents, in whole or in part, 16 guidelines and related items (see Table A-1). Each example is preceded by an annotation indicating the principal information for the five variables just noted. In addition, a brief introduction highlights especially salient points about the item in terms of purpose, content, or presentation. These notes should in no way be considered a complete analysis or evaluation of the item in the example. At the end of each write-up is the complete reference or citation to the guideline.

Inclusion in this appendix does *not* imply endorsement of the content of these guidelines or of the process by which they were developed. Some of these materials are not, for example, the products of a systematic develop-

TABLE A-1   List of Examples, by Main Purpose

Screening and Prevention
  1. Screening for diminished visual acuity in children
  2. Vaccination for pregnant women who are planning international travel

Diagnosis and Pre-Diagnosis Management of Patients
  3. Triage of the injured patient
  4. Evaluating chest pain in the emergency room
  5. Using erythrocyte sedimentation rate tests in diagnosis

Indications for Use of Surgical Procedures
  6. Indications for carotid endarterectomy
  7. Indications for percutaneous transluminal coronary angiography
  8. Managing labor and delivery after previous cesarean section

Appropriate Use of Specific Technologies and Tests as Part of Clinical Care
  9. Using autologous or donor blood for transfusions
 10. Detecting or tracking deteriorating metabolic acidosis

Guidelines for Care of Clinical Conditions
 11. Using oral contraceptives to prevent pregnancy and manage fertility
 12. Deciding on treatment for low back pain
 13. Managing patients following coronary artery bypass graft
 14. Guidelines for the management of patients with psoriasis
 15. Acute dysuria in the adult female
 16. Management of acute pain

ment process. Others may result from such a procedure but do not include references to the scientific literature used in development.

FORMATTING GUIDELINES

Formatting is a step beyond the development of a guideline. It can be executed in many ways and at many stages in the process of moving guidelines from development to application. Congress, for instance, recognized the importance of formatting by requiring the Agency for Health Care Policy and Research (AHCPR) to present its guidelines in formats that are appropriate for use by practitioners, medical educators, and medical care reviewers.

Many formatting activities of most relevance to the persuasive and effective presentation of guidelines may occur *after* the initial formatting and dissemination of a set of guidelines by its sponsor or developer. For example, a professional society may initially present its guidelines in one format in a journal but then rework them into another format for use in continuing medical education. The initial guidelines may also be converted by target users—hospitals, clinics, utilization review firms, health maintenance organizations, patient groups, and others—into formats ranging from a sophisticated computer-based algorithm to a simple chart that the patient can put on the refrigerator door or bathroom mirror. Voluntary associations such as the American Cancer Society and American Heart Association, as well as commercial firms, may reformat guidelines in various ways for dissemination to different groups.

Guidelines can vary quite dramatically, both logically and graphically, in their modes of presentation. The major approaches are free-text and formalized presentations, including if-then statements, algorithms, flowcharts, and decision trees. More recently, some clinical researchers and medical informatics experts are moving to more complex computer-based approaches. These approaches are discussed briefly below.

Free Text

The most common format for guidelines is free text; this report, for example, is presented in free text. Generally, free text is the starting point for most other formats and itself has many variants.

Shortened free-text versions of guidelines documents can be tailored for specific uses by specific types of practitioners. For instance, guidelines for the diagnosis and management of acute myocardial infarction might well be rendered into several different versions and formats depending on whether the target audience was to be emergency room physicians needing quick reference or cardiac specialists managing a patient over several weeks.

Narrative information may be collapsed into tables or graphs or summarized in highly technical terms with liberal use of acronyms, abbreviations, or symbols.[3]

To cite one example of a series of formatting steps, the U.S. Preventive Services Task Force took its guidelines to a commercial publisher, which created and copyrighted the graphic design and produced the guidelines for general publication. In addition to the basic text, that publication includes eight small, plasticized pull-out charts summarizing screening, counseling, and immunization schedules for different patient age groups. These tables include abbreviated references to nonroutine situations for which physicians may consider deviations from the schedules.

Guidelines can also be rendered into much simpler, less technical documents for use by patients, consumers, and their families. Although the free-text approach is likely to be preserved, some use may be made of lay terms (including colloquialisms), simple drawings, and such heuristic devices as introductory questions. One would expect such versions of guidelines to differ, depending on the target audience.

Formalized Presentations

Apart from translations into shorter, simpler, nontechnical versions, which may still be in a free-text format, guidelines documents may be formatted into stylized graphic representations such as flowcharts or decision trees. These, in turn, may become programs for computer-based clinical decision-making tools.

One reason for translating free text into other formats is that some guidelines identify dozens, if not hundreds, of specific criteria for care; even creative free-text presentations may not allow practical, quick access to this volume of information. Instead, the free text may be reconfigured (or, less often, the initial guidelines may be drafted) using various related or overlapping formal approaches including flowcharts, decision tables, and if-then rules.

---

[3] Guidelines may be translated from English into other languages to reach users, particularly patients and families, who do not use standard English comfortably. For instance, AHCPR plans a Spanish language translation, for at least the consumer versions, of certain of its guidelines. Guidelines may also diffuse internationally. Translation of guidelines into other languages may pose both technical and cultural difficulties because some terms and concepts may not have counterparts in other languages. For example, discussions of patient preferences and informed consent reflect policy and ethical concepts that are not equally salient across nations (see Miller, 1987). Not surprisingly, given the confusion over terminology in this country, it is also not immediately obvious how best to translate the term guidelines into other languages.

Algorithms

Typically, a preliminary step in the development of many such formats is the development of a clinical algorithm. Algorithms were invented in the ninth century by a Persian mathematician, Al-khaforizmi, to solve arithmetic problems. They were first applied to practical problem solving by the U.S. Army in job-training manuals, and they have been fundamental to the programming of electronic computers. More specifically in the health field, algorithms have been used since at least the 1960s to aid clinical problem solving (Gottlieb, 1990).

Strictly speaking, an algorithm is not a graphic representation but rather a presentation of information for decisionmaking using step-by-step conditional logic rather than ordinary prose or lists of factors to be considered. This distinction is frequently ignored.

The clinical algorithm, even when not used as the format of choice for disseminating guidelines, may be used to compare guidelines and to identify missing or conflicting decision "branches." In developing methods for analyzing and comparing guidelines, Margolis et al. (1991) have identified categories of logical error in guideline construction and have described the complexity of different guidelines in quantitative terms. Applying such a process could lead to the significant reworking of a set of guidelines, not just a repackaging or interpretation of the same content.

Constructing algorithms and translating them into flowsheets and other tools can be a powerful learning process for practitioners. The process can (1) highlight differences in practice patterns and values that may need to be explored, (2) clarify key characteristics and weaknesses of processes of care, (3) identify gaps in clinical knowledge, and (4) contribute to redesign of systems of care.

Free-text versions of guidelines or review criteria usually precede the development of algorithms and similar formats, but one exception is worth noting. The Health Standards and Quality Bureau of the Health Care Financing Administration (HCFA) is developing quality-of-care and appropriateness algorithms for collecting and analyzing clinical data in its Uniform Clinical Data Set (UCDS; Krakauer, 1990; Krakauer and Bailey, 1991). The agency believes that the application of these computer-based algorithms will be a major tool for quality review for the Medicare peer review organizations (PROs), improving on the manual review of hospital charts by PRO nurse reviewers.

The UCDS development process began in the late 1980s with more than 3,000 complex software algorithms for direct collection of data and identification of hospital admissions that did not meet certain admission or quality-of-care criteria. However, little documentation of the programming or clinical logic was performed. Consequently, the procedures and rules against which practitioners and hospitals may be judged to have provided poor or unnecessary care cannot be easily explained to clinicians or institutions. HCFA has sponsored some work to prepare free-text versions of the fraction of these algorithms that can generate "flags" about potential quality-of-care deficiencies.

Flowcharts and Similar Formats

Graphic representations of algorithms are of various kinds. They include flowcharts, decision tables (sometimes used to indicate appropriate health screening), protocol charts (e.g., for handling medical problems by telephone), and so-called influence diagrams (a decision clarification tool imported from the business world and now being adapted to medicine).

As used to assist clinical problem solving, flowcharts (which are commonly called algorithms) begin with a clinical condition or patient symptom and lead the reader through a series of branching, dichotomous choices based on the patient's risk status, medical history, or clinical findings. They also include action steps such as testing, treating, or scheduling further examinations. This appendix presents two flowcharts, one for patients (Example 12 on the treatment of low back pain) and one for practitioners (Example 15 on the treatment of dysuria). In clinical practice, flowcharts may help practitioners choose from among alternative actions the most efficient sequence (as in a diagnostic workup); they may also aid in reducing the likelihood of overlooking uncommon but important elements of care for specific patients.

The basic elements of flowcharts include boxes and arrows; the latter connect the boxes or direct the user to other parts of the algorithm. The boxes may be numbered and have internal text, and they may come in several shapes, depending on whether they describe a clinical state, ask a question (diagnostic assessment), or describe an action to be taken. Prose may be used to annotate the boxes. Experts recommend that flowcharts read from left to right and top to bottom and that only two arrows exit from a given box, corresponding to a yes or no response to the clinical question posed. (Further rules for creating flowcharts and algorithms are proposed below.)

Practitioners differ widely in their attitude toward flowcharts, decision trees, and other shorthand, visual formats for guidelines. Some see them as helpful reminders and a useful tool for assimilating or quickly locating information. Others are emphatic in their dislike of these formats, maintaining that the sequences do not represent the experienced clinician's mental processes or that the necessary complexity makes them impractical to use during care of a patient. Alternatively, they may argue that simplified formats do not adequately account for all the factors present in patient care.

Some practitioners are concerned that algorithms make patient care appear cut and dried and that they will become a series of rules to be applied, with mindless rigidity, by those without clinical expertise. As can happen with any format, some physicians may view any guidelines for familiar clinical conditions as insults that imply that without such a guideline they would not know what care to provide.

Proposed Standards

As noted, the clinical algorithm map, a type of practice guideline, has received increased attention in recent years and appears more frequently in various medical journals. However, format, style, graphics, and uses vary widely, posing an obstacle to widespread use and dissemination. To overcome this difficulty, Margolis, Gottlieb, and their associates (Margolis et al., 1991) advanced some suggestions for standardization of algorithms, which are briefly presented here. The proposals involve use of boxes, including clinical state boxes, decision boxes, action boxes, and link boxes; arrows; a numbering scheme; pagination; abbreviations; and various aspects of annotations.

TITLE

The title should define the clinical topic and intended users. Under it, the authors, their degrees, and institutional affiliations should be listed. The date of publication and revision (if applicable) should be specified. A footnote to the title should state the process by which the algorithm logic was decided; this might be, for instance, group consensus after literature review, individual recommendation based on clinical experience, or some other technique.

BOXES

Clinical state box—rounded rectangle or elliptical box. This box defines the clinical state or problem. It has only one exit path and may or may not have an entry path. This box always appears at the beginning of an algorithm. The initial clinical state box should describe the clinical problem to be addressed. Clinical state boxes in the body of the algorithm are used to clarify the status of the patient or diagnosis along the path of the algorithm (i.e., to describe a subset of patients with a particular clinical condition).

Decision box—hexagon. This box requires a branching decision, whose response will lead to one of two alternative paths. It always has an entry path and two exit paths. Statements in decision boxes should be phrased as questions punctuated with question marks. If two assessments are to be determined, then the developers should specify whether both ("and") or one ("or") must be positive for a "yes" response. Multiple questions can be asked in one box, and criteria are specified for a "yes" response to the entire box—for instance, whether two of three criteria must be present, whether all must be present, or whether any must be present.

Action box—rectangle. This box indicates an action, commonly either therapeutic or diagnostic. Several rules are suggested for action boxes, as follows: A single phrase within a box should not be punctuated with a period. Multiple actions that do not need to be sequenced in time may be listed in one box. When multiple actions are presented in one box, each action is to be listed on a separate line (preceded with an optional number, dash, or bullet). When two statements are to be joined by "and" or "or," the conjunction should be placed on a separate line for emphasis.

Link box—small oval. This box is used in place of an arrow, to link boxes for graphic clarity. This might be useful at page breaks or between separated nodes to maintain path continuity. The box itself should read "Go to Page . . . Box . . . ."

ARROWS

Several rules for arrows have also been advanced. The flow should be from top to bottom. In general, the flow should be from left to right, except when a side branch rejoins the main stem. Arrows should never intersect. Link boxes (see above) can be used to avoid crossing paths. Arrows originating from decision boxes should be labelled "yes" or "no." No other text should be used over an arrow. Wherever possible (i.e., where clinical content will not be obscured), "yes" arrows should point to the right, and "no" arrows should point down.

NUMBERING SCHEME

Clinical state boxes, decision boxes, and action boxes should be numbered sequentially from left to right and from top to bottom. Link boxes are *not* numbered.

PAGING

Whenever possible, it is advisable to consolidate the algorithm so that it can be presented on one page. Page breaks are inserted where clinical logic indicates, and a single box should not be isolated on a page. For complex algorithms, the first page could best serve as a directory to clinical subsets of patients. In this case, each subset is identified as a clinical state box.

ANNOTATIONS

Citation of the annotation. Annotations are an intrinsic part of the algorithm. They are used to clarify the rationale of the decisions, cite the supporting literature, and expand on less essential details of the clinical information contained in the box. Annotations would be cited following a single phrase using a capital letter at the end of the phrase. When multiple statements are contained in a single box, annotation(s) should appear at the end of the phrase(s) to which it is applicable. If an annotation is applicable to the entire box with multiple statements, then it should be cited using a capital letter centered on a separate line at the bottom of the box.

Annotation format. Annotations should be written in text format and should appear on pages that are separate from the algorithm. They should be referenced according to standard medical reference format, with references numbered using superscripts within the text.

ABBREVIATIONS

Except for units of measurement, abbreviations are discouraged.

Computer-based Formats

Some clinical researchers argue that clinical flowcharts are inefficient representations of algorithms because they are limited by yes/no branch points to arbitrary sequences and thus cannot accommodate the richer choices common to medicine. They have been looking for ways to avoid flowcharts and to move toward a "meta-language" by using a standard syntax to convert algorithms to different kinds of computer-based decision aids. The Arden Syntax, developed in medical centers with private-sector support, is an effort to create such a system (McDonald et al., 1991; Megargle, 1991).

Using this syntax, a well-defined algorithm can be transformed into various kinds of computer programming statements such as if-then statements or for-loop statements. Use of the Arden Syntax allows easy transfer of understandable contraindication alerts, management suggestions, data interpretations, treatment protocols, and similar aids from one computer system to another. Example 10, on detecting deteriorating metabolic acidosis, and Example 11, on the use of oral contraceptives, illustrate specific computer-based formats.

The rest of the appendix presents 16 examples of guidelines and related materials. A range of topics, formats, sponsors and users, clinical orientations and purposes, and levels of complexity are presented and discussed; cross-comparisons within the appendix are noted. As stated above, these discussions should not be taken as complete analyses of the items in question, nor should inclusion in this appendix be taken as endorsement of the content or development process of these guidelines.

Example 1

SCREENING FOR DIMINISHED VISUAL ACUITY

Clinical orientation: Clinical condition
Clinical purpose: Screening and prevention
Complexity: Medium
Format: Free text and a stand-alone reference chart
Intended users: Practitioners, perhaps patients

In 1989, the U.S. Preventive Services Task Force (USPSTF) published a 419-page document intended mainly for primary care providers. The task force's objective was to develop comprehensive recommendations addressing preventive services for all age groups for 60 target conditions, using a systematic process and explicit criteria to review evidence and develop recommendations. The work of the task force was discussed extensively in Chapter 2 and elsewhere in the report.

This particular guideline is presented, in the USPSTF book, as part of a larger course of preventive care. It is one of 169 guidelines for specific preventive interventions, each of which may include recommendations for preventive care by age group (e.g., in favor of vision screening for children of younger ages and possibly for the elderly but not for adolescents and adults). Reproduced here are (1) the specific recommendations for vision screening and (2) the plasticized reference card for preventive care of children ages 2-6, which recommends vision screening.

In its concern with reliability of a particular test, this guideline is similar to the one on erythrocyte sedimentation rate tests (Example 5). As is true of several items in the appendix, this guideline cites the literature on which it is based. Educated patients might also make use of this guideline, as they could for the guidelines on, for instance, deciding what to do about low back pain or managing labor and delivery after a previous cesarean delivery (see Examples 12 and 8, respectively).

SOURCE: Reprinted (public domain) from: U.S. Preventive Services Task Force. *Guide to Clinical Preventive Services: An Assessment of the Effectiveness of 169 Interventions.* Baltimore, Md.: Williams & Wilkins, 1989.

Screening for Diminished Visual Acuity

Recommendation: Vision screening is recommended for all children once before entering school, preferably at age 3 or 4 (see *Clinical Intervention*). Routine vision testing is not recommended as a component of the periodic health examination of asymptomatic schoolchildren. Clinicians should be alert for signs of ocular misalignment when examining all infants and children. Vision screening of adolescents and adults is not recommended, but it may be appropriate in the elderly. Screening for glaucoma is discussed in Chapter 32.

Burden of Suffering

About 2–5% of American children suffer from amblyopia ("lazy eye") and strabismus (ocular misalignment), and nearly 20% have simple refractive errors by age 16.[1-4] Amblyopia and strabismus usually develop between infancy and ages 5–7.[3] Since normal vision from birth is necessary for proper eye development, failure to treat amblyopia and strabismus before school age may later result in irreversible visual deficits, permanent amblyopia, loss of depth perception and binocularity, cosmetic defects, and educational and occupational restrictions.[1,4,5] In contrast, refractive errors such as myopia become common during school age but rarely carry serious prognostic implications.[1,3,6,7] Experts disagree on whether uncorrected refractive errors cause diminished academic performance among schoolchildren.[1,3,5,7,8]

The majority of vision disorders occur in adults; over 8.5 million Americans suffer from visual impairment.[9] Visual disorders such as presbyopia (decreased ability to focus on near objects) become more common with age,[10] and therefore the prevalence of visual impairment is highest in those over age 65. Preliminary statistics from recent surveys suggest that nearly 13% of Americans age 65 and older have some form of visual impairment, and almost 8% of this age group suffer from severe impairment: blindness in both eyes or inability to read newsprint even with glasses.[11] Vision disorders in the elderly may be associated with injuries due to falls and motor vehicle accidents, diminished productivity, and loss of independence.[12] Many older adults are unaware of changes in their visual acuity, and up to 25% of them may be using an incorrect lens prescription.[12]

Efficacy of Screening Tests

Although screening for strabismus and amblyopia is most critical at an early age, screening tests to detect occult vision disorders in children under age 3 have generally been unsuccessful due to the child's inability to cooperate, the time required for testing, and the inaccuracy of the tests.[13-15] Promising techniques such as alternate stimulation (cover testing), preferential-looking, grating acuity cards, and refractive screening are currently being developed for this age group.[14,16,17] Although refractive errors detected during infancy can predict some cases of amblyopia and strabismus, the sensitivity of this form of screening is quite poor.[2]

Screening tests for detecting strabismus and amblyopia in preschool children over age 3 include simple inspection, visual acuity tests, and stereograms. Visual acuity tests include the Snellen eye chart, the Landolt C, the tumbling E, the Sheridan-Gardner STYCAR test, Allen picture cards, grating cards, and other techniques.[15] The specificity of most acuity tests, however, is imperfect for detecting strabismus and amblyopia because diminished visual acuity can occur in other conditions, such as simple refractive error or visual immaturity.[2] In addition, many children with nonamblyopic strabismus often have normal visual acuity but are at risk for serious complications.[2,18] Thus, although simple acuity tests are inexpensive and easy to administer, they may miss many cases. Snellen letters, for example, are estimated to have a sensitivity of only 25–37%.[2,18,19] Refractive screening has also been criticized as not being a direct test for either amblyopia or strabismus.[2]

Stereograms such as the Random Dot E (RDE) have been proposed as more effective than visual acuity tests in detecting strabismus and amblyopia in preschool children.[2,18,20,21] The test, in which the patient views test cards through Polaroid glasses, requires about one minute to perform.[18,20] When compared with a battery of visual tests, the RDE has an estimated sensitivity of 64%, specificity of 90%, positive predictive value of 57%, and negative predictive value of 93%.[18]

A more effective but less efficient strategy is the combination of more than one visual test.[2,19] The Modified Clinical Technique (MCT), for example, includes retinoscopy, cover and Hirschberg tests, the Snellen acuity test, a color vision test, and external observation of the eye. The MCT has gained acceptance among optometrists since its introduction in the Orinda Study of 1959.[18,22-24] Sensitivity and specificity in excess of 90% were found in that study and have since been reproduced in screening programs involving as many as 50,000 children.[18] The MCT cannot be used routinely by primary care physicians for screening purposes, however, because it requires about 12 minutes to perform and the examiner must be a skilled eye care specialist.[18,23]

Vision screening of older children and adults is a means of detecting unrecognized refractive errors. Tests of visual acuity are often used for this purpose, but few studies have examined the sensitivity, specificity, and predictive value of these tests in adult age groups.

Effectiveness of Early Detection

There is convincing evidence that early detection and treatment of vision disorders in infants and young children improve the prognosis for normal eye development.[21] A prospective study has demonstrated that preschool children who receive visual acuity screening have significantly less visual impairment than controls when reexamined 6–12 months later.[25] Detection and treatment of strabismus and amblyopia by age 1–2 can increase the likelihood of developing normal or near-normal binocular vision and may improve fine motor skills.[2,4] Interventions for amblyopia and strabismus are significantly less effective if started after age 5, and such a delay increases the risk of irreversible amblyopia, ocular misalignment, and other visual deficits.[1,3] It is widely held that clinical screening tests can detect these disorders earlier than parents or teachers; only about 50% of children with ocular misalignment have a cosmetically noticeable defect.[2,8]

There is little evidence that bilaterally equal refractive errors among older children and adolescents are associated with significant morbidity, such as diminished academic performance.[1,3,6,7] This is true in young adults as well, and, in addition, uncorrected vision disorders are quite uncommon among young adults.[26] Vision screening for older adults is defended on the grounds that the prevalence of abnormal visual acuity is considerably greater among the elderly[10] and these deficits are more commonly left uncorrected.[26] Among persons aged 65–74, a visual acuity of 20/50 or less has been measured in 11% of those who wear glasses and in 26% of those who do not.[26] Some forms of visual impairment in the elderly are associated with difficulties in ambulation,[27] and early correction of refractive errors may serve a role in preventing injuries and facilitating the performance of daily living functions. However, there have been no prospective studies documenting these benefits in an elderly cohort receiving vision screening.

Recommendations of Others

The American Academy of Ophthalmology recommends an ophthalmological examination of newborns who are premature or at risk for eye disease; an examination of fixation preference and ocular alignment by age 6 months; an examination of visual acuity, ocular alignment, and ocular disease at age 3–4; annual screening of schoolchildren for visual acuity and ocular alignment; occasional examinations from puberty to age 40; and an examination for presbyopia at age 40 and every two to five years thereafter.[1] The American Academy of Pediatrics recommends external examination and tests of following ability and the pupillary light reflex in the newborn period and once during the first six months.[5] Testing of visual acuity, ocular alignment, and ocular disease is recommended by the Academy at ages 4, 5–6, and at less frequent intervals thereafter.[5] The Canadian Task Force recommends an eye examination and cover test at ages 1 week, 2 months, and, along with a vision chart test, at age 2–3 years and 5–6 years. Testing at age 10–11 is considered discretionary, and no adult screening is recommended.[28] The American Optometric Association recommends screening schoolchildren every three years and annual eye examinations in adults after age 35.[29] Screening guidelines have also been issued by other organizations, such as the National Society to Prevent Blindness, the National Association of Vision Program Consultants, Volunteers for Vision, and the American Public Health Association.[2,8] Vision screening of preschool and school children is also required by law in some states and in a number of Federal programs.[2,22]

Discussion

Although it is established that early detection of strabismus and amblyopia is most beneficial for children under age 3, a practical and effective screening test is not yet available for this age group. Clinicians should, of course, be alert to signs of ocular misalignment when examining infants and young children. Screening tests for preschool children are available but, with the exception of a comprehensive battery (e.g., the MCT), most tests for amblyopia and strabismus lack the sensitivity, specificity, and predictive value that are expected of good screening tests. Of these, the Random Dot E stereogram appears to have the best performance and is recommended by many experts.[2,21] Due to the high rate of false-negative results with this test, however, it would need to be repeated throughout the preschool period to achieve optimal effectiveness.

Screening of schoolchildren by primary care clinicians is not recommended because the procedure is usually performed by the public school system, and there is little scientific evidence that early detection of myopia is of greater benefit than detection when symptoms first become apparent. Similarly, there is no basis for screening asymptomatic adolescents or adults below age 40 who lack specific risk factors for vision disorders. With increasing age, there is a stronger argument for the early detection of uncorrected visual impairment to help prevent injury and improve independent living. The performance characteristics of acuity tests at this age are poorly described, and the claimed benefits of screening have not been proved. Repeated acuity testing can, however, improve sensitivity with presumably little cost or inconvenience to the patient. There are no available data for any age group on the optimal interval for vision screening; recommended frequencies are selected arbitrarily on the basis of expert opinion.

Clinical Intervention

Testing for amblyopia and strabismus is recommended for all children once before entering school, preferably at age 3 or 4. Stereotesting (e.g., Random Dot E stereogram) is more effective than visual acuity testing (e.g., Snellen optotype cards) in detecting these conditions. Routine screening for refractive errors is not recommended as a component of the periodic health examination of asymptomatic schoolchildren. Clinicians should be alert for signs of ocular misalignment when examining all infants and children. Vision screening of asymptomatic adolescents and adults is not recommended. It may be appropriate in the elderly, but there is insufficient evidence to recommend an optimal interval. All patients with abnormal test results should be referred to an eye specialist for further evaluation. Screening for glaucoma is discussed in Chapter 32.

REFERENCES

1. American Academy of Ophthalmology. Infants and children's eye care. Statement by the American Academy of Ophthalmology to the Select Panel for the Promotion of Child Health, Department of Health and Human Services. San Francisco, Calif.: American Academy of Ophthalmology, 1980.
2. Ehrlich MI, Reinecke RD, Simons K. Preschool vision screening for amblyopia and strabismus: programs, methods, guidelines, 1983. Surv Ophthalmol 1983; 28:145–63.
3. Cross AW. Health screening in schools. Part I. J Pediatr 1985; 107:487–94.
4. Sanke RF. Amblyopia. Am Fam Physician 1988; 37:275–8.
5. American Academy of Pediatrics. Vision screening and eye examination in children. Committee on Practice and Ambulatory Medicine. Pediatrics 1986; 77:918–9.
6. Rosner J, Rosner J. Comparison of visual characteristics in children with and without learning difficulties. Am J Optom Physiol Opt 1987; 64:531–3.
7. Helveston EM, Weber JC, Miller K, et al. Visual function and academic performance. Am J Ophthalmol 1985; 99:346–55.
8. APHA resolution number 8203: children's vision screening. Am J Public Health 1983; 73:329.
9. National Center for Health Statistics. Prevalence of selected chronic conditions, United States, 1979–81. Vital and Health Statistics, series 10, no. 155. Washington, D.C.: Government Printing Office, 1986. (Publication no. DHHS (PHS) 86–1583.)
10. Idem. Monocular visual acuity of persons 4–74 years, United States, 1971–1972. Vital and Health Statistics, series 11, no. 201G. Washington, D.C.: National Center for Health Statistics, 1977:60. (Publication no. DHEW (HRA) 77–1646.)

11. Nelson KA. Visual impairment among elderly Americans: statistics in transition. J Vis Impair Blind 1987; 81:331–4.
12. Stults BM. Preventive health care for the elderly. West J Med 1984; 141:832–45.
13. Hall SM, Pugh AG, Hall DMB. Vision screening in the under-5s. Br Med J 1982; 285: 1096–8.
14. Jenkins PL, Simon JW, Kandel GL, et al. A simple grating visual acuity test for impaired children. Am J Ophthalmol 1985; 99:652–8.
15. Fern KD, Manny RE. Visual acuity of the preschool child: a review. Am J Optom Physiol Opt 1986; 63:319–45.
16. Jacobson SG, Mohindra I, Held R. Visual acuity of infants with ocular diseases. Am J Ophthalmol 1982; 93:198–209.
17. Brown AM, Yamamoto M. Visual acuity in newborn and preterm infants measured with grating acuity cards. Am J Ophthalmol 1986; 102:245–53.
18. Hammond RS, Schmidt PP. A Random Dot E stereogram for the vision screening of children. Arch Ophthalmol 1986; 104:54–60.
19. Lieberman S, Cohen AH, Stolzberg M, et al. Validation study of the New York State Optometric Association (NYSOA) vision screening battery. Am J Optom Physiol Opt 1985; 62:165–8.
20. Simons K. A comparison of the Frisby, Random-Dot E, TNO, and Randot Circles stereotests in screening and office use. Arch Ophthalmol 1981; 99:446–52.
21. Reinecke RD. Screening 3–year-olds for visual problems: are we gaining or falling behind? Arch Ophthalmol 1986; 104:33.
22. Nussenblatt H. Symposium on optometry's obligation in vision screening. Opening remarks. Am J Optom Physiol Opt 1984; 61:357–8.
23. Peters HB. The Orinda Study. Am J Optom Physiol Opt 1984; 61:361–3.
24. Woodruff ME. Vision and refractive status among grade 1 children of the province of New Brunswick. Am J Optom Physiol Opt 1986; 63:545–52.
25. Feldman W, Milner R, Sackett B, et al. Effects of preschool screening for vision and hearing on prevalence of vision and hearing problems 6–12 months later. Lancet 1980; 2:1014–6.
26. National Center for Health Statistics. Refraction status and motility defects of persons 4–74 years, United States, 1971–1972. Vital and Health Statistics, series 11, no. 206. Washington, D.C.: National Center for Health Statistics, 1978: 89–93. (Publication no. DHEW (PHS) 78–1654.)
27. *Idem*. Aging in the eighties, impaired senses for sound and light in persons age 65 and over. Advance Data from Vital and Health Statistics, no. 125. Hyattsville, Md.: National Center for Health Statistics, 1986:4–5. (Publication no. DHHS (PHS) 86–1250.)
28. Canadian Task Force on the Periodic Health Examination. The periodic health examination. Can Med Assoc J 1979; 121:1194–254.
29. Miller SC, American Optometric Association. Personal communication, October 1988.

Table 2.

Ages 2–6

Schedule: See Footnote*

Leading Causes of Death:
Injuries (nonmotor vehicle)
Motor vehicle crashes
Congenital anomalies
Homicide
Heart disease

SCREENING	PATIENT & PARENT COUNSELING	IMMUNIZATIONS & CHEMOPROPHYLAXIS

Height and weight
Blood pressure
Eye exam for amblyopia and strabismus[1]
Urinalysis for bacteriuria
HIGH-RISK GROUPS
  Erythrocyte protoporphyrin[2] (HR1)
  Tuberculin skin test (PPD) (HR2)
  Hearing[3] (HR3)
	Diet and Exercise
	Sweets and between-meal snacks, iron-enriched foods, sodium
	Caloric balance
	Selection of exercise program
	
	Injury Prevention
	Safety belts
	Smoke detector
	Hot water heater temperature
	Window guards and pool fence
	Bicycle safety helmets
	Storage of drugs, toxic chemicals, matches, and firearms
	Syrup of ipecac, poison control telephone number
	
	Dental Health
	Tooth brushing and dental visits
		Diphtheria-tetanus-pertussis (DTP) vaccine[4]
		Oral poliovirus vaccine (OPV)[4]
		HIGH-RISK GROUPS
		  Fluoride supplements (HR5)

This list of preventive services is not exhaustive. It reflects only those topics reviewed by the U.S. Preventive Services Task Force. Clinicians may wish to add other preventive services on a routine basis, and after considering the patient's medical history and other individual circumstances. Examples of target conditions not specifically examined by the Task Force include:
  Developmental disorders
  Speech problems
  Behavioral and learning disorders
  Parent/family dysfunction
	Other Primary Preventive Measures
	Effects of passive smoking
	HIGH-RISK GROUPS
	  Skin protection from ultraviolet light (HR4)	

		Remain Alert For: Vision disorders Dental decay, malalignment, premature loss of teeth, mouth breathing Signs of child abuse or neglect Abnormal bereavement

*One visit is required for immunizations. Because of lack of data and differing patient risk profiles, the scheduling of additional visits and the frequency of the individual preventive services listed in this table are left to clinical discretion (except as indicated in other footnotes).

1. Ages 3–4. 2. Annually. 3. Before age 3, if not tested earlier. 4. Once between ages 4 and 6.

Table 2. Ages 2–6   High-Risk Categories

HR1   Children who live in or frequently visit housing built before 1950 that is dilapidated or undergoing renovation; who come in contact with other children with known lead toxicity; who live near lead processing plants or whose parents or household members work in a lead-related occupation; or who live near busy highways or hazardous waste sites.

HR2   Household members of persons with tuberculosis or others at risk for close contact with the disease; recent immigrants or refugees from countries in which tuberculosis is common (e.g., Asia, Africa, Central and South America, Pacific Islands); family members of migrant workers; residents of homeless shelters; or persons with certain underlying medical disorders.

HR3   Children with a family history of childhood hearing impairment or a personal history of congenital perinatal infection with herpes, syphilis, rubella, cytomegalovirus, or toxoplasmosis; malformations involving the head or neck (e.g., dysmorphic and syndromal abnormalities, cleft palate, abnormal pinna); birthweight below 1500 g; bacterial meningitis; hyperbilirubinemia requiring exchange transfusion; or severe perinatal asphyxia (Apgar scores of 0–3, absence of spontaneous respirations for 10 minutes, or hypotonia at 2 hours of age).

HR4   Children with increased exposure to sunlight.

HR5   Children living in areas with inadequate water fluoridation (less than 0.7 parts per million).

Example 2

VACCINATION FOR PREGNANT WOMEN

Clinical orientation:	Clinical states (protection against certain disorders, in the context of pregnancy, an existing clinical condition); use of a technology (vaccination guidelines)
Clinical purpose:	Prevention, in the context of managing a clinical condition
Complexity:	Low
Format:	Free text; summary tables; maps (excerpts included)
Intended users:	Practitioners, perhaps patients

This is an example of guideline development by a federal agency—here the Centers for Disease Control (CDC) of the U.S. Public Health Service (PHS)—as a direct product of its mandate. Example 1 on screening vision also came from a PHS agency and Example 9 on blood transfusions is the product of a state mandate. Chapter 2 discusses more fully the development of various guidelines at CDC and other federal agencies. Although aimed at clinicians, this guideline could be used by well-informed patients and consumers.

Of interest is the inclusion in the guideline of maps indicating areas in the world that are probably infected with specific diseases. An example concerning yellow fever in the Americas is included here. Since yellow fever vaccination is contraindicated except in cases of likely exposure, this map provides additional information for pregnant women to consider as they contemplate travel outside the United States. This guideline is the only one in the appendix to categorize levels of care according to "socio-geographic" considerations (i.e., level of health, common health perils, or socioeconomic level of a particular locale)—a reflection of its concern with providing advice for international travel and with controlling the entry of infectious diseases into the United States.

Finally, this guideline was also included because it has two very different orientations: it can be seen as a guideline for a broadly defined technology (immunization) that includes information for the care of quite specific patients, or as a guideline combining two clinical states (pregnancy and potential exposure to disease) and providing recommendations on the intersecting territory.

SOURCE: Reprinted (public domain) from: Centers for Disease Control. *Health Information for International Travel, 1990.* Washington, D.C.: U.S. Government Printing Office, 1990.

VACCINATION DURING PREGNANCY

On the grounds of a theoretical risk to the developing fetus, live, attenuated-virus vaccines are not generally given to pregnant women or to those likely to become pregnant within the next 3 months after receiving vaccine(s). With some of these vaccines—particularly rubella, measles, and mumps—pregnancy is a contraindication. Both yellow fever vaccine and OPV can be given to pregnant women at substantial risk of exposure to natural infection. When a vaccine is to be given during pregnancy, waiting until the second or third trimester is a reasonable precaution to minimize any concern over teratogenicity. Although there are theoretical risks, there has been no evidence of congenital rubella syndrome in infants born to susceptible mothers who inadvertently received rubella vaccine during pregnancy.

Since persons given measles, mumps, or rubella vaccine viruses do not transmit them (although virus shedding does occur), these vaccines can be administered safely to children of pregnant women. Although live polio virus is shed by persons recently immunized with OPV (particularly following the first dose), this vaccine also can be administered to children of pregnant women. Polio immunization of children should not be delayed because of pregnancy in close adult contacts. Experience to date has not revealed any risks of polio vaccine virus to the fetus.

There is no convincing evidence of risk to the fetus from immunization of pregnant women using inactivated viral or bacterial vaccines, or toxoids. A previously unimmunized pregnant woman who may deliver her child under unhygienic circumstances or surroundings should receive two properly spaced doses of Td before delivery preferably during the last two trimesters. Incompletely immunized pregnant women should complete the three-dose series. Those immunized more than 10 years previously should have a booster dose.

There is no known risk to the fetus from passive immunization of pregnant women with IG (see above).

TABLE 5. Vaccination during pregnancy

	Vaccine	Indications for vaccination during pregnancy
Live virus vaccines		
Measles Mumps Rubella	Live-attenuated	Contraindicated.
Yellow fever	Live-attenuated	Contraindicated except if exposure is unavoidable.
Poliomyelitis	Trivalent live-attenuated (OPV)	Persons at substantial risk of exposure may receive live-attenuated virus vaccine.
Inactivated virus vaccines		
Hepatitis B	Plasma derived or recombinant produced, purified hepatitis B surface antigen	Pregnancy is not a contraindication.
Influenza	Inactivated type A and type B virus vaccines	Usually recommended only for patients with serious underlying disease. It is prudent to avoid vaccination during the first trimester. Consult health authorities for current recommendations.
Poliomyelitis	Killed virus (IPV)	OPV not IPV, is indicated when immediate protection of pregnant females is needed.
Rabies	Killed virus Rabies IG	Substantial risk of exposure.
Inactivated bacterial vaccines		
Cholera Typhoid	Killed bacterial	Should reflect actual risks of disease and probable benefits of vaccine.
Plague	Killed bacterial	Selective vaccination of exposed persons.
Meningococcal	Polysaccharide	Only in unusual outbreak situations.
Pneumococcal	Polysaccharide	Only for high-risk persons.
Toxoids		
Tetanus-diphtheria (Td)	Combined tetanus-diphtheria toxoids, adult formulation	Lack of primary series, or no booster within past 10 years. It is prudent to avoid vaccination during first trimester.
Immune globulins, pooled or hyperimmune	Immune globulin or specific globulin preparations	Exposure or anticipated unavoidable exposure to measles, hepatitis A, hepatitis B, rabies, or tetanus.

YELLOW FEVER ENDEMIC ZONES

IN THE AMERICAS

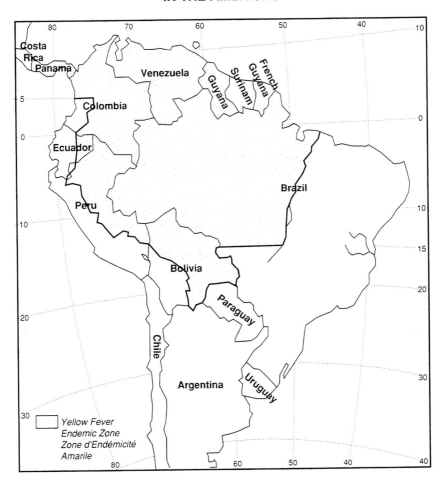

NOTE: Although the "yellow fever endemic zones" are no longer included in the International Health Regulations, a number of countries (most of them being not bound by the Regulations or bound with reservations) consider these zones as infected areas and require an International Certificate of Vaccination against Yellow Fever from travelers arriving from those areas. The above map based on information from WHO is therefore included in this publication for practical reasons.

In addition to areas shaded, CDC recommends vaccination for entire state of Mato Grasso in Brazil.

Example 3

TRIAGE OF THE INJURED PATIENT

Clinical orientation: Clinical conditions
Clinical purpose: Evaluation and management
Complexity: Medium
Format: Triage decision chart, free text, and trauma scoring
                              table (Chapter 3 is provided as an excerpt)
Intended users: Practitioners and prehospital care personnel

This item is actually a chapter from a longer document that is concerned with optimal care of the injured patient. It was produced by the American College of Surgeons' Committee on Trauma. The excerpt deals with field triage (essentially the decision of whether to move an injured patient to a trauma center or to evaluate and manage the patient at a local hospital) and with calculation of a well-known, widely used trauma score (which can be the first step in the triage decision as well as a factor in deciding on interhospital transfers).

This guideline was chosen for several reasons. First, the formatting facilitates quick evaluation of a patient and timely decisionmaking—critical elements for the circumstances in which the guideline would be used. Second, the report also explicitly notes that it "replaces similar documents published in 1976, 1979, 1983, and 1986/87. It is generally recognized that this document is a set of guidelines representing current thinking for optimal care of the injured patient. Further revisions will be published at timely intervals as new information becomes available" (p. 1). In keeping with the emphasis on providing up-to-date information, the book arrives with a sheet of emendations on self-sticking label paper and directions for placing them in the report.

Third, the guideline addresses a broad category of clinical conditions—those that result from injury. The full report focuses on reducing preventable deaths, and it notes the need to balance surgical education and the provision of optimal care. The text also offers discussion of such issues as: systems development; treatment protocols; specific subspecialties of trauma care such as musculoskeletal, pediatric, or eye care; and issues more closely related to policy than to clinical care such as quality assurance concerns, geographically disparate resources, populations, and personnel, and cost-effectiveness considerations. As an example of the last (policy) category, see the discussion in the excerpted free text (p. 18) of acceptable levels of undertriage and overtriage and the relationship between the two—the stated assumption being that in minimizing undertriage (i.e., minimizing the provision of inadequate care to injured patients), some level of overtriage (and therefore overuse of resources) may be inevitable.

SOURCE: American College of Surgeons, Committee on Trauma. *Resources for Optimal Care of the Injured Patient.* Chicago, Ill.: American College of Surgeons, 1990. Used with permission.

CHAPTER 3

FIELD CATEGORIZATION OF TRAUMA PATIENTS (FIELD TRIAGE)

Triage is the classification of patients according to medical need. There are three applications of this process in the early management of the trauma patient: 1) field triage; 2) interhospital triage to specialized care facilities; and 3) mass casualty triage.

Trauma patients who, because of injury severity, require care at Level I or Level II trauma centers, constitute a fraction of all patients hospitalized each year for trauma. In 1983, approximately 3.75 million patients were hospitalized for injury. In the same year, a study revealed 450 patients per million had an Injury Severity Score (ISS) of 15 or more, accounting for only 5.7 percent of all patients who were discharged from the hospital. Only 8.9 percent of the patients had severities greater than ISS 10, which incorporates just one serious body injury. Even with high over-triage rates, it is unlikely that the number of patients entering trauma centers will exceed 1,000 per million per year.

It is a substantial challenge for field personnel to identify that small proportion of patients who require prompt access to trauma centers. Furthermore, time is critical. Of the trauma victims who are going to die, 50 to 60 percent do so before reaching a hospital. Of the remaining who die in-hospital, about 60 percent do so within the first four hours.

The following factors must be considered in field triage: 1) the actual or potential level of severity of the injured patient; 2) medical control; and 3) the regional resources available to treat the patient, including time and distance.

ASSESSMENT OF PATIENT SEVERITY

For the purpose of field triage, assessment of patient severity is based on examination of the patient for 1) abnormal physiologic signs; 2) obvious anatomic injury; 3) mechanism of injury; and 4) concurrent disease.

A triage decision scheme based on current scientific knowledge is illustrated in Table 1.

MEDICAL CONTROL

The triage decision determines the level and intensity of initial management of the major or multiple trauma patient. The vast majority of trauma deaths occur within a few hours of injury. The triage decision is often germane to patient survival or death. It is for this reason that the highest available level of medical expertise should be brought into the triage decision-making process. Usually this process will involve advice and guidance from physicians who provide medical control to prehospital personnel. On-line physician medical control is vitally important in emergency medical systems for the trauma patient.

Surgeons, emergency physicians, and prehospital-care personnel should work together to develop prehospital triage protocols for trauma patients. In most instances of triage based on potentially severe injuries, the patient is unable to make an informed decision in selecting appropriate hospital care. The "system" is often responsible for this decision. The system must, therefore, make surrogate decisions. In no instance may these decisions prejudice patient outcome. Disposition decisions at the scene must hold the patient's interests and needs paramount.

RANGE OF RESOURCES; TIME AND DISTANCE FACTORS

Both the level of available hospital resource and time/distance factors also are considered in making the triage decision. It must be recognized that Level I through III trauma facilities are stratifications in a continuum of capability of commitment to trauma patient care. The system for trauma triage in an urban environment is considerably different from that in a rural environment. In the latter case access to any level of trauma care may involve a significant distance and time.

TABLE 1

TRIAGE DECISION SCHEME

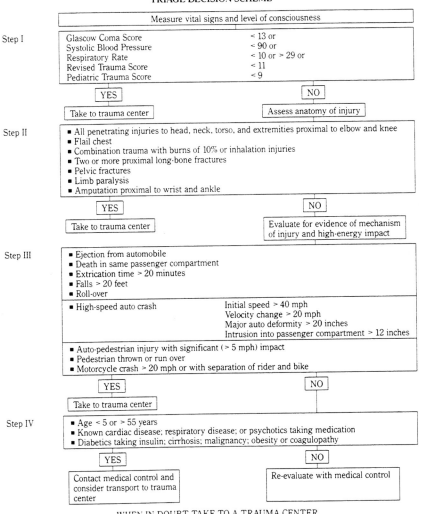

Measure vital signs and level of consciousness	

Step I

Glascow Coma Score	< 13 or
Systolic Blood Pressure	< 90 or
Respiratory Rate	< 10 or > 29 or
Revised Trauma Score	< 11
Pediatric Trauma Score	< 9

YES — Take to trauma center   NO — Assess anatomy of injury

Step II

- All penetrating injuries to head, neck, torso, and extremities proximal to elbow and knee
- Flail chest
- Combination trauma with burns of 10% or inhalation injuries
- Two or more proximal long-bone fractures
- Pelvic fractures
- Limb paralysis
- Amputation proximal to wrist and ankle

YES — Take to trauma center   NO — Evaluate for evidence of mechanism of injury and high-energy impact

Step III

- Ejection from automobile
- Death in same passenger compartment
- Extrication time > 20 minutes
- Falls > 20 feet
- Roll-over

- High-speed auto crash   Initial speed > 40 mph
Velocity change > 20 mph
Major auto deformity > 20 inches
Intrusion into passenger compartment > 12 inches

- Auto-pedestrian injury with significant (> 5 mph) impact
- Pedestrian thrown or run over
- Motorcycle crash > 20 mph or with separation of rider and bike

YES — Take to trauma center   NO

Step IV

- Age < 5 or > 55 years
- Known cardiac disease; respiratory disease; or psychotics taking medication
- Diabetics taking insulin; cirrhosis; malignancy; obesity or coagulopathy

YES — Contact medical control and consider transport to trauma center   NO — Re-evaluate with medical control

WHEN IN DOUBT TAKE TO A TRAUMA CENTER

Each region must, therefore, structure a trauma system in a manner that ensures the prompt access to appropriate care and minimizes the risk of delay in diagnosis, delay in surgical intervention, and inadequately focused care, which are responsible for most of the preventable deaths that occur.

URBAN TRIAGE

In most urban communities in the United States, prompt access to a Level I or Level II trauma center should be feasible within 30 minutes of activation of the EMS system. Many urban populations have more than reasonable access to sophisticated care because of the distribution of tertiary care hospitals that function as Level I trauma centers. Other hospitals that do not offer this level of care or commitment should be bypassed in favor of access to a trauma center.

RURAL TRIAGE

In the rural environment, an injured patient may be at substantial distances from a trauma center. Such patients should be initially treated at a Rural Trauma Hospital. In more remote rural areas, where Level III facilities are not available, staff should at least be trained in ATLS. Patients with major severe injuries should then be secondarily triaged to Level I or II trauma centers, should local resources prove inadequate for continued care (see chapter 15).

Just as the Level II trauma center provides the highest level of care available within most communities across the country, the importance of the Level III trauma facility cannot be overemphasized. Between rural and urban environments, there are geographic areas with increasing distances between hospitals and decreasing population density. Some patients may require initial triage and resuscitation at a Level III Rural Trauma Hospital. This action may be preferred to primary patient transport from the scene to an urban tertiary care referral center. The EMS system should be structured to provide the patient timely access to the best available level of care indicated by the extent and nature of injuries received.

NOTES TO TABLE 1

Step I Physiologic status thresholds are values of the Glascow Coma Score, blood pressure, and respiratory rate from which further deviations from normal are associated with less than a 90 percent probability of survival. Used in this manner, prehospital values can be included in the admission trauma score and the quality assessment process.

A variety of physiologic severity scores have been used for prehospital triage and have been found to be accurate. The scores contained in the triage guidelines, however, are believed to be the simplest to perform, and provide an accurate basis for field triage based on physiologic abnormality.

Step II Even in the presence of normal physiology, it is important to evaluate the likely presence of injuries that should be treated in a trauma center. A patient who has normal vital signs at the scene of the accident may still have a serious or lethal injury. Accurate diagnosis of life-threatening injury at the accident scene is unlikely. Thus, it is essential to look for indications that significant forces were applied to the body.

Evidence of damage to the automobile can be a helpful guideline to the change in velocity ('V). A 'V of 20 mph will produce an ISS of greater than 15 in 90 percent of automobile crash occupants. 'V can be estimated if one inch of vehicular deformity is equated to approximate one mph of 'V.

Step III Certain other factors that might lower the threshold at which patients should be treated in trauma centers must be considered in field triage. These include the following:

A. Age Patients over age 55 have an increased risk of death from even moderately severe injuries. Patients younger than age 5 have certain characteristics that may merit treatment in a trauma center with special resources for children.

B. Co-morbid Factors The presence of significant cardiac, respiratory, or metabolic diseases are additional factors that may merit the triage of patients with moderately severe head injury to trauma centers.

Step IV It is the general intention of these triage guidelines to select patients with an ISS of greater than 15 for trauma center care. Patients with this level of ISS have at least a 10 percent risk of dying from a single severe or multiple serious injuries. When there is doubt, the patient is often best evaluated in a trauma center.

CONTINUING EDUCATION AND EVALUATION

Because of acknowledged imperfections of current field triage and the importance of this process in the delivery of trauma patient care, it is essential to involve surgeons in the continuing education of prehospital care personnel, as well as in feedback to those personnel on the accuracy of their patient triage decisions. Undoubtedly, as decision rules are reviewed, and the results are reported back to the prehospital care personnel, the process of triage will improve.

OVER-TRIAGE AND UNDER-TRIAGE

A system has yet to be developed that reliably and correctly selects the patients for appropriate levels of care that might be available in a given region. As a result, there will always be a certain number of patients selected for trauma center care who could very adequately be handled at a community hospital (85 to 90 percent of all injured patients do not need trauma center care). These patients are referred to as over-triaged. Conversely, patients who are in need of trauma center care but fail to gain timely access to such care are referred to as under-triaged. Together, over-triaged and under-triaged patients combine to form a misclassification rate for any triage decision scheme or rule.

Over-triage and under-triage are interdependent. Considerable medical effort should be made to minimize the number of patients who are under-triaged in a trauma system, because these patients are at risk of dying. Lives may be saved or cost of care may be reduced by prompt access to the needed level of definitive care. There is also concern about the over-triage of patients; over-triage can produce overuse of trauma centers and may divert patients away from community hospitals.

Not all patients with apparent minor injuries can clearly be grouped as not needing trauma center evaluation. For example, a patient who suffers high-deceleration injuries is found to have a wide mediastinum on X-ray film in a rural emergency department. Because of the risk of a ruptured aorta, the standard of care would dictate that such a patient be promptly evaluated in a trauma center where an arteriogram and necessary surgical care were immediately available. A large number of patients who undergo X-ray studies for a wide superior mediastinum after trauma will not have a ruptured aorta. These patients might eventually exhibit only minimal injuries. They could represent an over-triage on trauma system statistics, yet the medical prudence of transferring such a patient group for trauma center evaluation could not be argued.

Studies have shown that a 35 to 50 percent over-triage may be required to maintain a minimum level of under-triage in a community. It also has been estimated that because of the small number of patients who really need to be in trauma centers, the impact of patient flow on an individual institution will be minimal, should this degree of over-triage exist. Clearly, the surgical community needs to be more concerned about under-triage and the medical consequences that result from inadequate use of a trauma system.

Example 4

EVALUATION OF CHEST PAIN IN THE EMERGENCY ROOM

Clinical orientation:	Clinical condition (symptom state)
Clinical purpose:	Diagnosis
Complexity:	Medium
Format:	Free text, tables, and algorithm (excerpts provided)
Intended users:	Emergency room physicians and other physicians; patients and families

In 1984, the Massachusetts chapter of the American College of Emergency Physicians (MACEP) developed a set of guidelines focused on continuous monitoring of patient care in high-risk clinical areas as a part of the Massachusetts Emergency Medicine Risk Management Program. The guideline reproduced here is part of this large-scale effort (which includes medical record auditing, data analysis, and feedback) to obtain a malpractice discount for emergency room physicians insured by the state's Joint Underwriters Association. The guidelines, which are developed by consensus, are published as one-page summaries with commentary and/or references from the literature and as individual algorithms. The algorithms are meant to indicate the critical actions that physicians in the emergency room should document for the high-risk diagnostic problem covered by the algorithm.

The excerpt given here is for the assessment of chest pain in the diagnosis of (possible) ischemic heart disease (see the guideline's "Appendix A. MI/Unstable Angina/New Onset Angina"). It indicates what the physician should take account of and document; it is basically intended to "alert the emergency physician to think of ischemic chest pain in the adult patient in terms of ischemic equivalents in addition to pain itself" (p. 289). It also includes an instruction sheet for those patients for whom ischemic disease has presumptively been ruled out and who are therefore being discharged (the "Chest Pain Instruction Sheet" of the guideline's Appendix A). Finally, a separate portion of the guideline gives the algorithm related to this particular guideline (the guideline's "Appendix B. Chest Pain Algorithm").

SOURCE: Karcz, A., and Holbrook, J. The Massachusetts Emergency Medicine Risk Management Program. *QRB (Quality Review Bulletin)* 17:267-292. 1991. Used with permission.

Chest Pain Algorithm

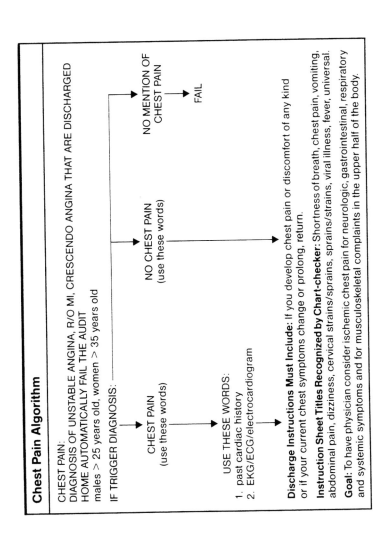

CHEST PAIN:
DIAGNOSIS OF UNSTABLE ANGINA, R/O MI, CRESCENDO ANGINA THAT ARE DISCHARGED HOME AUTOMATICALLY FAIL THE AUDIT
males > 25 years old, women > 35 years old

IF TRIGGER DIAGNOSIS:

CHEST PAIN
(use these words)

USE THESE WORDS:
1. past cardiac history
2. EKG/ECG/electrocardiogram

NO CHEST PAIN
(use these words)

NO MENTION OF
CHEST PAIN

FAIL

Discharge Instructions Must Include: If you develop chest pain or discomfort of any kind or if your current chest symptoms change or prolong, return.

Instruction Sheet Titles Recognized by Chart-checker: Shortness of breath, chest pain, vomiting, abdominal pain, dizziness, cervical strains/sprains, sprains/strains, viral illness, fever, universal.

Goal: To have physician consider ischemic chest pain for neurologic, gastrointestinal, respiratory and systemic symptoms and for musculoskeletal complaints in the upper half of the body.

MI/Unstable Angina/New Onset Angina

History:
Pain in chest, jaw, upper abdomen (indigestion), arms
Quality: burning, crushing, tight, pleuritic, sharp
Radiation: left/right arm, jaw, back
OR neurologic, respiratory, gastrointestinal symptoms without pain.

Associated symptoms: SOB, nausea, diaphoresis, syncope, vomiting

Risk factors: smoking, ASVD, hypertension, family history, obesity, diabetes, cocaine use, cardiac history

Physical examination:
Chest wall abnormalities/tenderness
Lungs: rubs, adventitial sounds
Cardiac: rubs, clicks, murmurs

EKG: Helpful if abnormal or changed from previous EKG. All bets are off if EKG normal.

Defend your diagnosis: Support your diagnosis from history, physical examination, associated symptoms, and risk factors.

Watch out for: pneumothorax, aortic dissection, pulmonary embolus.

If sending home: Document history, physical exam, and EKG as appropriate for discharge diagnosis. Give specific followup instructions.

Assessment of Chest Pain as the Presentation of Ischemic Heart Disease

It needs to be stated from the outset that at the present state of the art, it is not possible to diagnose ischemic heart disease with 100% accuracy. The best of clinicians will miss a certain percentage of cases and will undoubtedly admit many cases in which acute myocardial infarction will be ruled out. Given this, perhaps the most important element relating to proper evaluation of chest pain in the Emergency Department is a thorough and thoroughly documented history, physical examination, and appropriately evaluated EKG. The decision to admit a patient should not be dependent on an abnormal electrocardiogram, since, in fact, a normal electrocardiogram does not rule out acute ischemic heart disease.

History

The history should specifically note the presence or absence of the following:
Chest pain: (or its equivalent, e.g., heartburn, indigestion, discomfort, arm or jaw pain.)
Associated symptoms: Diaphoresis, nausea, anxiety, palpitations, shortness of breath, "sense of doom," weakness.
Other symptoms without chest pain or equivalent: Syncope, shortness of breath, weakness, dizziness.
Past medical history: Known coronary artery disease (history of angina or myocardial infarction), nitroglycerin use.

It may also be useful to elicit information regarding the duration, type, location, radiation and aggravating/relieving factors relating to the pain. Risk factors (sex, age, hypertension, family history, cigarette smoking, diabetes mellitus, cholesterol) may also be elicited and recorded.

Physical Examination

Physical examination should focus on the heart, lungs, chest wall and abdomen, as well as the general appearance of the patient. The presence or absence of murmurs, rubs, extra sounds, irregularities, gallop, or rales should be noted. Probably the most important clues of acute ischemia will be found in the vital signs; the respiratory rate, heart rate and blood pressure are uncommonly all normal during acute ischemia.

The electrocardiogram should be examined carefully for signs of acute ischemia or infarction. Comparison should be made to old electrocardiograms when available.

The diagnosis should follow naturally and logically from the history and physical examination and should be consistent with the findings. A differential diagnosis and documentation of the thought process used in determining the final diagnosis is useful.

Further history, physical exam and lab may be useful in evaluating the total picture of the patient's problem, but should not be allowed to obscure the basic findings.

In the Emergency Department, ischemic heart disease is frequently a clinical diagnosis, which relies more heavily on the thoughtful judgment of the clinician than any single finding or laboratory test.

Treatment/Disposition

When it has been determined that a patient does not appear to have ischemic chest pain, nor any other significant illness requiring immediate treatment or hospitalization, appropriate discharge instructions should be given to the patient and/or the patient's family. The patient should be encouraged to follow-up with his or her physician as soon as possible.

Summary

Determination of ischemic cause for chest pain (or its equivalent), is generally a clinical judgment. The physician should have a very high index or suspicion, with a low threshold for admission in those patients with chest pain and a history suggestive of a cardiac cause (associated symptoms, risk factors, etc.). In general, the history is essential and the electrocardiogram should be viewed as only an adjunct to the clinical evaluation.

References

1. Pozen, M,W, et al., A Predictive Instrument to Improve Coronary Care Unit Admission Practices in Acute Ischemic Heart Disease. NEJM, 310;20:1273–78.
2. Zaring, et al., Failure to Diagnose Acute Myocardial Infarction, JAMA, 250;9:1177–81.
3. Selker, H.P., Sorting Out Chest Pain, Emergency Decisions, June, 85; pp. 8–17.
4. Hedges, et al., Use of Cardiac Enzymes Identifies Patients with Acute MI Otherwise Unrecognized in the Emergency Department, Ann Emerg. Med, 16;3:248–252. 1987.
5. Goldman, L., et al., A Computer-Based Protocol to Aid in the Diagnosis of Emergency Room Patients with Acute Chest Pain, NEJM, 307;10:588–96. 1983.
6. Prior, D.B., et al., Estimating the Likelihood of Significant Coronary Artery Disease, Am. J. Med., 75:771, Nov. 1983.
7. Rude, R.E., et al., Electrocardiographic and Clinical Criteria for Recognition of Acute MI Based on Analysis of 3,697 Patients, Am. J. Card., 52:936–42, 1983.
8. Hoffman, J.R., et al., Influence of EKG Findings on Admission Decisions in Patients with Acute Chest Pain, Am. J. Med., 79:699–707, 1985.

MI/Unstable Angina/New Onset Angina (continued)

Chest Pain Instruction Sheet

You have been evaluated for chest discomfort and even though you are being allowed to go home, please follow the instructions below.

Rest at home today. Take medications prescribed as instructed.

Return to the Emergency Department by ambulance:
1. If chest pains, heaviness or pressure should develop and lasts longer than several minutes.
2. If you have known Angina and your chest discomfort is worse, lasts longer, comes on with less exertion, or is not relieved by the usual amounts of Nitroglycerin.
3. If you develop any shortness of breath, sweats, vomiting or nausea with your chest discomfort.
4. If your chest discomfort seems to travel into either of your arms, neck, back, jaw or stomach or otherwise changes in nature.

Even if you feel better and have no further discomfort, you should follow up with your own doctor tomorrow.

Example 5

USING ERYTHROCYTE SEDIMENTATION RATE TESTS IN DIAGNOSIS

Clinical orientation:	Technology (diagnostic test)
Clinical purpose:	Diagnosis
Complexity:	Medium
Format:	Free text, tables, and figures (excerpts provided)
Intended users:	Practitioners

This item, which consists of excerpts from a longer piece, is taken from a landmark monograph published by the American College of Physicians, *Common Diagnostic Tests*, which was discussed in Chapter 2. As is true of the entire monograph in its original 1987 version and in the revised edition of 1990, the intent of this guideline is to clarify the appropriate use of a long-established (and perhaps overused) test.

The recommendations are organized according to different patient states or characteristics: asymptomatic persons; problems of interpretation in symptomatic patients; patients with vague, unsubstantiated illness; cancer; temporal arteritis and polymyalgia rheumatica; estimating iron stores; inflammatory arthritis; suspected infection; an extreme or unexplained increase; and monitoring disease activity. Like certain of the other items in the appendix, it specifically focuses on the questions of when the service (here a diagnostic test) is indicated and when it is not.

Apart from its clinical significance, this guideline is of interest for formatting, as it makes use of free text, graphics, and tables. As is true of several other items in the appendix, it cites directly the literature on which its conclusions and recommendations are based. Shown here are the discussion of problems of interpretation in symptomatic patients and in patients with vague, unsubstantiated illness; a figure; and a summary table.

SOURCE: Sox, H.C., Jr., and Liang, M.C. The Erythrocyte Sedimentation Rate. Guidelines for Rational Use. In H.C. Sox, Jr., ed. *Common Diagnostic Tests*. Philadelphia, Pa.: American College of Physicians, 1987; 2nd ed., 1990. (Excerpts are from pages 209–212, 214.) Used with permission.

PROBLEMS OF INTERPRETATION IN SYMPTOMATIC PATIENTS

The ESR is sometimes used to provide confirmation when the history and physical findings point toward a diagnosis. The test is also used when the patient's chief complaint is not supported by evidence for a specific disease. In this situation, the physician uses the ESR to screen for any serious disease that may be present. Clinical studies have not provided sufficient information to define the role of the test in these two applications.

To evaluate the ESR in symptomatic patients, one must ask how well it predicts disease. The probability of a disease corresponding to an ESR result may be calculated with a Bayes theorem (14). Bayes theorem requires that the pretest probability of the disease and the sensitivity and specificity of the ESR for the disease be known. Unless both sensitivity and specificity are known, a test cannot be interpreted in all situations.

The sensitivity of the ESR has been measured in many diseases, but its specificity has been measured accurately only a few times (15,16). To understand why past studies are so limited, consider the design of an ideal study. The ESR is measured in all patients suspected of having a disease. All patients, regardless of the ESR results, undergo a definitive diagnostic procedure. Some study patients have the disease and the sensitivity of the test is measured in them. The specificity of the ESR is measured in study patients who do not have the disease. In contrast to this ideal study design, the study populations in past studies have comprised only patients with a disease and have not included patients who were suspected of having the disease but did not. Because the specificity of the ESR for a disease has seldom been measured in the appropriate population, the frequency of a normal ESR in healthy persons is sometimes used as a proxy. This approach leads to error because the specificity of the ESR for a disease will be higher in healthy persons than in patients suspected of having the disease, who often have other diseases that increase the ESR. In one study, the frequency of an ESR greater than 20 mm per hour was zero in 32 normal reference subjects, 0.42 in 149 cancer-free reference subjects, and 0.62 in 68 patients with cancer (17). The frequency of an increased ESR in the cancer-free reference subjects shows the lack of specificity of an increased ESR in sick people.

The shortcomings of studies of the ESR affect only the interpretation of an abnormal ESR. As shown in Figure 1A, test specificity largely determines the probability of disease when the ESR is abnormal. Because the specificity of the ESR for most diseases is not known, the post-test probability when the ESR is abnormal cannot be calculated. When the ESR is normal, the sensitivity of the test determines the post-test probability of a disease (Figure 1B). Because the sensitivity of the ESR for many diseases is known, a normal ESR can be interpreted, even if its specificity is not known.

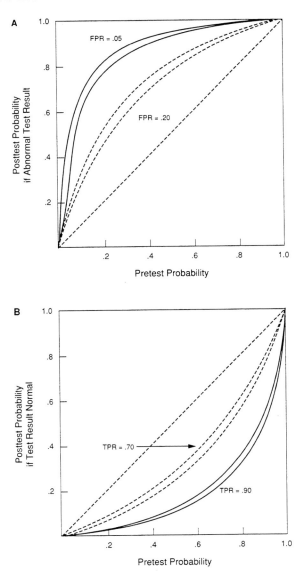

FIGURE 1.   Relation between pretest probability of disease and post-test probability. The post-test probability was calculated with Bayes theorem. **Figure 1A.** The probability of disease in a patient with an abnormal test result. Two values for the false-positive rate (*FPR*) were assumed. For each value, the sensitivity of the test was assumed to be 0.9 (*top curve*) and 0.7 (*bottom curve*). **Figure 1B.** The probability of disease for a normal (or negative) test result. Two values for the sensitivity of the test (true-positive rate, *TPR*) were assumed. For each value, the false-positive rate of the test was assumed to be 0.2 (*top curve*) and 0.05 (*bottom curve*).

PATIENTS WITH VAGUE, UNSUBSTANTIATED ILLNESS

Physicians often obtain an ESR in patients whose history and physical findings do not suggest any cause for their illness. These patients' pretest probability of serious disease is presumably very low, perhaps nearly as low as that in asymptomatic persons. Although too little is known to be certain, several considerations suggest that the ESR is generally not useful in these patients.

In principle, either a normal or an increased ESR could be diagnostically useful. In practice, neither result is very useful. A normal ESR can exclude temporal arteritis, but the test is too often normal in other diseases to be of much value in excluding serious disease. An increased ESR is a clue to unsuspected serious disease but it is seldom present in patients with vague, poorly characterized complaints. As discussed in the preceding section, too little is known to interpret an increased ESR with confidence. However, when the pretest probability of disease is low, the post-test probability will be low unless the ESR is markedly elevated. The probability of some form of serious disease is probably relatively high when the ESR exceeds 50 mm/h, because a markedly increased ESR seldom occurs in healthy people. For example, in one population survey the ESR exceeded this rate in only 4 of 1462 apparently healthy women (15). However, the probability of a markedly increased ESR is very low when the pretest probability of disease is very low (14). This reasoning is substantiated by the very low frequency of an increased ESR in persons with unsuspected disease (Table 3).

These considerations suggest that the ESR is not very useful when the patient's symptom is unsubstantiated by the other clinical data. However, clinical studies of the ESR have not been done in such patients, and a precise recommendation cannot be made at present. Many diagnosticians will choose to focus on possible psychophysiologic explanations for the symptom and allow the evolution of the symptom over time to determine the need for diagnostic testing.

Table 3. Effects of Doing the Erythrocyte Sedimentation Rate (ESR) as a Screening Procedure

Study Description (Reference)	Definition of Abnormal ESR	Patients with Increased ESR	ESR as Only Clue to Diagnosis
	mm/h	n/n (%)	n(%)
Random sample of Swedish women; 6-year follow-up (9)	>30	78/1462 (5.3)	0
Clinic patients: 10-year follow-up (10)	>30 (men) >35 (women)	790/9140 (8.6)	5* (0.06)
Male clinic patients: no follow-up (11)	>20	Not given	1† (0.05)
Surgical admissions: 6 to 42-month follow-up (12)	‡	99/6148 (6.0)	1§ (0.06)
Israeli airmen age 18-33; yearly follow-up for 15 years (13)	‖	44/1000 (4.4)	10¶ (1.0)

* Colonic cancer, pancreatic cancer, tuberculosis (in two patients) and systemic lupus erythematosus.

† Multiple myeloma.

‡ An abnormal ESR was defined as ≥ 15 mm/h for men < 50 years, ≥ 20 mm/h for women < 50, and ≥ 30 mm/h for women > 50.

§ Patient died of prostate cancer 28 months after the index visit, at which there was no evidence of cancer and the ESR was 28 mm/h.

‖ An abnormal ESR was defined as one elevated to at least 2 SD above the mean for the same age group on at least three of four consecutive annual examinations.

¶ Ankylosing spondylitis (in three patients), myocardial infarction (in four patients), inflammatory bowel disease, psoriasis, and benign gammopathy were diagnosed several years after the abnormal ESR was first noted.

Example 6

INDICATIONS FOR APPROPRIATE USE OF
CAROTID ENDARTERECTOMY

Clinical orientation: Clinical condition
Clinical purpose: Evaluation
Complexity: High
Format: Free text, tables, and diagrams (excerpts provided)
Intended users: Health sciences researchers, policy analysts, and practitioners

In the mid-1980s, the RAND Corporation developed appropriateness criteria for the use of six specific clinical procedures; indications for carotid endarterectomy were one of the six topics. The procedures were chosen for evaluation according to the following criteria: they are frequently performed, use substantial medical resources, and exhibit significant variation in rates of use across large geographic areas of the United States.

The immense array of possible indications for carotid endarterectomy (excerpts of which are shown in the example) is not, strictly speaking, a guideline; rather it is a detailed analysis and categorization of indications for use of the procedure. Thus, it is closer to being a set of medical review criteria than a tool for shared decisionmaking by physician and patient (the IOM definition of practice guidelines). Using these indicators requires translating the indications into computer algorithms, or learning to read tens of pages of charts such as those included here, or both.

Several of the examples in this appendix are products of a consensus or expert panel; in this case, the process also involved significant analytic and logistical support from the sponsoring organization. The development process included rigorous analysis of all the literature in the subject area, although individual recommendations (indications) are not tied directly to that literature. Like Example 3, on triage of injured patients, and Example 5, on the use of erythrocyte sedimentation rates, this guideline implicitly considers the cost-effectiveness of resource use. Finally, the initial definitions of clinical conditions, the literature analysis, and the process of getting data from practicing physicians are carefully and extensively documented.

SOURCE: Merrick, N.J., Fink, A., Brook, R.H., et al. *Indications for Selecting Medical and Surgical Procedures—A Literature Review and Ratings of Appropriateness: Carotid Endarterectomy.* R-3204/6-CWF/HF/PMT/RWJ. Santa Monica, Calif.: RAND, 1986. (Excerpts are from pages 48-55.) Used with permission.

RESULTS

The following is the final list of rated indications for carotid endarterectomy. Figure 3 provides a key to reading the results. Note that the first indication for carotid endarterectomy is for a patient with a single episode of carotid TIA or amaurosis fugax whose surgical risk is low and whose angiogram demonstrates an occlusion of the ipsilateral artery and less than 50 percent stenosis of the opposite artery.

This indication received a rating of 1 (extremely inappropriate) by all nine panelists; the median rating was 1.0. Because of the unanimity of the rating the dispersion was 0.0, and panelists agreed on the rating.

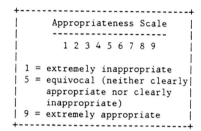

Clinical Presentation:

I. Carotid TIA and/or Amaurosis Fugax--Single episode

APPROPRIATENESS OF
OPERATING IPSILATERALLY
IF ANGIOGRAPHY SHOWS:

	Low Surgical Risk	Elevated Surgical Risk	High Surgical Risk

Ipsi: Degree of
stenosis of
ipsilateral artery

Contra: Degree of
stenosis of contra-
lateral artery

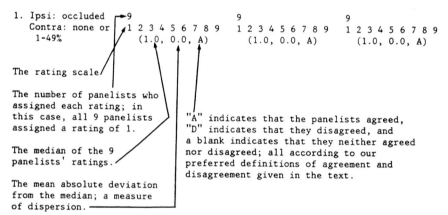

1. Ipsi: occluded   9   9   9
   Contra: none or   1 2 3 4 5 6 7 8 9   1 2 3 4 5 6 7 8 9   1 2 3 4 5 6 7 8 9
   1-49%   (1.0, 0.0, A)   (1.0, 0.0, A)   (1.0, 0.0, A)

The rating scale

The number of panelists who
assigned each rating; in
this case, all 9 panelists
assigned a rating of 1.

The median of the 9
panelists' ratings.

The mean absolute deviation
from the median; a measure
of dispersion.

"A" indicates that the panelists agreed,
"D" indicates that they disagreed, and
a blank indicates that they neither agreed
nor disagreed; all according to our
preferred definitions of agreement and
disagreement given in the text.

Fig. 3—A key to reading the final results of appropriateness ratings
for each indication for carotid endarectomy

INDICATIONS AND RATINGS

DEFINITIONS USED BY THE PANELISTS AT THE TIME THEY RATED THE INDICATIONS FOR CAROTID ENDARTERECTOMY

1. *Carotid Transient Ischemic Attack and/or Amaurosis Fugax—Single Episode*: The patient's symptoms are consistent with hemispheric ischemia, the TIA episode occurred within the past three months, and the symptoms resolved within 24 hours of onset. The patient may or may not have been placed on medical therapy.

2. *Carotid TIAs and/or Amaurosis Fugax—Multiple Episodes, Never Tried on Medical Therapy*: The patient's symptoms are consistent with hemispheric ischemia, the most recent TIA episode occurred within the past three months, the symptoms resolved within 24 hours of onset, and the symptoms are different from those grouped separately as "crescendo TIAs." The patient has never been placed on platelet inhibitors or anticoagulation for cerebrovascular symptoms in the past.

3. *Carotid TIAs and/or Amaurosis Faugax—Multiple Episodes, At Least One Recurrence Since Initiation of Medical Therapy*: As above, the symptoms are consistent with hemispheric ischemia, the most recent TIA occurred within the past three months, the symptoms resolved within 24 hours and are different from "crescendo TIAs." The patient had at least one TIA subsequent to the initiation of treatment with platelet inhibitors or anticoagulation.

4. *Carotid TIAs and/or Amaurosis Fugax—Multiple Episodes, No Recurrence Since Initiation of Medical Therapy*: The symptoms are the same as those in #2. The patient has been without TIA recurrence while on platelet inhibitors or anticoagulation.

5. *Vertebrobasilar TIAs*: The patient has suffered symptoms that are not consistent with hemispheric ischemia, but that are consistent with a TIA episode; the most recent TIA episode occurred within the past one year; the symptoms resolved within 24 hours of onset; and the symptoms are different from those grouped separately as "crescendo TIAs." We group patients who have experienced only a single TIA episode with those who have experienced more than one. This category excludes isolated, nonspecific symptoms of dizziness or confusion.

6. *Post-Atherothrombotic Stroke*: The patient has suffered an atherothrombotic stroke at least three weeks previously. We assume that the patient has not suffered an incapacitating or profound neurologic deficit, but rather is a functional adult living within the community; the patient's symptoms are not consistent with the separately described category "stroke in evolution," and neurologic symptoms have fully stabilized.

7. *Stroke in evolution*: We used Goldstone and Moore's[1] definition: Stroke in evolution is an acute neurological deficit of modest degree that may, within hours or days of the initial event, progress in a sequential series of acute exacerbations to a major stroke. Alternatively, after the initial episode, the neurological deficit may improve temporarily, only to reappear later, often with more widespread involvement, leading to a pattern of waxing and waning of signs and symptoms that occurs over hours to days with an incomplete recovery.

8. *Crescendo TIAs*: We used Goldstone and Moore's[2] definition: Crescendo TIAs are those attacks abruptly increasing in frequency to at least more than one per day.

9. *Ipsilateral artery (ipsi)*: The artery on the same side as the cerebral hemisphere with symptoms.

   Contralateral (contra) artery: The artery on the side opposite the symptomatic cerebral hemisphere.

   Example: For a patient whose TIA has resulted in a weakness in the right leg, a left-sided TIA, ipsi = left and contra = right.

10. *Vessel diameter*: The degree of stenosis of both carotid arteries is specified as none or 0%, 1–49%, 50–99%, or 70–99% reduction in luminal diameter.

11. *Ulceration categories*: Multicentric refers to a large ulceration having multiple cavities or more than one ulcer in a plaque or possessing a cavernous appearance on angiography.

12. *Asymptomatic*: We include all asymptomatic patients here (other than those undergoing other surgery) whether screening was on the basis of a carotid bruit, other peripheral vascular disease, or a contralateral carotid lesion. We also include here patients with vague symptoms (such as dizziness) not meeting the previous definitions of TIAs.

13. *Asymptomatic, Patient to Undergo Other Surgery*: Patients undergoing carotid endarterectomy prophylactically before other surgery. Separate ratings were made for two subgroups: intra-abdominal or intra-thoracic excluding coronary artery bypass surgery, and coronary artery bypass surgery.

14. *"Dementia of Vascular Origin"*: Any patient whose primary indication for endarterectomy is "dementia" that the physician feels is amenable to surgery. "Multi-infarct dementia" is included here.

15. *Surgical Risk*: Surgical risk is classified as low, elevated, or high. Our classifications come from an index developed by Goldman, Caldera, Nussbaum et al.[3] and the Dripps-American Surgical Association Classification.[4] The first groups patients according to their scores on the following variables:

---

[1] J. Goldstone and W. S. Moore, "A New Look at Emergency Carotid Artery Operations for the Treatment of Cerebrovascular Insufficiency," *Stroke*, 1978; 9:599–602.

[2] Ibid.

[3] L. Goldman, D. L. Caldera, S. R. Nussbaum, et al., "Cardiac Risk Factors and Complications in Non-cardiac Surgery," *New England Journal of Medicine*, 1977; 57:357–370.

[4] R. D. Dripps, A. Lamont, J. E. Eckenhoff, "The Role of Anaesthesia in Surgical Mortality," *Journal of the American Medical Association*, 1961; 178:261–266.

Patient Characteristics	Score
Age greater than 70 years	5
Myocardial infarction in previous 6 months	10
S3 gallop or jugular venous distention	11
Significant valvular aortic stenosis	3
Rhythm other than sinus, or premature atrial contractions on last EKG	7
More than five premature ventricular contractions per minute	7
Poor general medical status[a]	3
Emergency operation	4
Intraperitoneal, intrathoracic, or aortic operation	3

[a]$PO2 < 60$, $PCO2 > 50$mm Hg, $K < 3.0$ or $HCO3 < 20$ mg/L, $BUN > 50$ or $Creatinine > 3.0$, abnormal SGOT, signs of chronic liver disease or patient bedridden from noncardiac causes.

Class I patients are those with total scores of 0–5 points; Class II, 6–12 points; Class III, 13–25 points; and Class IV, 26 points or greater. Class I is described as "low surgical risk," Class II and III as "elevated surgical risk," and Class IV as "high surgical risk."

The Dripps-American Surgical Association Classification also correlates well with surgical outcome. Patients are categorized as follows by the Dripps system:

DRIPPS I   Normal healthy person.

DRIPPS II   Person with mild systemic disease (hypertension, asthma, etc.).

DRIPPS III Person with severe systemic disease that is not incapacitating (e.g., insulin-requiring diabetes, chronic obstructive pulmonary disease without CO2 retention).

DRIPPS IV   Person with an incapacitating systemic disease that is a constant threat to life.

DRIPPS V   Person who is moribund and not expected to survive for 24 hours with or without an operation. (No such patients were apparently found in the population studied by Goldman, Caldera, Nussbaum, et al. [3]).

We considered patients in Dripps Classes I and II to represent low surgical risk; Classes III and IV, elevated; and Class V, high surgical risk.

16. *Risk of stroke is either high or normal:* High stroke risk is defined as a probability of greater than 100 per 1000 patients of developing an atherothrombotic brain infarction in eight years based on data from the Framingham Study, 18 year follow-up.[5] Calculations of probability take into account a patient's age, sex, presence of left ventricular hypertrophy, whether the patient is diabetic, a smoker, and his or her diastolic blood pressure and cholesterol level.

---

[5]D. Shurtleff, *The Framingham Study: An Epidemiological Investigation of Cardiovascular Disease*, Section 26, GPO, 1970.

CLINICAL PRESENTATION:
1. CAROTID TIA and/or AMAUROSIS FUGAX - Single Episode

	Low Surgical Risk	Elevated Surgical Risk	High Surgical Risk

APPROPRIATENESS OF
OPERATING IPSILATERALLY
IF ANGIOGRAPHY SHOWS:

Ipsi: Degree of stenosis
 of ipsilateral artery
Contra: Degree of stenosis
 of contralateral artery

1. Ipsi: Occluded
Contra: None or 1-49%

	Low	Elevated	High

	`                9`
	 `1 2 3 4 5 6 7 8 9`
	 (1.0, 0.0, A)
		`                9`
		 `1 2 3 4 5 6 7 8 9`
		 (1.0, 0.0, A)
			`                9`
			 `1 2 3 4 5 6 7 8 9`
			 (1.0, 0.0, A)

2. Ipsi: Occluded
Contra: 50-99%

	Low	Elevated	High

	`                9`
	 `1 2 3 4 5 6 7 8 9`
	 (1.0, 0.0, A)
		`                9`
		 `1 2 3 4 5 6 7 8 9`
		 (1.0, 0.0, A)
			`                9`
			 `1 2 3 4 5 6 7 8 9`
			 (1.0, 0.0, A)

3a. Ipsi: 50-69%
Contra: None, 1-49%, or 50-99%

	Low	Elevated	High

	`1         1 4   3`
	 `1 2 3 4 5 6 7 8 9`
	 (7.0, 1.3,)
		`1     2 3   2   1`
		 `1 2 3 4 5 6 7 8 9`
		 (5.0, 1.6,)
			`5     3   1`
			 `1 2 3 4 5 6 7 8 9`
			 (1.0, 1.1, A)

3b. Ipsi: 70-99%
Contra: None, 1-49%, or 50-99%

	Low	Elevated	High

	`1   1 2 5`
	 `1 2 3 4 5 6 7 8 9`
	 (9.0, 0.9, A)
		`1 2 1 2 1 2`
		 `1 2 3 4 5 6 7 8 9`
		 (7.0, 1.4,)
			`2 2 2   1       2`
			 `1 2 3 4 5 6 7 8 9`
			 (3.0, 2.0, D)

4a. Ipsi: 50-69%
Contra: Occluded

	Low	Elevated	High

	`1   1   1 3 3`
	 `1 2 3 4 5 6 7 8 9`
	 (8.0, 1.3,)
		`1   1 1 2 1 1 2`
		 `1 2 3 4 5 6 7 8 9`
		 (6.0, 1.8,)
			`2 4   1 1 1`
			 `1 2 3 4 5 6 7 8 9`
			 (2.0, 1.2,)

4b. Ipsi: 70-99%
Contra: Occluded

	Low	Elevated	High

	`1 1   1 6`
	 `1 2 3 4 5 6 7 8 9`
	 (9.0, 0.9,)
		`2   2 1 1 3`
		 `1 2 3 4 5 6 7 8 9`
		 (7.0, 1.7,)
			`1 2 1 1 2   2`
			 `1 2 3 4 5 6 7 8 9`
			 (4.0, 1.8, D)

5. Ipsi: 1-49%
Contra: None or 1-49%

	Low	Elevated	High

	`5 1 2             1`
	 `1 2 3 4 5 6 7 8 9`
	 (1.0, 1.4, A)
		`7 1               1`
		 `1 2 3 4 5 6 7 8 9`
		 (1.0, 1.0, A)
			`8   1`
			 `1 2 3 4 5 6 7 8 9`
			 (1.0, 0.2, A)

6. Ipsi: 1-49%
Contra: 50-99%

	Low	Elevated	High

	`4 1 1   1   1   1`
	 `1 2 3 4 5 6 7 8 9`
	 (2.0, 2.2, D)
		`6   2             1`
		 `1 2 3 4 5 6 7 8 9`
		 (1.0, 1.3, A)
			`7 1       1`
			 `1 2 3 4 5 6 7 8 9`
			 (1.0, 0.6, A)

7. Ipsi: 1-49%
Contra: Occluded

	Low	Elevated	High

	`4 1 1   2           1`
	 `1 2 3 4 5 6 7 8 9`
	 (2.0, 2.0,)
		`6   2             1`
		 `1 2 3 4 5 6 7 8 9`
		 (1.0, 1.3, A)
			`8           1`
			 `1 2 3 4 5 6 7 8 9`
			 (1.0, 0.4, A)

8a. Ipsi: 1-49% with large ulcerative lesion
Contra: None, 1-49% or 50-99%

	Low	Elevated	High

	`1       2 1 2 3`
	 `1 2 3 4 5 6 7 8 9`
	 (8.0, 1.4,)
		`1 1         1 5   1`
		 `1 2 3 4 5 6 7 8 9`
		 (7.0, 1.6, D)
			`4 3   1 1`
			 `1 2 3 4 5 6 7 8 9`
			 (2.0, 1.0,)

8b. Ipsi: 50-69% with large ulcerative lesion
Contra: None, 1-49% or 50-99%

	Low	Elevated	High

	`1       2 1 5`
	 `1 2 3 4 5 6 7 8 9`
	 (9.0, 1.2, A)
		`1           5 1 2`
		 `1 2 3 4 5 6 7 8 9`
		 (7.0, 1.0, A)
			`2 1   2 3 1`
			 `1 2 3 4 5 6 7 8 9`
			 (4.0, 1.4,)

9a. Ipsi: 1-49% with multicentric ulcerative lesion
Contra: None, 1-49%, or 50-99%

	Low	Elevated	High

	`1       1 1 1 5`
	 `1 2 3 4 5 6 7 8 9`
	 (9.0, 1.3,)
		`1     2   3 2 1`
		 `1 2 3 4 5 6 7 8 9`
		 (7.0, 1.4,)
			`4 1 2   2`
			 `1 2 3 4 5 6 7 8 9`
			 (2.0, 1.3,)

9b. Ipsi: 50-69% with multicentric ulcerative lesion
Contra: None, 1-49%, or 50-99%

	Low	Elevated	High

	`1   1 2 5`
	 `1 2 3 4 5 6 7 8 9`
	 (9.0, 0.9, A)
		`1       1 3 1 3`
		 `1 2 3 4 5 6 7 8 9·`
		 (7.0, 1.4,)
			`2   2 2 2   1`
			 `1 2 3 4 5 6 7 8 9`
			 (4.0, 1.4,)

10a. Ipsi: 1-49% with small ulcerative lesion
Contra: None, 1-49% or 50-99%

	Low	Elevated	High

	`5 1 1         1 1`
	 `1 2 3 4 5 6 7 8 9`
	 (1.0, 2.2, D)
		`6 1 1             1`
		 `1 2 3 4 5 6 7 8 9`
		 (1.0, 1.4,)
			`7 1 1`
			 `1 2 3 4 5 6 7 8 9`
			 (1.0, 0.6, A)

CLINICAL PRESENTATION:
1. CAROTID TIA and/or AMAUROSIS FUGAX - Single Episode

	Low Surgical Risk	Elevated Surgical Risk	High Surgical Risk
10b. Ipsi: 50-69% with small ulcerative lesion Contra: None, 1-49% or 50-99%	4 1 11 11 1 2 3 4 5 6 7 8 9 (3.0, 2.7, D)	5 1 2 1 1 2 3 4 5 6 7 8 9 (1.0, 2.3,)	6 1 2 1 2 3 4 5 6 7 8 9 (1.0, 1.1,)

APPROPRIATENESS OF
OPERATING CONTRALATERALLY
IF ANGIOGRAPHY SHOWS:

	Low Surgical Risk	Elevated Surgical Risk	High Surgical Risk
11. Ipsi: None Contra: 1-49%	9 1 2 3 4 5 6 7 8 9 (1.0, 0.0, A)	9 1 2 3 4 5 6 7 8 9 (1.0, 0.0, A)	9 1 2 3 4 5 6 7 8 9 (1.0, 0.0, A)
12a. Ipsi: None or 1-49% Contra: 50-69%	4 1 1 2 1 1 2 3 4 5 6 7 8 9 (2.0, 1.8,)	6 1 1 1 2 3 4 5 6 7 8 9 (1.0, 0.8, A)	8 1 2 3 4 5 6 7 8 9 (1.0, 0.0, A)
12b. Ipsi: None or 1-49% Contra: 70-99%	2 3 1 1 2 1 2 3 4 5 6 7 8 9 (5.0, 2.3, D)	4 1 1 2 1 1 2 3 4 5 6 7 8 9 (4.0, 2.6, D)	6 1 2 1 2 3 4 5 6 7 8 9 (1.0, 0.6, A)
13. Ipsi: None or 1-49% Contra: Occluded	9 1 2 3 4 5 6 7 8 9 (1.0, 0.0, A)	9 1 2 3 4 5 6 7 8 9 (1.0, 0.0, A)	9 1 2 3 4 5 6 7 8 9 (1.0, 0.0, A)
14. Ipsi: Occluded Contra: 1-49%	7 1 1 1 2 3 4 5 6 7 8 9 (1.0, 0.4, A)	8 1 1 2 3 4 5 6 7 8 9 (1.0, 0.1, A)	9 1 2 3 4 5 6 7 8 9 (1.0, 0.0, A)
15a. Ipsi: Occluded Contra: 50-69%	3 1 2 1 1 1 1 2 3 4 5 6 7 8 9 (5.0, 2.4, D)	3 1 2 3 1 2 3 4 5 6 7 8 9 (5.0, 1.9,)	6 1 1 1 2 3 4 5 6 7 8 9 (1.0, 0.6, A)
15b. Ipsi: Occluded Contra: 70-99%	2 1 1 5 1 2 3 4 5 6 7 8 9 (9.0, 2.3, D)	1 2 1 1 3 1 1 2 3 4 5 6 7 8 9 (6.0, 1.9, D)	5 2 2 1 2 3 4 5 6 7 8 9 (1.0, 1.1,)

Example 7

INDICATIONS FOR PERCUTANEOUS TRANSLUMINAL CORONARY ANGIOPLASTY

Clinical orientation:	Technology (surgical procedure)
Clinical purpose:	Treatment
Complexity:	Medium
Format:	Free text
Intended users:	Practitioners

This guideline on percutaneous transluminal coronary angioplasty (PTCA) is the result of a collaboration between the American College of Cardiology and the American Heart Association (ACC/AHA); it was noted in the discussion in Chapter 2 on multiorganizational efforts at guidelines development. The guideline illustrated here builds on earlier ACC/AHA work on PTCA generally; this one focuses on indications for angioplasty in patients with acute myocardial infarction (AMI) and makes further clinical distinctions concerning, for example, evolving AMI.

Interestingly, this guideline classifies patients (as opposed to clinical symptoms or technologies) into subgroups, and recommendations are expressed in reference to those subgroups. (This can be contrasted with the subgroup approach to appropriateness indicators as illustrated in Example 6 on carotid endarterectomy from the RAND Corporation.)   As is true for several items in this appendix, this guideline cites the relevant literature for its recommendations.

Like most journals the *Journal of the American College of Cardiology* uses a double column format. In order to include this example, however, it has been reproduced in a single column format. This clearly changes its appearance but probably does not affect its basic utility.

SOURCE: Gunnar, R.M., Passamani, E.R., Bourdillon, P.D., et al. Guidelines for the Early Management of Patients with Acute Myocardial Infarction. ACC/AHA Task Force Report. *Journal of the American College of Cardiology* 16:249-292, 1990. (Excerpt taken from pages 273-276.) Used with permission.

Percutaneous Transluminal
Coronary Angioplasty

Introduction. The guidelines for the use of percutaneous transluminal coronary angioplasty have been previous published in an ACC/AHA Task Force Report (129). That report outlines the immediate and long-term effects of elective angioplasty, its risks and contraindications, the selection of patients and current indications for its use. The present report will elaborate on the indications for angioplasty in patients with acute infarction. The use of angioplasty alone in evolving acute myocardial infarction will be considered separately from the use of angioplasty as an adjunct to thrombolytic therapy.

Primary coronary angioplasty. Along with the increasing interest in thrombolysis for the treatment of acute myocardial infarction, there has been interest in mechanical reperfusion by coronary angioplasty. There have been a number of reports (130–135) describing the use of angioplasty alone in the treatment of acute myocardial infarction. These have all been relatively small series and only one (134) has been randomized in comparison with an alternative therapy (streptokinase). These studies have generally reported a beneficial effect on left ventricular function, but there has been no good large scale randomized study comparing this form of treatment with either conventional supportive therapy or the most effective forms of thrombolytic therapy given early during acute infarction.

Percutaneous transluminal coronary angioplasty as the primary treatment strategy suffers from the need to have facilities and personnel for cardiac catheterization and a physician qualified to perform angioplasty available at all times. Because of this, intravenous thrombolysis has become established as the first line of therapy in acute myocardial infarction in suitable patients.

With this background, angioplasty should be considered as primary therapy in acute myocardial infarction only when facilities are available for expeditious transfer to a cardiac catheterization laboratory and where the personnel have the technical expertise and experience in performing angioplasty in this acute situation. Primary coronary angioplasty may appropriately be considered when a hospitalized patient has acute myocardial infarction, a patient presents within 4 h after onset of symptoms to an institution where adequate facilities and personnel are available or when thrombolytic therapy is contraindicated. Patients presenting in cardiogenic shock are a special group that may benefit from emergency angioplasty (vide infra).

Although intracoronary thrombolytic therapy is not usually as practical as primary therapy, the use of adjunctive intracoronary thrombolytic therapy during or after an angioplasty procedure may be appropriate when there is evidence of residual thrombus in the artery. In this situation, a smaller dose can be used than that used intravenously (such as 50,000 to 500,000 U of streptokinase or urokinase). Using a smaller dose, particularly <100,000 U, has the advantage of avoiding a systemic lytic effect, therefore minimizing bleeding complications resulting from thrombolytic therapy.

Recommendations for Primary Angioplasty of Infarct-Related Artery Only

Class I
1. Patients presenting within 6 h of onset of pain and who meet the criteria for thrombolysis but in whom thrombolytic therapy is clearly contraindicated and only if facilities and personnel are immediately available. This recommendation is operative only when data indicate a large amount of myocardium is at risk.

Class IIa
1. Intermittent continuous pain indicating the possibility of "stuttering" infarction, especially if there are ECG changes, but without clear indication for thrombolytic therapy.
2. Within 18 h of acute infarction in patients developing cardiogenic shock or pump failure.
3. Patients who have had previous coronary artery bypass graft surgery in whom recent occlusion of a vein graft is suspected.

Class IIb
1. Patients with known coronary anatomy in whom thrombolytic therapy is not contraindicated, but who develop symptoms and ECG evidence of acute infarction in hos-

pital at a time when rapid access to a catheterization laboratory with personnel experienced in performing expeditious angioplasty for acute myocardial infarction is available (completion within 1 h).

2. Patients in whom thrombolytic therapy is not contraindicated who present within 4 h of onset of symptoms of acute infarction at a facility where rapid access to a catheterization laboratory with personnel experienced in performing expeditious angioplasty for acute myocardial infarction is available (completion within 1 h).

Class III

This category applies to patients with acute myocardial infarction who do not fulfill the Class I or II criteria. For example:

1. Patients with severe left main coronary artery disease when instrumentation of a more distal occluded artery may be hazardous.

2. Patients in whom only a small area of myocardium is involved, as evidenced by clinical data or previously known coronary anatomy.

3. Dilation of vessels other than the infarct-related artery within the early hours of infarction. (This may not apply to the patient in shock or pump failure.)

Angioplasty after thrombolytic therapy. *Immediate angioplasty.* Although intravenous thrombolysis offers the promise of early reperfusion in up to 75% of patients (136), more complete reperfusion may be possible by performing angioplasty in those with a high grade residual stenosis of the infarct-related artery and those who failed intravenous thrombolysis. Three well-controlled, relatively large prospective trials (79,136,137) have, however, cast doubt on the utility of this strategy when applied early after thrombolysis and in the absence of continued or recurrent ischemia. The TAMI trial (136), European Cooperative Study (137) and TIMI-IIA (79) trial of urgent angioplasty failed to demonstrate a significant improvement in global or regional ventricular function in patients undergoing emergency (immediate) angioplasty of infarct-related vessels with a residual stenosis after administration of tissue plasminogen activator compared with patients receiving intravenous tissue plasminogen activator alone and undergoing elective angioplasty (TAMI trial), delayed angioplasty (TIMI-IIA trial) or no angioplasty (European Cooperative Study). The incidence of complications and death associated with emergency angioplasty was significantly greater in those undergoing emergency angioplasty after intravenous rt-PA than in those undergoing intravenous rt-PA administration without emergency angioplasty in the summed results of the three trials. It therefore appears that urgent angioplasty of infarct-related vessels with a residual stenosis after rt-PA therapy has no significant benefit, but does have a significant increase in risk. The failure of angioplasty immediately after thrombolysis may be related to an increased risk of hemorrhagic infarction when angioplasty is performed after administration of tissue plasminogen activator or to an increased risk of rethrombosis. Thrombolytic agents such as streptokinase, urokinase or tissue plasminogen activator have been shown to cause platelet activation and release of thromboxane A_2 (138,139).

Because thrombolysis is incomplete 1.5 to 3 h after the administration of an intravenous thrombolytic agent such as tissue plasminogen activator, it is not surprising that angioplasty performed under these circumstances may further predispose to platelet deposition on the residual thrombosis, with subsequent, distal platelet embolization, reocclusion and death. Whether a similar risk exists with other thrombolytic agents remains to be determined.

Delayed angioplasty. In view of the increased risk of urgent angioplasty after thrombolysis, attention has focused on the role of delayed and elective angioplasty. The need for further revascularization after intravenous thrombolysis relates to the often incomplete thrombolysis and the high incidence of residual stenosis in the infarct-related artery after intravenous thrombolysis. This is in part due to the presence of residual thrombosis and in part to the underlying atherosclerotic lesion. Patients undergoing thrombolysis alone, such as in the GISSI trial (9) or the Western Washington trial (96), had a higher incidence of reocclusion and reinfarction than those not given a thrombolytic agent. The significant advantages of early reperfusion in patients with anterior myocardial infarction in the Western Washington trial of intracoronary streptokinase were lost over a year follow-up as a result of reocclusion of the infarct-related artery and reinfarction. In a recent study, Mathey et al. (140) reported that patients undergoing coronary artery bypass graft surgery after reperfusion with streptokinase had a better survival rate than patients undergoing thrombolysis alone. *The ISIS-2 study,* in which aspirin was given in conjunction with intravenous streptokinase, suggested a reduced incidence of reinfarction compared with that from intravenous streptokinase alone (10). The beneficial result of the use of aspirin in conjunction with intravenous streptokinase in regard to survival, reocclusion and reinfarction may modify the need for delayed angioplasty. Nevertheless, a high grade residual stenosis with the potential for recurrent ischemia and infarction persists in many patients after intravenous thrombolysis, suggesting a potential role for delayed or elective angioplasty.

In the Johns Hopkins University trial (121) of delayed angioplasty, patients were first randomized to receive tissue plasminogen activator or placebo and then after 48 to 72 h were rerandomized to undergo or not undergo angioplasty. At follow-up study before hospital discharge, patients undergoing angioplasty had a significant improvement in exercise ejection fraction but not rest left ventricular ejection fraction compared with those not undergoing angioplasty. The risk of angioplasty under these circumstances 48 to 72 h after infarction does not appear to be appreciably greater than that for elective angioplasty. The advantages of this strategy include avoiding the risk of early angiography, avoiding the risk of emergency angioplasty and achieving a high incidence of final reperfusion, a decrease in the incidence of recurrent ischemic events and an improvement in exercise-stressed ventricular function. A disadvantage of this strategy is the possible overuse of angioplasty in low risk individuals.

The TIMI-IIB investigators (79) examined the strategy of delayed angioplasty in a relatively large number of patients and demonstrated that there was no advantage of this strategy on rest left ventricular ejection fraction or survival compared with a noninvasive strategy in which angioplasty was performed only for postinfarction angina or the development of ischemia on stress testing before hospital discharge (79). The noninvasive strategy avoids the risk of early angiography and urgent angioplasty. It restricts the use of coronary angioplasty to those at increased risk of ischemic events. The disadvantage of this strategy relates to the failure to identify coronary anatomy and the argument that a submaximal prehospital discharge stress test may not reliably predict recurrent ischemic events, reinfarction and death.

In view of the failure of available data to demonstrate an advantage of salvage or rescue angioplasty and the failure to show a benefit of routine urgent or delayed angioplasty after successful thrombolysis, it appears that an elective or noninvasive strategy is preferred. Until further data are available from prospective controlled trials, a conservative approach after intravenous thrombolytic therapy seems indicated. This would reserve angiography and angioplasty for patients with postinfarction angina, severe left ventricular dysfunction or stress-induced myocardial ischemia detected before hospital discharge.

Recommendations for Angioplasty After Intravenous Thrombolysis

Class I
Dilation of a significant lesion suitable for coronary angioplasty in the infarct-related artery in patients who are in the low risk group for angiographic-related morbidity and mortality who have a type A lesion (see ACC/AHA Task Force Report on coronary angioplasty [129]) and:
1. Have recurrent episodes of ischemic chest pain particularly if accompanied by ECG changes (postinfarction angina).
2. Show evidence of myocardial ischemia while on optimal medical therapy during submaximal stress testing performed before hospital discharge or on maximal stress testing in the early posthospital period.
3. Have recurrent ventricular tachycardia or ventricular fibrillation, or both, convincingly related to ischemia while on antiarrhythmic therapy.

Class IIa
Dilation of significant lesions in patients who:
1. Are similar to those in class I but who have type B lesions (anticipated success rate 60% to 85%) (see ACC/AHA Task Force Report on coronary angioplasty [129]).
2. Are within 18 h of onset of acute infarction and have

cardiogenic shock or pump failure. These patients should be studied and undergo reperfusion as soon as possible.

3. Before hospital discharge in those who have survived cardiogenic shock or pump failure.

Class IIb

Dilation of a lesion in patients who:

1. Have an occluded coronary artery after attempted thrombolytic therapy.
2. Require multivessel angioplasty.
3. Have >90% diameter proximal narrowing of an infarct-related artery with a large area of viable myocardium still at risk.

Class III

All patients in the immediate postinfarct period (during initial hospitalization) who do not fulfill Class I or II criteria. For example:

1. Dilation in patients who are within the early hours of an evolving myocardial infarction and have <50% residual stenosis of the infarct-related artery after receiving a thrombolytic agent.
2. Dilation of lesions in vessels other than the infarct-related artery within the early hours of infarction.
3. Dilation of residual lesions that are borderline in severity (50% to 70% diameter narrowing) of the infarct-related artery without demonstration of ischemia on functional testing.
4. Dilation of type C lesions (see ACC/AHA Task Force Report on coronary angioplasty for definition [129]).
5. Undertaking angioplasty in patients in the high risk group for morbidity and mortality (see ACC/AHA Task Force Report on coronary angioplasty for definition [129]).

Example 8

MANAGEMENT OF LABOR AND DELIVERY AFTER A
PREVIOUS CESAREAN SECTION

Clinical orientation:	Clinical condition
Clinical purpose:	Management of birth after previous cesarean birth
Complexity:	Low
Format:	Free text condensed from an extensive computer data base on CD-ROM disks (excerpt provided)
Intended users:	Practitioners (and perhaps educated patients)

This guideline is one of many in the 400-page *A Guide to Effective Care in Pregnancy and Childbirth.* The book is a synopsis of the main conclusions of a systematic, 10-year analysis of clinical data conducted by physicians and researchers at Oxford University, England. The analysis was based on a large, continuously updated data base of information (managed and stored using computer systems), which led to a 1,500-page, two-volume reference book called *Effective Care in Pregnancy and Childbirth.* This example, therefore, is drawn from a summarizing publication that is independent of the data base and reference document.

The guideline was chosen chiefly for two reasons: (1) its relation to the CD-ROM data base and (2) the unusual amount of time and the rigor of analysis that went into its development. In addition, it addresses an area of care about which, in the United States at least, malpractice concerns are great (see the discussions of malpractice and the anesthesia guidelines developed by the American Society for Anesthesiology in Chapters 2 and 5 and case study 4 of Chapter 3). Malpractice is explicitly considered in Example 4 on evaluation of chest pain in the emergency room.

The excerpts shown here might be usefully contrasted with several others in the appendix that also concern the management of a clinical condition but that are presented in quite varied formats (e.g., Example 12 on low back pain and Example 13 on post-bypass surgery care).

SOURCE: Enkin, M., Keirse, M.J.N.C., and Chalmers, I. *A Guide to Effective Care in Pregnancy and Childbirth.* Oxford: Oxford University Press, 1990. Used with permission.

——————— 39 ———————

Labour and delivery after previous caesarean section

This chapter is derived from the chapter by Murray Enkin (70) in EFFEC-TIVE CARE IN PREGNANCY AND CHILDBIRTH.

1 Introduction

Although in recent years the dogma of 'once a caesarean always a caesarean' has come under both professional and public scrutiny, in many countries the practice is still carried out, and remains a stated policy in many institutions.

Two general propositions underlie the widespread practice of repeat caesarean section: that trial of labour, with its inherent risk of uterine rupture, represents a significant hazard to the wellbeing of mother and baby; and that planned repeat caesarean operations are virtually free of risk. It is important to examine the validity of these propositions.

2 Results of a trial of labour

No controlled trials have compared the results of elective caesarean section versus trial of labour for women who have had a previous caesarean section. In the absence of such trials, the best available data on the relative safety of trial of labour comes from the prospective comparative studies that have been reported. In these studies, including a total of almost 9000 pregnant women with a history of one caesarean section, over two-thirds were allowed a trial of labour. Of these women almost 80 per cent gave birth vaginally. Thus, for the series for which total data are available, well over half of all women with a previous caesarean section gave birth vaginally.

A large number of retrospective studies have also compared the effects of elective caesarean section versus trial of labour in women who have had one previous caesarean section. There is far greater potential for bias in these retrospective studies than in the prospective studies, and one should be cautious in drawing conclusions from them; nevertheless, it is interesting to note that their results are similar to, and support the conclusions from the prospective studies.

Uterine dehiscence (wound breakdown) or rupture (the data available do not allow these two conditions to be quantified separately) occurred in 0.5 to 2.0 per cent of the women who had elective caesarean sections, and in 0.5 to 3.3 per cent of the women in the trial of labour groups in the prospective cohort studies. Most of these dehiscences were minor in nature, and had no sequelae.

Data from the prospective studies show that febrile morbidity rates were consistently and substantially higher in the groups of women who underwent elective caesarean section (range 11 to 38 per cent) than in the groups of women who had a trial of labour, including both those who had an emergency caesarean section and those who had a vaginal delivery (range 2 to 23 per cent). Although the febrile morbidity rates were highest among women who underwent caesarean section after a trial of labour, these were more than counterbalanced by the lower rate in the two-thirds of women who give birth vaginally after a trial of labour.

Blood transfusions, endometritis, abdominal wound infections, thrombo-embolic phenomena, anaesthetic complications, pyelonephritis, pneumonia, and septicemia were also less common in women who had a vaginal delivery following low transverse caesarean section than in women who underwent a repeat caesarean section.

Perinatal mortality and morbidity rates were similar with trial of labour and elective caesarean section in the studies that report these data. Such comparisons, however, are of little value, because the groups compared are not equivalent. The decision to perform a repeat caesarean section or to permit a trial of labour may be made on the basis of whether or not the fetus is living or dead, anomalous, or immature.

3 Risks of caesarean section

3.1 Risks to the mother

Large series of caesarean sections have been reported with no associated maternal mortality. One should not be lulled into a false sense of security by this. The risk of a mother dying with caesarean section is small, but is still considerably higher than with vaginal delivery.

The rate of maternal death associated with caesarean section (approximately 40 per 100 000 births) is four times that associated with vaginal delivery (10 per 100 000 births). The maternal death rate associated with elective repeat caesarean section (18 per 100 000 births), although lower than that associated with caesarean sections overall, is still almost twice the rate associated with all vaginal deliveries, and nearly four times the mortality rate associated with normal vaginal delivery (5 per 100 000 births).

The rate of maternal mortality attributable to caesarean section *per se* is difficult to estimate, as some of the deaths observed are caused by the condition which necessitated the caesarean section in the first place. While it is not possible to quantitate exactly the extent of increased risk of death to the mother from elective caesarean section, the data available suggest that it is between two and four times that associated with vaginal delivery.

Most forms of maternal morbidity are higher with caesarean section than with vaginal delivery. In addition to the risks of anaesthesia attendant on all surgery, there are risks of operative injury, febrile morbidity, and effects on subsequent fertility, and of psychological morbidity as well.

3.2 Risks to the baby

The major hazards of caesarean section for the baby relate to the risks of respiratory distress contingent on either the caesarean delivery itself, or on preterm birth as a result of miscalculation of dates. Babies born by caesarean section have a higher risk of respiratory distress syndrome than babies born vaginally at the same gestational age.

The availability of more accurate and readily available dating with ultrasound may decrease the risk of unexpected preterm delivery. Nevertheless, it is unlikely that this risk can ever be completely eliminated.

4 Factors to consider in the decision about a trial of labour

A mathematical, utilitarian approach comparing the balance of risks and benefits of trial of labour with those of planned caesarean section will not always be the best way to choose a course of action. Such an approach can, however, provide important data that may be helpful in arriving at the best decision.

The technique of decision analysis has been used to determine the optimal delivery policy after previous caesarean section. The probabilities and utilities of a number of possible outcomes, including the need for hysterectomy, uterine rupture, iatrogenic 'prematurity', need for future repeat caesarean sections, prolonged hospitalization and recovery, additional cost, failed trial of labour, discomfort of labour, and inconvenience of awaiting labour can be put into a mathematical model comparing different policies. Over a wide range of probabilities and utilities, which included all reasonable values, trial of labour proved to be the logical choice.

4.1 *More than one previous caesarean section*

Data on the results of trials of labour in women who have had more than one previous caesarean section tend to be buried in studies of trial of labour after previous caesarean section as a whole. The available data on delivery outcome for trial of labour in women who have had more than one previous caesarean section show that the overall vaginal delivery rate is little different from that seen in women who have had only one previous caesarean section. Successful trials of labour have been carried out on women who have had three or more previous caesarean sections.

The rate of uterine dehiscence (wound breakdown) in women who have had more than one previous caesarean section is slightly higher than the dehiscence rate for women with only one previous caesarean, but all dehiscences in the reported series were without symptoms and without serious sequelae. There was no maternal or perinatal mortality associated with any of the trials of labour after more than one previous caesarean section reported in these series. No data have been reported on other maternal or infant morbidity specifically associated with multiple previous caesarean sections.

While the number of cases reported is still small, the available evidence does not suggest that a woman who has had more than one previous caesarean section should be treated any differently from the woman who has had only one caesarean section.

4.2 *Reason for the primary caesarean section*

The greatest likelihood of vaginal delivery is seen when the first caesarean section was done because of breech presentation; vaginal delivery rates are lowest when the initial indication was failure to progress in labour, dystocia, or cephalopelvic disproportion. Even when the indication for the first caesarean section was disproportion, dystocia, or failure to progress, successful vaginal delivery occurred over 50 per cent of the time in most published series, and the rate was over 75 per cent in the largest series reported. It is clear that a history of caesarean section for dystocia is not a contraindication to a trial of labour, and has only a small effect on the likelihood of vaginal birth when a trial of labour is permitted.

4.3 *Previous vaginal delivery*

Mothers who have had a previous vaginal delivery in addition to their previous caesarean sections are more likely to deliver vaginally after trial of labour than mothers with no previous vaginal deliveries. This advantage is increased even further in those mothers whose previous vaginal delivery occurred after rather than before the primary caesarean section.

4.4 *Type of previous incision in the uterus*

Modern experience with operative approaches other than the lower segment operation for caesarean section is limited. There is, however, a growing trend towards the use of vertical incisions in preterm caesarean sections. This, and the inverted T incision sometimes necessary to allow delivery, show that consideration of the type of uterine scar is still relevant.

The potential dangers of uterine rupture are related to the rapid 'explosive' rupture which is most likely to be seen in women who have a classical midline scar. The majority of dehiscences found following lower segment transverse incisions are 'silent', 'incomplete', or incidentally discovered at the time of repeat caesarean section. While scars found at repeat caesarean section can be described as 'dangerous' (meaning thin or 'windowed'), only a small proportion of them actually demonstrated a rupture. What the fate of these 'dangerous' scars would actually have been, had labour been permitted, can only be surmised.

Following a classical caesarean section, rupture of the scar is not only more serious than rupture of a lower segment scar, it is also more likely to occur. Rupture may occur suddenly during the course of pregnancy, prior to labour, and before a repeat caesarean section can be scheduled. A review of the literature at a time when classical caesarean section was still common showed a 2.2 per cent rate of uterine rupture with previous classical caesarean, and a rate of 0.5 per cent with previous lower segment caesarean sections. That is, the scar of the classical operation was more than four times more likely to rupture in a subsequent pregnancy than that of the lower segment incision.

Unfortunately, even in the older literature, there are very few data on the risk of uterine rupture of a vertical scar in the lower segment.

One 1966 study reported an incidence of rupture of 2.2 per cent in classical incision scars, 1.3 per cent in vertical incision lower segment scars and 0.7 per cent in transverse incision lower segment scars. The distinction between the risk of rupture of vertical and transverse lower segment scars may be related to extension of the vertical incision from the lower segment into the upper segment of the uterus.

The uncertain denominators in the reported series make it difficult to quantify the risk of rupture with a previous classical or vertical incision lower segment scar. It is clear, however, that the risk that such a rupture may occur, that it may occur prior to the onset of labour, and that it may have serious sequelae, are considerably greater with such scars than with transverse incision lower segment scars. It would seem reasonable that women who have had a hysterotomy, a vertical uterine incision, or an 'inverted T' incision should be treated in subsequent pregnancies in the same manner as women who have had a classical caesarean section, and that trial of labour, if permitted at all, should be carried out with great caution, and with acute awareness of the increased risks likely to exist.

4.5 *Gestational age at previous caesarean section*

During the past decade improved neonatal care has increased the survival rate of preterm babies, and this in turn has led to a reduction in the stage of gestation at which obstetricians are prepared to perform caesarean sections for fetal indications. This has resulted in caesarean sections being used to deliver babies at or even before 26 weeks. At these early gestations the lower segment is poorly formed, and so-called 'lower segment' operations at this period of gestation are, in reality, transverse incisions in the body of the uterus. Whether or not such an incision confers any advantage over a classical incision remains in doubt. Indeed, some obstetricians now recommend performing a classical incision under these circumstances.

Whichever of these incisions is used at these early gestational ages, their consequences for subsequent pregnancies are currently unknown. It is quite possible, in theory at least, that they may result in a greater morbidity in future pregnancies than that associated with the lower segment operation at term.

4.6 *Integrity of the scar*

The decision to advise for or against a trial of labour may be influenced by an assessment of the integrity of the scar. This assessment may be helped by knowledge of the operative technique used at the previous caesarean section, the operative findings at the time of surgery, whether an extension of the operative incision had occurred, and the nature of the postoperative course.

5 Care during a trial of labour

5.1 *Use of oxytocics*

The use of oxytocin or prostaglandins for induction or augmentation of labour in women who have had a previous caesarean section has remained controversial, because of speculation that there might be an increased risk of uterine rupture or dehiscence. This view is not universally held, nor is it strongly supported by the available data. A number of series have been reported in which oxytocin or prostaglandins were used for the usual indications with no suggestion of increased hazard. Review of the reported case series shows that any increased risk of uterine rupture with the use of oxytocin is likely to be extremely small.

Such comparisons, of course, are rendered invalid by the fact that the cohorts of women who received, or did not receive, oxytocin may have differed in many other respects in addition to the use of oxytocin. Nevertheless, the high vaginal delivery rates and low dehiscence rates noted in these women suggest that oxytocin can be used for induction or augmentation of labour in women who have had a previous caesarean section, with the same precautions that should always attend its use.

5.2 *Regional analgesia and anaesthesia*

The use of regional (caudal or epidural) analgesia in labour for the woman with a previous caesarean section has been questioned because of fears that it might mask pain or tenderness, which are considered to be early signs of rupture of the scar. The extent of the risk of masking a catastrophic uterine rupture is difficult to quantify. It must be minuscule; only one case report of this having occurred was located. In a number of reported series regional block is used whenever requested by the woman for pain relief, and no difficulties were encountered with this policy.

There does not appear to be any increased hazard from uterine rupture associated with the use of regional anaesthesia for women who have had a previous caesarean section. It is sensible, safe, and justified to use analgesia for the woman with a lower segment scar in the same manner as for the woman whose uterus is intact.

5.3 *Manual exploration of the uterus*

In many reports of series of vaginal births after previous caesarean section, mention is made of the fact that the uterus was explored postpartum in all cases, in a search for uterine rupture or dehiscence without symptoms. The wisdom of this approach should be seriously challenged.

Manual exploration of a scarred uterus immediately following a vaginal delivery is often inconclusive. It is difficult to be sure whether or not the thin, soft lower segment is intact. In any case, in the absence of bleeding or systemic signs, a rupture without symptoms discovered postpartum does not require any treatment, so the question of diagnosis would be academic.

No studies have shown any benefit from routine manual exploration of the uterus in women who have had a previous caesarean section. There is always a risk of introducing infection by the manual exploration, or of converting a dehiscence into a larger rupture. A reasonable compromise consists of increased vigilance in the hour after delivery of the placenta, reserving internal palpation of the lower segment for women with signs of abnormal bleeding.

6 Rupture of the scarred uterus in pregnancy and labour

Complete rupture of the uterus can be a life-threatening emergency. Fortunately the condition is rare in modern obstetrics despite the increase in caesarean section rates, and serious sequelae are even more rare. Although often considered to be the most common cause of uterine rupture, previous caesarean section is involved in less than half the cases.

Excluding symptomless wound breakdown, the rate of reported uterine rupture has ranged from 0.09 per cent to 0.22 per cent for women with a singleton vertex presentation who underwent a trial of labour after a previous transverse lower segment caesarean section. To put these rates into perspective, the probability of requiring an emergency caesarean section for other acute other conditions (fetal distress, cord prolapse, or antepartum haemorrhage) in any woman giving birth, is approximately 2.7 per cent, or 30 times as high as the risk of uterine rupture with a trial of labour.

Treatment of rupture of a lower segment scar does not require extraordinary facilities. Hospitals whose capabilities are so limited that they cannot deal promptly with problems associated with a trial of labour are also incapable of dealing appropriately with other obstetrical emergencies. Any obstetrical department that is prepared to look after women with much more frequently encountered conditions such as placenta praevia, abruptio placentae, prolapsed cord, and acute fetal distress should be able to manage a trial of labour safely after a previous lower segment caesarean section.

7 Gap between evidence and practice

Obstetric practice has been slow to reflect the scientific evidence confirming the safety of trial of labour after previous caesarean section. The degree of opposition to vaginal birth after caesarean section, in North America in particular, is difficult to explain, considering the strength of the available evidence that trials of labour are, under proper circumstances, both safe and effective. Two national consensus statements and two national professional bodies, in Canada and the United States, have recommended policies of trial of labour after previous caesarean section.

Increasing numbers of pregnant women, as well as professionals, are vehemently protesting the status quo. For a variety of reasons many women prefer to attempt a vaginal birth after a caesarean section. Their earlier caesarean experience may have been emotionally or physically difficult. They may be unhappy because they were separated from their partners or from their babies. They may wonder if it was all necessary in the first place. They may be aware of the accumulated evidence on the relative safety and advantages of trial of labour, and simply be looking for a better experience this time.

In recent years a number of consumer 'shared predicament' groups have appeared, with the expressed purposes of demythologizing caesarean section, of combatting misinformation, and of disseminating both accurate information and their own point of view. Special prenatal classes are available for many parents who elect to attempt a vaginal birth after a caesarean section.

8 Conclusions

A trial of labour after a previous caesarean section should be recommended for women who have had a previous lower segment transverse incision caesarean section, and have no other indication for caesarean section in the present pregnancy. The likelihood of vaginal birth is not significantly altered by the indication for the first caesarean section (including 'cephalopelvic disproportion' and 'failure to progress'), nor by a history of more than one previous caesarean section.

A history of classical, low vertical, or unknown uterine incision or hysterotomy carries with it an increased risk of uterine rupture, and in most cases is a contraindication to trial of labour.

The care of a woman in labour after a previous lower segment caesarean section should be little different from that for any woman in labour. Oxytocin induction or stimulation, and epidural analgesia, may be used for the usual indications. Careful monitoring of the condition of the mother and fetus is required, as for all pregnancies. The hospital facilities required do not differ from those that should be available for all women giving birth, irrespective of their previous history.

Example 9

USE OF AUTOLOGOUS OR DONOR BLOOD
FOR TRANSFUSIONS

Clinical orientation:	Technology
Clinical purpose:	Treatment
Complexity:	Low
Format:	Free-text table
Intended users:	Patient or family, health care practitioners

In 1990, the California legislature enacted a bill requiring that any patient undergoing treatment that might involve a blood transfusion be presented with written information about benefits, risks, and options. The written document used must be the standardized document approved by the state's Department of Health Services; furthermore, physicians are required to buy supplies of the guideline to make it available to patients.

This guideline is of interest for several reasons. First, its use was mandated by a state, a relatively unusual occurrence with guidelines (although see Example 4 on diagnosis of chest pain and its relationship to events in Massachusetts). Second, it is intended for use by both practitioners and patients and thus implicitly assumes that patient preferences are a critical factor in providing appropriate care. Like the guideline on deciding about low back pain (Example 12), this guideline is designed primarily for patient use, but its purpose is to convey a fairly sophisticated set of advantages and trade-offs so that any decisions patients make about the course of treatment are based on adequate information and their preferences. Finally, the formatting as a table is clear and concise. This guideline was referred to in Chapter 5 in the discussion on ethics and informed consent.

SOURCE: Reproduction of a public domain brochure from the State of California Department of Health Services, Sacramento, California.

The Safest Blood is Your Own.
Use It Whenever Possible.

Many surgeries do not require blood transfusions. However, if you need blood, you have several options. Although you have the right to refuse a blood transfusion, this decision may hold life-threatening consequences. Please carefully review this brochure and decide with your doctor which option(s) you prefer.

PLEASE NOTE: Your options may be limited by time and health factors, so it is important to begin carrying out your decision as soon as possible.

A Patient's Guide to Blood Transfusions

- ASK YOUR PHYSICIAN ABOUT NEW DEVELOPMENTS IN TRANSFUSION MEDICINE.

- CHECK WITH YOUR INSURANCE COMPANY FOR THEIR REIMBURSEMENT POLICY.

This brochure was developed by
California Department of Health Services
714/744 P Street
Sacramento, CA 95814
Kenneth W. Kizer, M.D., M.P.H., Director
For information about the contents, please call:
(916) 445-1248

This brochure is distributed by
Medical Board of California
1426 Howe Avenue
Sacramento, CA 95825-3236
Kenneth J. Wagstaif, Executive Director

TO ORDER ADDITIONAL COPIES, PLEASE WRITE TO THE
FOLLOWING ADDRESS.

Office of Procurement
Publications Section
P.O. Box 1015
North Highlands, CA 95660

Ask for the publication: "IF YOU NEED BLOOD". Sold in bundles of 50 copies at $4.00 per bundle. [Note: This publication is not copyrighted. You may duplicate for distribution to your patients.]

IF YOU NEED BLOOD...

308

The methods of using your own blood can be used independently or together to eliminate or minimize the need for donor blood, as well as virtually eliminate transfusion risks of infection and allergic reaction

■ AUTOLOGOUS BLOOD - Using Your Own Blood

Option	Explanation	Advantages	Disadvantages
PRE-OPERATIVE DONATION Donating Your Own Blood Before Surgery	The blood bank draws your blood and stores it until you need it, during or after surgery. For elective surgery only.	✓ Eliminates or minimizes the need for someone else's blood during and after surgery.	• Requires advance planning. • May delay surgery. • Medical conditions may prevent pre-operative donation.
INTRA-OPERATIVE AUTOLOGOUS TRANSFUSION Recycling Your Blood During Surgery	Instead of being discarded, blood lost during surgery is filtered, and put back into your body during surgery. For elective and emergency surgery.	✓ Eliminates or minimizes need for someone else's blood during surgery. Large amounts of blood can be recycled.	• Not for use if cancer or infection is present.
POST-OPERATIVE AUTOLOGOUS TRANSFUSION Recycling Your Blood After Surgery	Blood lost after surgery is collected, filtered and returned. For elective and emergency surgery.	✓ Eliminates or minimizes the need for someone else's blood after surgery.	• Not for use if cancer or infection is present.

309

| HEMODILUTION
Donating Your
Own Blood During
Surgery | Immediately before surgery, some of your blood is taken and replaced with I.V. fluids. After surgery, your blood is filtered and returned to you. For elective surgery. | ✓ Eliminates or minimizes the need for someone else's blood during and after surgery. Dilutes your blood so you lose less concentrated blood during surgery. | • Limited number of units can be drawn.
• Medical conditions may prevent hemodilution. |
| APHERESIS
Donating Your
Own Platelets and
Plasma | Before surgery, your platelets and plasma, which help stop bleeding, are withdrawn, filtered, and returned to you when you need it. For elective surgery. | ✓ May eliminate the need for donor platelets and plasma, especially high blood-loss procedures. | • Medical conditions may prevent apheresis.
• Procedure has limited application. |

In some cases, you may require more blood than anticipated. If this happens and you receive blood other than your own, there is a possibility of complications, such as hepatitis or AIDS.

■ DONOR BLOOD - Using Someone Else's Blood

Donor blood and blood products can never be absolutely 100% safe, even though testing makes the risk very small.

Option	Explanation	Advantages	Disadvantages
VOLUNTEER BLOOD From the Community Blood Supply	Blood and blood products donated by volunteer donors to a community blood bank.	■ Readily available. Can be life-saving when your own blood is not available.	● Risk of disease transmission (such as hepatitis or AIDS), and allergic reactions.

Note: You may wish to check whether donors are paid or volunteer, since blood from commercial (paid) donors may not, in some cases, be as safe as blood from volunteers.

Option	Explanation	Advantages	Disadvantages
DESIGNATED DONOR BLOOD From Donors You Select	Blood and blood donors you select who must meet the same requirements as volunteer donors.	■ You can select people with your own blood type who you feel are safe donors.	● Risk of disease transmission (such as hepatitis or AIDS), and allergic reactions. ● May require several days of advanced donation. ● Not necessarily as safe, nor safer, than volunteer donor blood.

Note: Care should be taken in selecting donors. Donors should never be pressured into donating. Donations from certain family members may require irradiation of blood.

Example 10

DETECTION AND TRACKING OF METABOLIC ACIDOSIS

Clinical orientation:	Clinical conditions (physiologic states)
Clinical purpose:	Detection of worsening clinical status
Complexity:	High
Format:	Decision path with text
Intended users:	Practitioners

This guideline was developed by clinicians at a large academic medical center to clarify the appropriate use of serum bicarbonate levels as a means of alerting physicians to new or worsening metabolic acidosis. An alert is triggered when laboratory values for one or a series of these tests meet (or fall below or above) certain criteria; the guideline also alerts the physician to common causes of metabolic acidosis. This specific guideline does not go on to suggest any further diagnostic or therapeutic steps.

The guideline is a shortened version of a Medical Logic Module (MLM) being run at Columbia-Presbyterian Medical Center in New York; MLMs are essentially aggregations of the information necessary to make a single medical decision. Clinical alerts, management critiques, diagnostic scoring algorithms, protocols, and screening rules for research studies have been encoded in this fashion. An MLM is composed of a set of slots grouped into three larger categories: maintenance, library, and knowledge, of which only the knowledge slot is here presented. For clarity, comments on the slots and the three overall categories are imbedded within the guideline in italics—these comments would not appear on the practitioner's computer monitor.

The guideline was selected in part because it is written in Arden Syntax. This is a computer language specially designed to accommodate and promote the use of various health knowledge databases in the service of medical decisionmaking. Hence, it is an interesting sample of a computer-driven algorithm.

SOURCE: Hripcsak, G. Screen for worsening metabolic acidosis based on serum bicarbonate. In the annual *ASTM Book of Standards*, copyright ASTM, 1916 Race Street, Philadelphia, PA 19103, forthcoming 1992. Used with permission.

SCREEN FOR WORSENING METABOLIC ACIDOSIS
BASED ON SERUM BICARBONATE

KNOWLEDGE: *The knowledge category specifies the actual medical decision. The MLM is evoked whenever a serum bicarbonate is stored in the patient database, and the MLM alerts the health care provider to the development of worsening metabolic acidosis. If worsening acidosis is detected, then an alert is stored in the patient database where it can be seen by the provider. The first slot is the type slot, which will be used for future expansion of the syntax; it indicates which slots follow.*

type: data-driven;;

data: *The data slot maps the terms used in the rest of the MLM to entities in the patient database. The first statement is a query in which "current_bicarb," "sodium," "chloride," and "creatinine" are defined as laboratory values that are a part of the data that evoked this MLM (thus these are the data that have just been stored in the patient database). The second statement is a query that maps "raw_bicarbs" to the patient's last 10 bicarbonate values within the past year. The aggregation operator ("last 10 from") and the time constraint ("where they occurred within the past 1 year") are defined in the Arden Syntax. The part in curly brackets ("{serum_bicarbonate}") is specific to the institution in which the MLM is used. When an MLM is shared, this part must be altered to match the institution's patient database. The last statement defines "bicarb_storage" as an event in which a serum bicarbonate is stored in the patient database.*

```
/*————————————————————————————*/
/* get the data that evoked this MLM               */
/*————————————————————————————*/
(current_bicarb, sodium, chloride, creatinine) := READ last
      {serum_bicarbonate, serum_sodium, serum_chloride,
      serum_creatinine where they are evoking};

/*————————————————————————————*/
/* get the last 10 bicarbs (may or may not be valid)   */
/*————————————————————————————*/
raw_bicarbs := READ last 10 from
      ({serum_bicarbonate}
      where they occurred within the past 1 year;
```

```
/*————————————————————————————*/
/* define the storage of serum bicarbonate            */
/*————————————————————————————*/
    bicarb_storage := EVENT
        {insertion of serum_bicarbonate};

    ;;
```

evoke: *The evoke slot defines the context in which the MLM is executed. In this case the term "bicarb_storage" is used to specify that this MLM is evoked whenever a serum bicarbonate is stored. The serum bicarbonate is usually stored as part of a panel of tests that includes the sodium, chloride, and creatinine. If the bicarbonate is stored by itself, then the first query in the data slot would assign a value of "null" to "sodium," "chloride," and "creatinine," indicating that there are no valid values for these terms.*

```
/*————————————————————————————*/
/* this MLM is evoked by the storage of serum bicarbonate  */
/*————————————————————————————*/
    bicarb_storage;;
```

logic: *The logic slot decides whether or not an action needs to be taken. Processing occurs in the logic slot until a "conclude" statement is reached; "conclude true" indicates that the action defined in the action slot should be performed, and "conclude false" indicates that it should not. In this logic slot, there is first a check of whether there is a valid value for "current_bicarb;" this ensures that the sample was not hemolyzed. Then there is a check of whether the bicarbonate is below a threshold. The threshold varies with the patient's renal function, as indicated by the creatinine.*
Once it is determined that the bicarbonate is below a threshold, the rest of the logic slot checks whether the bicarbonate is worsening. The term "valid_bicarbs" is defined as only those "raw_bicarbs" that are valid numbers. There is a check to make sure that the data being stored is not significantly older (in terms of the time that the sample was drawn from the patient) than others in the database. Then "comparison_bicarbs" is defined as those bicarbonates that occurred before the current one and after the last time the bicarbonate was as low as the current one. Finally, there is a check to see whether the bicarbonate has

fallen by at least 20% within the search interval. Note that rather than look for a drop of 20%, the MLM looks for a drop of 10% plus 2 units; this accounts for the absolute variability of the reported bicarbonate value. If all these conditions have been satisfied, then the logic slot concludes true, and the action slot is executed. The original version of this MLM contained additional logic to avoid duplicate alerts and to tailor the alert message to the patient's condition.

```
/*————————————————————————————————————————*/
/* Decide whether to send an alert.                             */
/*————————————————————————————————————————*/


/*————————————————————————————————————————*/
/* Is there a valid bicarbonate value to check (vs. hemolyzed)?  */
/*————————————————————————————————————————*/
if current_bicarb is not number then
     conclude false;      /* no alert */
endif;


/*————————————————————————————————————————*/
/* Check for evidence of significant metabolic acidosis.        */
/*————————————————————————————————————————*/
if creatinine >= 3 then    /* check for renal insufficiency */

/*————————————————————————————————————————*/
/* If there is renal insufficiency, expect some acidosis.       */
/*————————————————————————————————————————*/
     if current_bicarb >= 15 then  /* lower threshold */
         conclude false; /* no significant acidosis so no alert */
     endif;
else                       /* BUN normal or unknown */
     if current_bicarb >= 18 then  /* higher threshold */
         conclude false; /* no significant acidosis so no alert */
     endif;
endif;
```

```
/*_____*/
/* Is the acidosis worsening?                      */
/*_____*/


/*_____*/
/* Define valid bicarbonates (vs. hemolyzed, . . .). */
/*_____*/
  valid_bicarbs := raw_bicarbs where they are number;


/*_____*/
/* Find out whether there are more recent bicarbonates */
/* than the current one being stored.  If so, then do  */
/* not alert on old data.  Define "more recent" as more */
/* than the half time of the bicarbonate changing or of */
/* seeing an alert (about 1 hour).                 */
/*_____*/
      if current_bicarb occurred before
      (1 hour before the time of last of valid_bicarbs) then
      conclude false;      /* do not alert */
  endif;


/*_____*/
/* Generate a list of bicarbonates for comparison to */
/* decide whether the value has fallen enough to merit */
/* an alert.  Pick a search window that ends at the  */
/* current bicarb and that begins at the last bicarb */
/* that was less than or equal to the current bicarb. */
/*_____*/
  previous_bicarbs := valid_bicarbs  /* previous = before current */
      where they occurred before the time of the current_bicarb;
  start_time := time of last(      /* last time it was <= current */
      previous_bicarbs where they <= current_bicarb);
  if start_time is present then
      comparison_bicarbs :=       /* comparison = after start */
          previous_bicarbs
          where they occurred not before start_time;
  else                  /* none of previous bicarbs is this low */
      comparison_bicarbs :=
          previous_bicarbs; /* so use them all */
  endif;
```

```
/*─────────────────────────────────────────────*/
/* Make sure the value is dropping and that it has          */
/* dropped by at least 20% since the last alert or since     */
/* it was last this low.  Note that 10%-2 mEq/l is used      */
/* in place of 20% to better account for variability          */
/* at very low bicarbs.  If there are no comparison          */
/* bicarbs, then an alert is sent.                           */
/*─────────────────────────────────────────────*/
if (max(comparison_bicarbs)*0.90)-2 < current_bicarb then
        conclude false;        /* has not dropped by 20% so no alert */
else
        conclude true;         /* drop 20% or no comparison, so alert */
endif;

;;
```

action: *The action slot defines what the MLM should do if the logic
               slot's criteria are satisfied. Possible actions include storing a
               message in the patient database, sending an electronic mail message,
               printing a message, and evoking other MLMs. In this MLM the
               bicarbonate value and time are inserted into an alert message,
               and then they are stored in the patient database.*

```
/*─────────────────────────────────────────────*/
/* send an alert warning new or worsening metabolic acidosis    */
/*─────────────────────────────────────────────*/
write "The patient's serum bicarbonate level " ‖ current_bicarb ‖ " mEq/l
        at " ‖ time of current_bicarb ‖ ") shows evidence of new or worsening
        metabolic acidosis.  Common causes of metabolic acidosis in-
        clude:  ketoacidosis (diabetic, alcoholic, starvation), lactic aci-
        dosis (sepsis, shock, toxins), poisoning (salicylates, ethylene glycol,
        methanol), renal failure, renal tubular dysfunction (RTA), loss
        of alkali (diarrhea, ureterosigmoidoscopy), medication, compen-
        sation for respiratory alkalosis.";

;;

end:
```

Example 11

USE OF ORAL CONTRACEPTIVES

Clinical orientation:	Technology (pharmaceutical agent)
Clinical purpose:	Prevention of pregnancy, management of fertility
Complexity:	Medium
Format:	If-then decision statements
Intended users:	Practitioners

This guideline was included mainly for reasons relating to formatting. Specifically, it clearly demonstrates the use of both a computer-based guideline and an if-then series of statements. As a guideline displayed on a screen and incorporated in computer software, its advantages lie in ease of use, likely frequency of use, feasibility of frequent or continuous updating, ability to print out specific information for patient reference or patient records, and the ability to bring important information to the physician's attention for needed action in a timely way. In addition, because the guideline is recorded in the computer, it can easily be updated or used to print out patient references or patient records. Note that the citations in parentheses (such as R:2255, R:2097) are to references listed in the computer system (not reproduced here). This approach might easily be employed to generate medical review criteria, such as those used for quality assurance purposes.

Another reason for including this guideline was that it involves a technology (here, a pharmaceutical agent) that raises questions of whether and how to manage a clinical condition with long-term therapy that may have significant harmful side effects.

SOURCE: Reprinted, with permission, from Regenstrief Institute and Wishard Memorial Hospital, Indianapolis, Indiana.

ESTROGENS AND ORAL CONTRACEPTIVES

BEGIN BLOCK ESTROGEN CONTROL

If begun within a few years after the onset of menopause, treatment with exogenous estrogens greatly retards the development of osteoporosis (R:2255, R:2097). Estrogen therapy poses a high risk of endometrial cancer to menopausal women with intact uteri, but there is no such risk if the uterus has been removed. The following rule suggests estrogen replacement for "young" women who have had hysterectomy and oophorectomy. The risk of disabling osteoporosis is all the greater because of their young age, and estrogens have the additional advantage of improving their sense of well-being and preventing vaginal atrophy.

    IF NO "ESTROGEN USE"
    AND NO "ORAL CONTRACEPTIVE USE"
    AND NO "ESTROGENS VAG USE"
        THEN IF NO "PREVIOUS VISIT"
            AND (("HYSTERECTOMY SURG"
            AND "CERVICAL PAP LAST" WAS =
            "ATROPHIC PATTERN")
            OR "SURGICAL HX" WAS = "OOPHORECTOMY")
            AND "AGE" IS LT 45
            AND NO "CAD RISK FACTORS"
            AND NO "DX" IS = "BREAST CA"
                THEN If patient had both ovaries removed, "estro-
                    gens" (with cycling) should be considered to
                    retard osteoporosis. R:2255
            AND EXIT
        ELSE EXIT

Only patients who are currently using estrogens or oral contraceptives are admitted to the protocols below.

    IF "ESTROGEN USE" EXISTS
    OR "ORAL CONTRACEPTIVE USE" EXISTS
        THEN CONTINUE
        ELSE EXIT

The use of oral contraceptives is associated with an increased risk of stroke, myocardial infarction, and thromboembolic phenomena. The risk is proportional to the patient's age and is amplified by cigarette smoking. The medical community has long assumed that the estrogen half of the birth control pill caused this increased risk (R:1168). Estrogens do tend to raise the blood pressure, and to increase low-density and very-low-density lipo-proteins (R:1159). In young women they increase cholesterol levels and decrease the activity of antithrombin III. However, in postmenopausal women, pure estrogens decrease cholesterol levels and have no effect on the cardiovascular risk (R:2840, R:2815). Could it be that the progesterone half is the villain? A study performed at the Kaiser Permanente Clinics (R:3163) suggests this possibility.

Whatever the underlying mechanism, birth control pills have a substantial influence on the cardiovascular risk in women in their middle and upper reproductive years, particularly if they are smokers. The following warning protocol has 3 branches. The first deals with known smokers above the age of 40 in whom the cardiovascular risk of oral contraceptives is severe. The second deals with women over 35 in whom the smoking history is unknown. It generates a reminder once a year per patient. The third branch calls attention to the fact that the birth control pills could be causing the patient's hypertension.

IF "ORAL CONTRACEPTIVE USE" WAS ON_AFTER "MOST RECENT VISIT"
  THEN IF "AGE" IS GT 40
  AND "CIGARETTE SMOKER"
    THEN Smokers on "B/C" pills" over age 40 have a CV mortality risk 10X that of patients on traditional birth control & 2.5X the mortality risk of expected pregnancies off all birth control. Nonsmokers on B/C pills have a risk 3X that of nonsmokers on IUD's. Alternative contraception should be sought [494]. R:2229
  AND EXIT
  ELSE IF "MOST RECENT VISIT" WAS BEFORE 1/1
  AND LAST "SMOKER 0-1" WAS NOT = 0
  AND "AGE" IS GT 35
    THEN If patient is a smoker, her CV mortality risk from "B/C pills" is 6X that of the mortality risk of patients on IUD's & 2X that of patients using traditional birth control and therefore alternative birth control method should be considered. R:2229
  AND EXIT
  ELSE IF
  "DIAS BP SITTING LAST" WAS GT 100
    THEN "oral contraceptives" may cause or aggravate hypertension (R:1168). Alternative contraceptive method should be sought.
  AND EXIT

Estrogens are contraindicated in some forms of porphyria. This protocol simply reminds the clinician of that fact.

IF LAST "COPROPORPH T-URINE" WAS GT HIGH_NORMAL
& ON_AFTER "MOST RECENT VISIT"
OR LAST "UROPORPHYRIN" WAS GT HIGH_NORMAL &
ON_AFTER "MOST RECENT VISIT" OR "PORPHYRINS QUAL"
WAS NE "NEG" & ON_AFTER "MOST RECENT VISIT"
OR "PORPHYRIA DX" EXISTS
> **THEN if lab results suggesting porphyria are verified, "estrogens" are contraindicated. R:12**

The basis of the following rule is the clinical maxim that the least treatment is the best. In younger women, the most important adverse effect of birth control pills is venous thrombosis and pulmonary embolism. Some empirical data suggest that the risks of these complications are less with 50-μg than with 80 μg doses of mestrinol. Extrapolating from these observations it seems likely (but is not certain) that the risk could be reduced even further by use of the 30 μg pills that are currently available.

IF "ESTRGN B/C'S LRG USE" WAS ON_AFTER "MOST
RECENT VISIT"
> **THEN Note of interest: B/C pills with 30 mcg estrogen (e.g. "Lo/OVRAL 28") provide as effective birth control as patient's current B/C pills and may have less CV risk. R:803.**

Replacement estrogens increase the risk of endometrial cancer (R:3101).

IF "ESTROGEN USE" WAS ON_AFTER "MOST RECENT
VISIT" AND "AGE" IS GT 50
AND NO "HYSTERECTOMY SURG" EXISTS
> **THEN "Estrogens" increase the risk of endometrial ca 4-8 fold, yielding a net cancer risk greater than that of smoking. (If hysterectomy has been done, please disregard message and note date of hysterectomy = _____here.) R:1349**

AND EXIT

The following is just a simple reminder about the potential causal effect of estrogens on trigylceride elevations (R:1159).

IF "HYPERTRIGLYCERIDE DX" OCCURRED ON_AFTER
"MOST RECENT VISIT"
> **THEN Reconsider need for "estrogens" in presence of hyperlipidemia since estrogens may be a contributing factor.**

END BLOCK ESTROGEN CONTROL

END BLOCK GYNECOLOGY

Example 12

DECIDING ON TREATMENT FOR LOW BACK PAIN

Clinical orientation:	Clinical condition (symptom state)
Clinical purpose:	Management
Complexity:	Low
Format:	Decision path graphic
Intended users:	Patients

This simple guideline was designed specifically for patient use and is taken from a well-known book designed to help individuals decide whether to consult a physician, apply home treatment, or do nothing.

Like other items in the appendix aimed at patients, it uses formatting and graphics effectively, and the decision steps are depicted serially. It is oriented toward a clinical situation (actually, the symptom state of pain in the lower back as the patient would experience it), not toward the technologies (drugs, procedures, etc.) that clinicians might eventually use to care for the patient if the patient decided to seek care.

SOURCE: Vickery, D.M. and Fries, J.F. *Take Care of Yourself.* Copyright 1990, Reading, Pa.: Addison-Wesley Publishing Company. Used with permission.

Low Back Pain

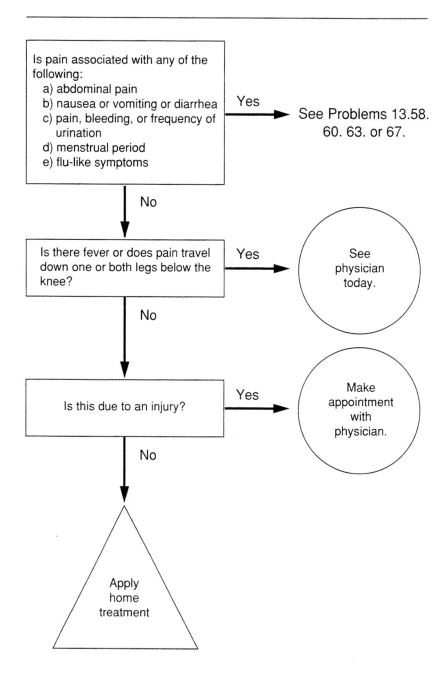

Is pain associated with any of the following:
    a) abdominal pain
    b) nausea or vomiting or diarrhea
    c) pain, bleeding, or frequency of urination
    d) menstrual period
    e) flu-like symptoms

Yes → See Problems 13. 58. 60. 63. or 67.

No

Is there fever or does pain travel down one or both legs below the knee?

Yes → See physician today.

No

Is this due to an injury?

Yes → Make appointment with physician.

No

Apply home treatment

Example 13

MANAGEMENT OF PATIENTS FOLLOWING CORONARY ARTERY BYPASS GRAFT

Clinical orientation: Clinical condition (care needed after a specific surgical procedure)

Clinical purpose: Management

Complexity: Medium

Format: Critical pathway

Intended users: Practitioners, particularly nurses

Critical pathways for care are intended to indicate appropriate and efficient steps and timing of care. Typically, they reflect more the established practice norms—that is, the clinical experience and consensus—at the institution developing the pathway than conclusions based on rigorous review and analysis of the scientific literature. They usually cover (explicitly or otherwise) multiple caregivers and services in the institution or practice; in the case of pathways developed by inpatient medical centers, they may (as in this case) provide some guidance on the posthospitalization services to be arranged before discharge. Specific steps in the pathway such as drug therapy may then be covered by more detailed protocols.

Like several of the items in the appendix dealing with the management of a patient with a specific clinical state, this guideline is explicitly sequential in its approach to care; intermediate evaluations of the patient's state are necessary before a patient "moves" to the next step in the process. Presumably because of its intended audience (physicians and nurses within a single institution), it makes liberal use of specialized abbreviations.

This guideline provides a concrete example of the importance of formatting. What is here represented on four pages was originally a single 8.5″ × 11″ page printed sideways. Not only is the original easier to consult in an actual cardiac care unit, it provides a sense of progress as the plan of care moves across the page from many activities (DAY 1) to fewer (DAY 9). The formatting requirements of this book have in effect compromised the clarity of this guideling example.

Finally, this guideline illustrates how guidelines or protocols may be diffused; the staff of Holston Valley Hospital adapted (but only slightly) a guideline developed by the New England Medical Center in Boston.

SOURCE: Holston Valley Hospital and Medical Center, Kingsport, Tennessee. Used with permission.

HOLSTON VALLEY HOSPITAL AND MEDICAL CENTER
CABG CRITICAL PATH

PATIENT ___
PHYSICIAN ___
DATE REVIEWED ___

RM ___

CASE MANAGER ___
DRG 107
EXPECTED LOS ___

	Day 1	Day 2	Day 3	Day 4
DATE	Admit PCICU, CICU, or Med Surg.	to OR, then CICU	POD 1	POD 2 transfer to PCICU
CONSULTS	Cardiologist, Anesthesiologist, Surgical PA, CICU RN			Discharge Planning Social Services as as needed
TESTS	Chest X-Ray, EKG, CBC, SMA 18, UA, TxX, ABG, Open Heart Coag panel, occasionally PFT and OPG Duplex Heparin Assay Direct Donal Blood offered	Immed. + In 4 hrs. port chest x-ray, CBC, SMA 18, cong screen; K + 2 and 4 hrs p admit; EKG	EKG, CBC, SMA 18, coag screen, port chest x-ray	CBC, SMA 7-18, port chest x-ray
ACTIVITY	up Ad Lib or BRP if monitored or with Heparin drip	12 hr bed rest HOB flat then turn every 2 hrs	HOB at 30-40° then dangle at bedside if tol, then up in chair	up in chair most of day, amb. 1-2 times after chest tubes pulled
TREATMENTS	Phisoplex showers or bed baths X 3 with shampoo X 1, prep chin to toe, mouth care in AM prior to OR, weight on CICU scales	Auto trans as ord. Q 15 min X 4, then with V.S. thigh length TED hose, vent. suction prn use Ambu with 100% oxygen, IV fluids, Foley, Pacer wires, Swan Ganz, NGT, wt. Immed. & repeat after MN	Dressing chg. Q day, wean from ventilator & extubate D/C NGT weight 12MN to 2AM, Incentive Spirometry Q 4 hrs.	V.S. 1-2 hrs. DC Foley

MEDS	Continue as per usual at home, DC all ASA salis. agents and anti-coag., preop-Kelzol, Persantine, Zantac, nasal O2	O2,IV vasopressor, antiarrythmics as ordered, analgesics, ASA, Persantine, Riopan, Cephalosporin unless allergic to PCN	Nasal O2, titrate & wean from vaso-pressors and K + drips	maint. IV fluids with K+, Oral Vit., Dulcolax Supp.
DIET	Low Na + and/or Low Sat. Fat Corn Oil NPO p MN	NPO	sips + ice chips	clear to full liquids
TEACHING	Teaching plans CABG, by Respiratory Dept. for disp. Spirometry Cardiac Rehab	pt + family about communication with ETT, pain, fluid restriction	reason for being up in chair to drain chest	Moving Right Along Booklet given, teaching regarding ambulation and need to be out of bed, reason for airing Geo Mat mattress
DISCHARGE PLANNING	screen and assess who will assist home care p OR Family Support/Assessment	transfer to CICU p OR		Transfer to PCICU

ADMISSION DATE_____ DISCHARGE DATE/TIME_____
VARIATIONS FROM STANDARD (RECORD ON BACK)

HOLSTON VALLEY HOSPITAL AND MEDICAL CENTER
CABG CRITICAL PATH

PATIENT _____ RM _____

PHYSICIAN _____ CASE MANAGER _____

DATE REVIEWED _____ DRG _107_

EXPECTED LOS _____

DATE	Day 5 POD 3	Day 6 POD 4	Day 7 POD 5	Day 8 POD 6
CONSULTS			Discharge by 6:00 p.m. or	D/C by 11:00 am
TESTS	Port, chest X-ray CBC, SMA 7-18	as ordered	pre discharge work up - EKG, PA & Lat Chest X-ray in dept., CBC, SMA 18 bed rest 2 hrs. after pacer wires pulled, then amb.	
ACTIVITY	ambulate 3-4 times Phase 1 Activity Program - Active ROM leg & arm Bid - 6 reps	8 reps		10 reps
TREATMENTS	V.S. 2-4 hrs. daily wt. at 5 am		stop dressings if staples removed	

MEDS	stop O2, IV to INT if eating well	stop antibiotic stop IMT if off monitor	
DIET	Low Na + and/or Low Sat Fat Corn Oil		
TEACHING	Discharge teaching started, Cardiac Rehab teaching started and Booklet given, need for warm up exercises and avoid sternal stress	diet class with Clinical Dietician CAD & Risk factor modification	Discharge teaching completed Exercises plan for home
DISCHARGE PLANNING	Discharge Planning In progress		D/P completed with teaching

copyright 1992
Holston Valley Hospital and Medical Group

Example 14

GUIDELINES FOR THE MANAGEMENT OF PATIENTS WITH PSORIASIS

Clinical orientation:	Clinical condition
Clinical purpose:	Management (referral to consultant, treatment) and quality assurance audit
Complexity:	Medium
Format:	Free text, tables, photographs, lists (excerpts provided)
Intended users:	Practitioners ("everyone. . .concerned in the management of patients with psoriasis" p. 829)

This rather comprehensive guideline uses varied formats: free text, quick reference boxes, color photographs, tables, and a list of yes/no questions that parallels the guidelines in structure and is used for quality assurance. The photographs in particular present useful examples of chronic plaque, guttate, localized and generalized pustular, and erythrodermic psoriases. The specific pharmaceutical agents, the necessary pretreatment assessment, contraindications, response time, and areas for monitoring are summarized in a table (reproduced here).

Like Example 11 on the use of oral contraceptives, this guideline addresses the treatment of an ongoing condition; for both the treatment is "suppressive." Like Examples 1, 7, and 8 it summarizes the current information about a clinical condition in an easily read, free-text version. Like the graphic representations of the guidelines on low back pain and dysuria (Examples 12 and 15) this guideline takes an explicitly cumulative approach to treatment—topical treatments are discussed, as a first level of care, then phototherapy and photochemotherapy. The guideline explicitly takes patient concerns and preferences into consideration; it also addresses the question of when to refer a patient from a general practitioner to a consultant dermatologist. Finally, an interesting facet is the quality assurance checklist, which appears to be designed for use by the individual physician rather than by a hospital or other review organization.

SOURCE: Workshop of the Research Unit of the Royal College of Physicians of London; Department of Dermatology, University of Glasgow; British Association of Dermatologists. Guidelines for management of patients with psoriasis. *British Medical Journal* 303:829-835, 1991. Used with permission.

Types of psoriasis

CHRONIC PLAQUE PSORIASIS

Figure 1 illustrates chronic plaque psoriasis. Depending on the patient's wishes, appropriate management includes the option of no active treatment or the use of a simple emollient. If active treatment is required then the vast majority of patients can be adequately managed with topical agents of proved efficacy such as tar[3] and dithranol.[4] Under carefully monitored conditions, which are fully recorded below, the use of topical corticosteroid preparations is also appropriate.

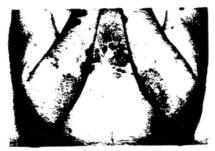

FIG 1—*Chronic plaque psoriasis*

Although each patient must be individually assessed, in general the larger the individual psoriatic plaques and the fewer their number the more appropriate is dithranol. The more numerous the lesions and the smaller they are, the more difficult the use of dithranol becomes, and tar and topical corticosteroids become more suitable. The effect of all topical treatments can be enhanced by suitably supervised treatment with ultraviolet B radiation.

Care must be exercised when a patient's psoriasis is in an inflammatory, eruptive, or unstable phase. In these circumstances the skin may display a general, non-specific irritancy to topical treatments, and therefore only emollients or low concentrations of tar or dithranol should be used.

Topical coal tar—Coal tar is extremely safe and can be used either as a refined product, of which there are many commercially available examples, or as cruder extracts such as crude coal tar in petroleum jelly. The cruder tar extracts are messier to use but are generally considered to be much more effective than more refined products such as coal tar solution. Although there is little published evidence to support the use of any particular concentration, a common treatment regimen is to start with concentrations of 0·5-1·0% of crude coal tar in petroleum jelly and increase the concentration every few days to a maximum of 10%.

Topical dithranol (anthralin)—Use of dithranol must be accompanied by adequate explanation of side effects, such as irritancy and staining of the skin and clothes. To minimise side effects treatment should normally be started at a concentration between 0·1% and 0·25% and increased in doubling concentrations as the response of psoriasis and development of drug induced irritancy allows. Great care should be taken with dithranol on sensitive body sites such as the face, flexures, and genitalia. It is reasonable to start treatment with a commercially available preparation, but for resistant lesions there may be an advantage in prescribing a similar concentration of dithranol in a different preparation such as modified Lassar's paste. The use of dithranol in the so called "short contact mode," in which the preparation is left on the skin for only 15 to 45 minutes every 24 hours, can be of great social advantage to the patient without a significant reduction in efficacy.[5]

Topical corticosteroids—Although effective, cosmetically acceptable, and safe under proper supervision, the use of topical corticosteroids in psoriasis is accompanied by a risk of side effects such as dermal atrophy, tachyphylaxis, fast relapse times, precipitation of unstable and pustular psoriasis,[6] and, in extreme cases, adrenal suppression due to systemic absorption. These risks are related to the potency and cumulative amount of steroid used and the concomitant use of occlusion. If appropriate guidelines are followed (box), however, the use of British National Formulary grade IV (mild) preparation on the face and a grade IV or grade III (moderately potent) preparation elsewhere remains a useful and acceptable therapeutic option.

Guidelines for the use of topical corticosteroids

● There should be regular clinical review

● No unsupervised repeat prescriptions should be made

● No more than 100 g of a British National Formulary grade III (moderately potent) preparation should be applied each month

● There should be periods each year when alternative treatment is employed

● Use of British National Formulary grade I (very potent) or grade II (potent) preparations should be under dermatological supervision

Systemic agents used in treatment of psoriasis

Systemic agent	Pretreatment assessment	Contraindications	Approximate response time	Precautions and monitoring
PUVA (psoralens + ultraviolet A)	History and examination, liver function tests + eye examination	Pregnancy or wish to conceive, clinically significant cataracts, age <18 years, previous cutaneous malignancy, previously received ionising radiation or arsenicals, concomitant methotrexate or cyclosporin. Hypersensitivity to psoralens, psoriasis on shielded sites — for example, scalp — previously received PUVA with cumulative lifetime dose of >1000 J/cm² ultraviolet A	Four weeks	Contraception, ultraviolet A eye protection, shielding of genitalia unless specific need to treat,[v,v] regular skin examination for premalignant and malignant changes
Methotrexate	History and examination, full blood count, liver function tests, serum urea and electrolytes, serum creatinine, creatinine clearance	Pregnancy, breast feeding, wish to conceive, wish to father children, significant hepatic damage, anaemia, leucopenia, thrombocytopenia, excessive alcohol consumption, acute infectious diseases, diabetes or extreme obesity, immunodeficiency, interactive drugs, renal impairment (reduce dose)	Two weeks	Contraception (men and women), avoid drugs which interact (for example, non-steroidal anti-inflammatory drugs and co-trimoxazole), full blood count, liver function tests, serum urea and electrolytes, serum creatinine, consider liver biopsy
Etretinate	History and examination, full blood count, liver function tests, fasting serum lipids, spine radiography, pregnancy test	Pregnancy or wish to conceive within two years of stopping treatment, severe hypercholesterolaemia or hypertriglyceridaemia, severe hepatic or renal impairment, concomitant methotrexate	Six weeks	Contraception, liver function tests and fasting serum lipids (one month after starting treatment and then every three to six months), annual lateral radiography of thoracic spine
Cyclosporin	History and examination, blood pressure, serum creatinine, measurement of glomerular filtration rate, serum urea and electrolytes, magnesium and uric acid	Abnormal renal function, uncontrolled hypertension (diastolic blood pressure >95 mm Hg), previous or concomitant malignancy, concomitant radiation therapy, pregnancy and breast feeding, immunodeficiency and immunosuppression, interactive drugs, drug or alcohol misuse	Three weeks	Contraception, blood pressure (reduce dose if diastolic >95 mm Hg), serum creatinine (reduce dose if value increases >30% of patient's own baseline value)
Hydroxyurea	History and examination, full blood count, serum urea and electrolytes, serum creatinine	Pregnancy and breast feeding, severe anaemia or leucopenia or thrombocytopenia, hypersensitivity to hydroxyurea	Four weeks	Contraception, full blood count, liver function tests (weekly during first month and then monthly)
Azathioprine	History and examination, full blood count, serum urea and electrolytes, serum creatinine, liver function tests	Pregnancy and breast feeding, severe anaemia, significant hepatic damage, interactive drugs	Four weeks	Contraception, full blood count, liver function tests (weekly during first two months and then with decreasing frequency), avoid drugs which interact
Systemic steroids	Used only in extreme and very rare circumstances			

*Estimate of how long any particular treatment should be tried before deciding it is ineffective.
†Measurement of aspartate aminotransferase, alanine aminotransferase, alkaline phosphatase, γ-glutamyl transpeptidase, bilirubin, and albumin.

Use of guidelines to derive audit measures

Diagnosis, assessment, and initial management

(1) Is the diagnosis in clinical doubt? — Yes/No

(2) Is the patient receiving any treatment likely to precipitate or aggravate psoriasis? — Yes (What)/No

(3) What in the patient's view is the most distressing or disabling aspect of the psoriasis?

(4) Has the nature of psoriasis been explained to the patient? — Yes/No

(5) Have the treatment options been discussed in the light of (4)? — Yes/No

(6) Has the patient had an adequately documented 8-12 week trial of topical treatment? — Yes/No

(7) If topical steroids are included in the regimen is the potency and quantity used appropriate? — Yes/No

(8) Is referral to a consultant dermatologist appropriate? — Yes/No

Phototherapy

(9) Has the minimal erythema dose been estimated? — Yes/No

(10) Is the patient receiving an appropriate treatment regimen? — Yes/No

Systemic treatment

(11) Are the indications to move to systemic treatment appropriate? — Yes/No

(12) Have the options and side effects of possible regimens been fully discussed with the patient? — Yes/No

(13) If appropriate, has the need for contraception been fully discussed and appropriate provision arranged if required? — Yes/No

(14) Has the patient been given a psoriasis systemic treatment card? — Yes/No

(15) If yes, does the patient show this card to the general practitioner when receiving prescriptions for unrelated problems? — Yes/No

Photochemotherapy (PUVA)

(16) Has the patient been given advice about appropriate eye protection? — Yes/No

(17) Have men been given advice about screening genitalia during PUVA? — Yes/No

(18) Has the minimal phototoxic dose been estimated? — Yes/No

(19) Is there a clear record of individual treatments and cumulative ultraviolet A dosage? — Yes/No

(20) Is the patient receiving an appropriate review and follow up programme? — Yes/No

Methotrexate

(21) Have pretreatment investigations excluded haematological, biochemical, and hepatic contraindications? — Yes/No

(22) Is the patient taking any drug known to have an adverse interaction with methotrexate? — Yes/No

(23) Are the arrangements for regular review and haematological and biochemical monitoring appropriate? — Yes/No

Etretinate

(24) For women has the need for prolonged contraception (two years) after withdrawal of drug been fully discussed? — Yes/No

(25) Is the dosage regimen appropriate? — Yes/No

(26) Are review arrangements adequate? — Yes/No

Cyclosporin

(27) Has the serum creatinine concentration been measured? — Yes/No

(28) Have potential drug interactions been considered? — Yes/No

(29) Is the current dose of cyclosporin appropriate? — Yes/No

Example 15

ACUTE DYSURIA IN THE ADULT FEMALE

Clinical orientation: Clinical condition
Clinical purpose: Treatment and management
Complexity: Medium
Format: Algorithm
Intended users: Practitioners

The Harvard Community Health Plan (HCHP) is a multisite, group-model health maintenance organization. Over the past several years, HCHP has developed an extensive series of computer-accessible algorithms for ambulatory care management. Each algorithm is developed by a task force of clinicians based on a thorough review of the scientific literature. The task forces operate under the guidance of a research faculty and staff who are experienced in algorithm development. Each algorithm is followed by explanatory notes regarding options, patients at special risk, and recommended medications and dosages. Some are several pages long.

Like many of the items in this appendix, this guideline is designed for use by practitioners or other health care personnel in the patient's presence; the liberal use of abbreviations makes this easier. It also involves step-by-step decisionmaking, whether by a practitioner or a patient. The relative complexity of this graphic—which is intended for physicians—might usefully be contrasted with the simplicity of the graphic for low back pain (Example 12)—which is intended for lay persons. It also illustrates some of the points made in the text concerning rules for formatting flowcharts and algorithms.

SOURCE: Harvard Community Health Plan, Cambridge, Massachusetts. Used with permission.

ACUTE DYSURIA IN THE ADULT FEMALE (A)

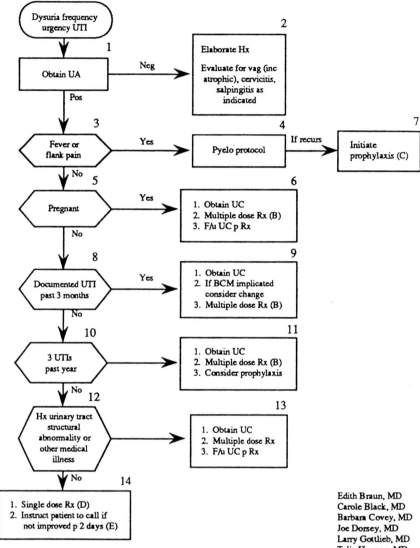

Dysuria frequency urgency UTI

1. Obtain UA
   - Neg → 2. Elaborate Hx / Evaluate for vag (inc atrophic), cervicitis, salpingitis as indicated
   - Pos ↓

3. Fever or flank pain
   - Yes → 4. Pyelo protocol
     - If recurs → 7. Initiate prophylaxis (C)
   - No ↓

5. Pregnant
   - Yes → 6.
     1. Obtain UC
     2. Multiple dose Rx (B)
     3. F/u UC p Rx
   - No ↓

8. Documented UTI past 3 months
   - Yes → 9.
     1. Obtain UC
     2. If BCM implicated consider change
     3. Multiple dose Rx (B)
   - No ↓

10. 3 UTIs past year
    - Yes → 11.
      1. Obtain UC
      2. Multiple dose Rx (B)
      3. Consider prophylaxis
    - No ↓

12. Hx urinary tract structural abnormality or other medical illness
    - Yes → 13.
      1. Obtain UC
      2. Multiple dose Rx
      3. F/u UC p Rx
    - No ↓

14.
1. Single dose Rx (D)
2. Instruct patient to call if not improved p 2 days (E)

Edith Braun, MD
Carole Black, MD
Barbara Covey, MD
Joe Dorsey, MD
Larry Gottlieb, MD
Talia Herman, MD
Beth Ingram, PA
Carl Isihara, MD
Mon Kim, MD
Tom Lawrence, MD
Carmi Margolis, MD
Marvin Packer, MD
Barbara Stewart, MD

HCHP clinical guidelines are designed to assist clinicians by providing an analytical framework for the evaluation and treatment of the more common problems of HCHP patients. They are not intended either to replace a clinician's clinical judgement or to establish a protocol for all patients with a particular condition. It is understood that some patients will not fit the clinical conditions contemplated by a guideline and that a guideline will rarely establish the only appropriate approach to a problem.

ACUTE DYSURIA IN THE ADULT FEMALE

A. A primary goal of this algorithm is to separate women with acute uncomplicated UTI that can be treated with single dose antibiotic therapy from women
with complicated UTI that will require further evaluation or longer duration of
therapy. Therefore, women who have symptoms longer than 2 or 3 days,
women who have fever or flank pain, pregnant women and women with frequent recurrences or other underlying medical problems need to be eliminated
from this algorithm. Initial steps in their management are suggested at branch
points of this algorithm, but other algorithms will be necessary to more fully
address the management of these groups of patients.

Stamm, W., Causes of the Acute Urethral Syndrome in Women, NEJM 1980; 303;
409-415.

B. Choices for multiple dose Rx include 7-10 day course of:

1. Trimethoprim sulfa DS BID (contraindicated in pregnancy, known G6PD
deficiency or allergic Hx).
2. Amoxicillin 250 mg po tid (lst choice in pregnancy).
3. Nitrofurantoin 50 mg QID (alternative for patient with multiple allergies
or pregnant patient with Hx Pen allergy).

C. Prophylaxis is usually continued for 6 months.

Options for prophylaxis include:

1. Trimethoprim sulfa 1/2 regular strength tab, QHS.
2. Nitrofurantoin 50 mg QHS (in pregnant patient or patient with Hx T/X
allergy or known G6PD deficiency).

Ronald, A. and Harding, G., Urinary Infection Prophylaxis in Women, Annals Int.
Med. 1981; 94(2) 268-269.

D. Options for single dose Rx include:

1. Trimethoprim sulfa DS 2 tabs x 1.
2. Amoxicillin 3 gm po x 1.

Kamaroff, A., Acute Dysuria in Women, NEJM 1984; 310; 368-375.

E. Patients who have failed single dose Rx should be considered to have upper
tract infection and treated per pyelo protocol.

Example 16

MANAGEMENT OF ACUTE PAIN

Clinical orientation: Clinical condition
Clinical purpose: Management of acute pain due to operative
procedures, medical procedures, or trauma
Complexity: Medium
Format: Free text, flow charts, tables, graphic pain scales
Intended users: Practitioners and patients

The following pages are excerpts from the 1992 guideline, *Acute Pain Management: Operative or Medical Procedures and Trauma*, commissioned by the Agency for Health Care Policy and Research (AHCPR). The guideline addresses the "widespread inadequacy of pain management" (AHCPR, February 1992, p. 1) by providing clinicians and patients with approaches and tools for assessing and managing pain.

An interdisciplinary panel developed the guideline. They focused on the need for pain management, clinical practice patterns, and clinical and technological options for pain management. The development process included an extensive literature search, evaluation of the quality of clinical data, peer review of drafts of the guideline, tests of the guidelines in clinical situations, an open meeting for testimony, and use of external consultants.

The guideline is available in four forms. In addition to the full guideline cited above, there are two "quick reference guides for clinicians"—*Acute Pain Management in Infants, Children, and Adolescents: Operative and Medical Procedures* and *Acute Pain Management in Adults: Operative Procedures*—and a patient's guide, *Pain Control After Surgery*, available in both English and Spanish. The guideline will also be incorporated into data bases at the National Library of Medicine and the National Technical Information Service and into the computer-based information systems.

The complete guide discusses: the need for aggressive postoperative control of pain; pain assessment and reassessment; options for preventing and controlling postoperative pain; control of site-specific pain; management of pain in infants, children, adolescents, and other patients with special needs (e.g., the elderly, known or suspected substance abusers); and institutional responsibility for effective pain relief. It also contains a significant list of references and appendices.

SOURCES: Reprinted (public domain) from: Acute Pain Management Guideline Panel. *Acute Pain Management: Operative or Medical Procedures and Trauma. Clinical Practice Guideline.* AHCPR Pub. No. 92-0032. Rockville, Md.: Agency for Health Care Policy and Research, Public Health Service, U.S. Department of Health and Human Services. February 1992. Acute Pain Management Guideline Panel. *Acute Pain Management in Adults: Operative Procedures. Quick Reference Guide for Clinicians.* AHCPR Pub. No. 92-0019. Rockville, Md.: Agency for Health Care Policy and Research, Public Health Service, U.S. Department of Health and Human Services. 1992.

Pain Treatment Flow Chart:
Postoperative Phase

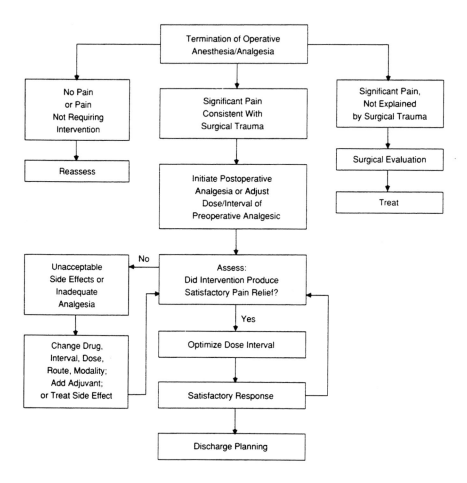

Options to Prevent and Control Postoperative Pain

Patient education and reduction of any preexisting pain should occur before the operation. Because the goal of the treatment plan is to prevent significant postoperative pain from the outset, treatment alternatives, potential risks, dosage adjustments, and adjunctive therapies should be described to the patient and family. Teaching emphasizes what the patient is likely to experience postoperatively, including the specific method(s) of pain assessment, intervention(s) the staff will employ, and the level of patient participation required. Staff also should inform patients that it is easier to prevent pain than to "chase" or treat it once it has become established, and that communication of unrelieved pain is essential to its relief.

Pain control options include:

- Cognitive-behavioral interventions such as relaxation, distraction, and imagery; these can be taught preoperatively and can reduce pain, anxiety, and the amount of drugs needed for pain control;

- Systemic administration of nonsteroidal anti-inflammatory drugs (NSAIDs) or opioids using the traditional "as needed" schedule or around-the-clock administration (American Pain Society, 1989);

- Patient controlled analgesia (PCA), usually meaning self-medication with intravenous doses of an opioid; this can include other classes of drugs administered orally or by other routes;

- Spinal analgesia, usually by means of an epidural opioid and/or local anesthetic injected intermittently or infused continuously;

- Intermittent or continuous local neural blockade (examples of the former include intercostal nerve blockade with local anesthetic or cryoprobe; the latter includes infusion of local anesthetic through an interpleural catheter);

- Physical agents such as massage or application of heat or cold; and

- Electroanalgesia such as transcutaneous electrical nerve stimulation (TENS).

Examples of Pain Intensity and Pain Distress Scales

Pain Intensity Scales

Simple Descriptive Pain Intensity Scale*

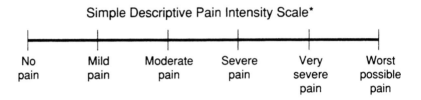

| No pain | Mild pain | Moderate pain | Severe pain | Very severe pain | Worst possible pain |

0 - 10 Numeric Pain Intensity Scale*

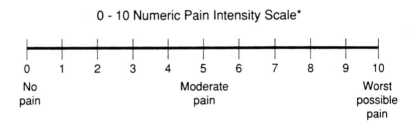

0   1   2   3   4   5   6   7   8   9   10

No pain   Moderate pain   Worst possible pain

Visual Analog Scale (VAS)**

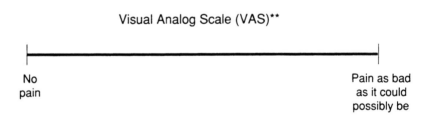

No pain

Pain as bad as it could possibly be

*If used as a graphic rating scale, a 10-cm baseline is recommended.
**A 10-cm baseline is recommended for VAS scales.

Institutional Responsibility for Pain Management

The institutional process of acute pain management begins with the affirmation that patients should have access to the best level of pain relief that may safely be provided. (See Table 3 for a summary of the scientific evidence for interventions to manage pain in adults.) Each institution should develop the resources necessary to provide the best and most modern pain relief appropriate to its patients and should designate who and/or which departments are responsible for the required activities.

Optimal application of pain control methods depends on cooperation among different members of the health care team throughout the patient's course of treatment. To ensure that this process occurs effectively, formal means must be developed and used within each institution to assess pain management practices and to obtain patient feedback to gauge the adequacy of pain control.

The institution's quality assurance procedures should be used periodically to assure that the following pain management practices are being carried out:

- Patients are informed that effective pain relief is an important part of their treatment, that communication of unrelieved pain is essential, and that health professionals will respond quickly to their reports of pain. They are also told that a total absence of pain is often not a realistic or even a desirable goal.

- Clear documentation of pain assessment and management is provided.

- There are institution-defined levels for pain intensity and relief that elicit review of current pain therapy, documentation of the proposed modifications in treatment, and subsequent review of their efficacy.

- Each clinical unit periodically assesses a randomly selected sample of patients who have had surgery within 72 hours to determine their current pain intensity, the worst pain intensity in the first 24 hours, the degree of relief obtained from pain management interventions, satisfaction with relief, and satisfaction with the staff"s responsiveness.

Table 3.   Scientific Evidence for Interventions to Manage Pain in Adults

Pharmacologic Interventions

Intervention[1]		Type of Evidence	Comments
NSAIDs	Oral (alone)	Ib, IV	Effective for mild to moderate pain. Begin preoperatively. Relatively contraindicated in patients with renal disease and risk of or actual coagulopathy. May mask fever.
	Oral (adjunct to opioid)	Ia, IV	Potentiating effect resulting in opioid sparing. Begin preop. Cautions as above.
	Parenteral (ketorolac)	Ib, IV	Effective for moderate to severe pain. Expensive. Useful where opioids contraindicated, especially to avoid respiratory depression and sedation. Advance to opioid.
Opioids	Oral	IV	As effective as parenteral in appropriate doses. Use as soon as oral medication tolerated. Route of choice.
	Intramuscular	Ib, IV	Has been the standard parenteral route, but injections painful and absorption unreliable. Hence, avoid this route when possible.
	Subcutaneous	Ib, IV	Preferable to intramuscular for low-volume continuous infusion. Injections painful and absorption unreliable. Avoid this route for long-term repetitive dosing.
	Intravenous	Ib, IV	Parenteral route of choice after major surgery. Suitable for titrated bolus or continuous administration (including PCA), but requires monitoring. Significant risk of respiratory depression with inappropriate dosing.
	PCA (systemic)	Ia, IV	Intravenous or subcutaneous routes recommended. Good, steady level of analgesia. Popular with patients but requires special infusion pumps and staff education. See cautions about opioids above.
	Epidural and intrathecal	Ia, IV	When suitable, provides good analgesia. Significant risk of respiratory depression, sometimes delayed in onset. Requires careful monitoring. Use of infusion pumps requires additional equipment and staff education.
Local Anesthetics	Epidural and intrathecal	Ia, IV	Limited indications. Expensive if infusion pumps employed. Effective regional analgesia. Opioid sparing. Addition of opioid to local anesthetic may improve analgesia. Risks of hypotension, weakness, numbness. Use of infusion pump requires additional equipment and staff.
	Peripheral nerve block	Ia, IV	Limited indications and duration of action. Effective regional analgesia. Opioid sparing.

Nonpharmacologic Interventions

Intervention[1]		Type of Evidence	Comments
Simple Relaxation (begin preoperatively)	Jaw relaxation Progressive muscle relaxation Simple imagery	Ia, IIa, IIb, IV	Effective in reducing mild to moderate pain and as an adjunct to analgesic drugs for severe pain. Use when patients express an interest in relaxation. Requires 3–5 minutes of staff time for instructions.
	Music	Ib, IIa, IV	Both patient-preferred and "easy listening" music are effective in reducing mild to moderate pain.
Complex Relaxation (begin preoperatively)	Biofeedback	Ib, IIa, IV	Effective in reducing mild to moderate pain and operative site muscle tension. Requires skilled personnel and special equipment.
	Imagery	Ib, IIa, IIb, IV	Effective for reduction of mild to moderate pain. Requires skilled personnel.
Education/ Instruction (begin preoperatively)		Ia, IIa, IIb, IV	Effective for reduction of pain. Should include sensory and procedural information and instruction aimed at reducing activity related pain. Requires 5–15 minutes of staff time.
TENS		Ia, IIa, III, IV	Effective in reducing pain and improving physical function. Requires skilled personnel and special equipment. May be useful as an adjunct to drug therapy.

[1] Insufficient scientific evidence is available to provide specific recommendations regarding the use of hypnosis, acupuncture, and other physical modalities for relief of postoperative pain.

Type of Evidence – Key

Ia   Evidence obtained from meta-analysis of randomized controlled trials.

Ib   Evidence obtained from at least one randomized controlled trial.

IIa   Evidence obtained from at least one well-designed controlled study without randomization.

IIb   Evidence obtained from at least one other type of well-designed quasi-experimental study.

III   Evidence obtained from well-designed nonexperimental descriptive studies, such as comparative studies, correlational studies, and case studies.

IV   Evidence obtained from expert committee reports or opinions and/or clinical experiences of respected authorities.

Note: References are available in the *Guideline Report. Acute Pain Management: Operative or Medical Procedures and Trauma.* AHCPR Pub. No. 92–0001. Rockville, MD: Agency for Health Care Policy and Research, Public Health Service, U.S. Department of Health and Human Services. In press.

Summary

Summary recommendations 1-5 and 7, below, should be implemented in every hospital where operations are performed on inpatients. The Acute Pain Management Guideline Panel recommends that any hospital in which abdominal or thoracic operations are routinely performed offer patients postoperative regional anesthetic, epidural or intrathecal opioids, PCA infusions, and other interventions requiring a similar level of expertise, under the supervision of an acute pain service as described in summary recommendation 6, below. For pain management to be effective, each hospital must designate who or which department will be responsible for all of the required activities.

There are a number of alternative approaches to preventing or relieving postoperative pain, many of which can give good results if attentively applied. The following elements, however, apply to most cases and might serve as a focus for assessing the results of these guidelines:

1. *Promise patients attentive analgesic care.* Patients should be informed before surgery, verbally and in printed format, that effective pain relief is an important part of their treatment, that talking about unrelieved pain is essential, and that health professionals will respond quickly to their reports of pain. It should be made clear to patients and families, however, that the total absence of any postoperative discomfort is normally not a realistic or even a desirable goal.

2. *Chart and display assessment of pain and relief.* A simple assessment of pain intensity and pain relief should be recorded on the bedside vital sign chart or a similar record that encourages easy, regular review by members of the health care team and is incorporated in the patient's permanent record. The intensity of pain should be assessed and documented at regular intervals (depending on the severity of pain) and with each new report of pain. The degree of pain relief should be determined after each pain management intervention, once a sufficient time has elapsed for the treatment to reach peak effect. A simple, valid measure of intensity and relief should be selected by each clinical unit. For children, age-appropriate measures should be used.

3. *Define pain and relief levels to trigger a review.* Each institution should identify pain intensity and pain relief levels that will elicit a review of the current pain therapy, documentation of the proposed modifications in treatment, and subsequent review of its efficacy. This process of treatment review and followup should include participation by physicians and nurses involved in the patient's care.

4. *Survey patient satisfaction.* At regular intervals defined by the clinical unit and quality assurance committee, each clinical unit should assess a randomly selected sample of patients who have had surgery within 72 hours. Patients should

be asked their current pain intensity, the worst pain intensity in the past 24 hours, the degree of relief obtained from pain management interventions, satisfaction with relief, and their satisfaction with the staff's responsiveness.

5. *Analgesic drug treatment should comply with several basic principles*:

a. *Non-opioid "peripherally acting" analgesics*. Unless contraindicated, every patient should receive an around-the-clock postoperative regimen of an NSAID. For patients unable to take medications by mouth, it may be necessary to use the parenteral or rectal route.

b. *Opioid analgesics*. Analgesic orders should allow for the great variation in individual opioid requirements, including a regularly scheduled dose and "rescue" doses for instances in which the usual regimen is insufficient.

6. *Specialized analgesic technologies*, including systemic or intraspinal, continuous or intermittent opioid administration or patient controlled dosing, local anesthetic infusion, and inhalational analgesia (e.g., nitrous oxide) should be governed by policies and standard procedures that define the acceptable level of patient monitoring and appropriate roles and limits of practice for all groups of health care providers involved. The policy should include definitions of physician and nurse accountability, physician and nurse responsibility to the patient, and the role of pharmacy.

7. *Nonpharmacological interventions*: Cognitive and behaviorally based interventions include a number of methods to help patients understand more about their pain and to take an active part in its assessment and control. These interventions are intended to supplement, not replace, pharmacological interventions. Staff should give patients information about these interventions and support patients in using them.

8. *Monitor the efficacy of pain treatment*: Periodically review pain treatment procedures as defined in summary recommendations 1-4 above, using the institution's quality assurance procedures.

B

A Provisional Instrument for Assessing Clinical Practice Guidelines

KATHLEEN N. LOHR AND MARILYN J. FIELD
Division of Health Care Services

The Institute of Medicine (IOM) of the National Academy of Sciences has been engaged since the beginning of 1990 in two projects relating to the development, implementation, and evaluation of clinical practice guidelines. One IOM committee defined practice guidelines as "systematically developed statements to assist practitioners and patients in choosing appropriate health care for specific clinical conditions." It also delineated several desirable attributes of guidelines that are intended to help users understand the elements of a sound guideline and to recognize good (or not-so-good) guidelines. These aspects of guidelines were discussed in *Clinical Practice Guidelines: Directions for a New Program* (IOM, 1990) and *Guidelines for Clinical Practice: From Development to Use* (this report).

The first IOM study committee discovered that no explicit method was available for assessing existing or emerging practice guidelines. At least one instrument was being tested to assess some aspects of guideline development (AMA, 1990), but nothing existed to judge the quality, reliability, and validity of the content of the guideline itself. Therefore, one task the second IOM committee undertook was to develop an "assessment instrument" that could be used by various parties in formal evaluations of guidelines.

The next sections of this document describe, first, the purposes of the "provisional" assessment instrument and, second, its development. The discussion covers several features of the instrument and its application, and notes several cautions and caveats about the present form, all of which warrant further consideration. Finally, the document presents the instrument itself, in three operational parts—a general information sheet, the full instrument, and a summary evaluation sheet. The instrument is termed provisional because the committee firmly believed that more experience needs to be accumulated by testing it on different kinds of guidelines.

PURPOSES OF THE ASSESSMENT INSTRUMENT

The central purpose of the IOM's instrument for assessing clinical practice guidelines is to provide an explicit method for examining the soundness of such guidelines and to encourage their systematic development. By assessment is meant a prospective judgment of the soundness of both the process used in developing a guideline *and* the resulting guideline. The intent is to avoid situations in which a guideline that is not consistent with the scientific evidence is nonetheless "rated" as good on procedural criteria alone.[1]

More concretely, the IOM intended to operationalize its attributes of good guidelines and to provide a standardized approach and structure for the assessment of a guideline document. The resulting form is not simple. Therefore, the IOM does not expect practicing physicians or other clinicians, patients, other nonprofessionals, or policymakers to apply this instrument. Rather it expects individuals (or groups) with three types of expertise to apply it—namely, those with clinical experience with patients who have the conditions or problems covered by the guideline document, those with research experience in the conditions or technologies covered, and those with methodologic skills in developing guidelines. Any final or overall judgments of a guideline document emerging from the application of this instrument would be reported in simpler, summary form in ways that would convey the relative soundness (or lack of it) of a given guideline document to all potential users of the guideline.

The IOM committee sees three possible uses of this instrument: as an educational tool, as a self-assessment tool, and as a means of judging guidelines before their adoption. The Agency for Health Care Policy and Research (AHCPR) may want to use this instrument, or one like it, in directing the work of its guidelines-development panels; the agency may also wish to employ it in judging the products of those panels or the guidelines developed by other groups, such as medical specialty societies. Furthermore, other groups may wish to review existing or draft guidelines of their own against this instrument, in an effort to identify guidelines warranting revision or defects in draft guidelines that warrant correction before they are put into final form. Finally, if an organization were to be created for the

---

[1] Evaluation of the eventual impact of guidelines is a separate step. Both IOM reports (1990 and this one) include discussions of evaluation.

express purpose of certifying or otherwise reporting on the soundness of particular guidelines, it might wish to employ the instrument as part of its review activities.

DEVELOPMENT PROCESS

The concept of the instrument originated during discussions with members of the AHCPR staff about their responsibilities for practice guidelines under the Omnibus Budget Reconciliation Act of 1989. In seeking to respond to those early ideas, the IOM committee went through four steps.

First, with the aid of an outside consultant, staff drafted a set of questions to operationalize the eight conceptual attributes of good practice guidelines identified in the IOM's 1990 report on guidelines.[2] (Discussions of these attributes introduce sections of the assessment instrument.) Second, these questions were combined with background information and instructions for users and subjected to considerable internal and external review, as described below. Members of the IOM committee twice reviewed drafts of the assessment instrument during this time.

Third, IOM staff used the critiques and suggestions of reviewers to revise the instrument, and it, together with background material, was subjected to external review according to IOM and National Research Council (NRC) procedures. Fourth, the instrument was revised in response to that external review, resulting in the provisional questionnaire and other forms incorporated into this document.

Initial Reviews

An interim draft of the instrument was sent to AHCPR in December 1990 and was subsequently forwarded to several professional societies that had volunteered to review and test the instrument against guidelines of their own. By June 1991, the committee had received more than 15 separate responses and commentaries. Responses included a lengthy summary review provided by IMCARE (Internal Medicine Center to Advance Research and Education), which had solicited reviews from the 231 internists then in its Guideline Network. IMCARE also sent the document to 147 physicians who requested more information and received 65 responses from network members who reviewed and, in many cases, applied the instruments to real guidelines.

Reactions to the draft instrument were extremely varied. With respect to format, instructions, ease of use, and similar issues, positive comments included the following:

---

[2] Anne-Marie Audet, M.D., of the Health Institute, New England Medical Center, Inc., served as consultant during the initial stage of the project.

- "Well written—concise."
- "The instrument was easy to apply and the definitions of attributes were helpful in driving the assessment."
- "The meaning of each attribute, the instructions, and response categories were generally clear."
- "Overall, the instrument provides a precise algorithm for examining the degree to which a clinical guideline meets defined aspects of seven attributes. In our opinion, the instrument can be used for its intended purpose. In addition, application of an instrument such as this is, in itself, a thought-provoking exercise for individuals active in developing clinical practice guidelines."

By contrast, negative comments were of the following kind:

- "The form seems excessively lengthy and not particularly user-friendly."
- "The instructions are verbose and redundant, and almost legalistic. They are not user-friendly."
- "This instrument was very confusing, almost 'impossible.'"
- "Instrument of intellectual torture. Beyond Bureaucracy! . . . This makes me feel stupid!"

A form that accompanied the instrument asked reviewers to indicate the time (in person-hours) needed to apply the assessment instrument to a guideline of their choice. Among 59 individuals in the IMCARE group who evidently applied the instrument to an actual guideline and completed the form, 13 said that the instrument took under two hours to apply, 38 said two to three hours, and 8 said four hours or more. Several commentators indicated that their learning curve was quite steep and that repeated use of the instrument would make it simpler and less time-consuming to apply.

In rating the overall difficulty of understanding or using the assessment instrument, the majority of respondents indicated that it was moderately to very difficult. In addition, the great majority found the instrument good or at least somewhat helpful in helping them reach an overall judgment of the strengths and weaknesses of the guideline they were evaluating. Finally, more than half indicated that the instrument definitely should be revised; most of the rest were uncertain or had no opinion, and only about 1 in 10 advised abandoning the effort.

Among the more concrete recommendations for revisions were the following: (1) add more "don't know" or "not applicable" responses to certain questions; (2) simplify and shorten the instructions; (3) include a "prologue" containing pertinent information from the first IOM (1990) report on guidelines, which defines key terms and similar concepts; (4) consider adding an attribute related to endorsement by appropriate affiliated or outside organizations; and (5) clarify exactly who the intended users are. In addition, many reviewers offered comments on the draft instrument itself, chiefly observations about the wording of questions and the addition of response categories. More general suggestions included employing the instrument to help generate guidelines (rather than rate them) and using the instrument to guide an assessment process (without necessarily requiring that the instrument be completed in full).

Final Reviews

In accordance with IOM and NRC procedures, the revised instrument was subjected to an external, anonymous review by a panel similar to the full IOM committee. The "provisional" form in this document reflects the reactions of this group of seven experts, and many of their comments have been incorporated into the discussion presented here.

IMPORTANT FEATURES OF THE PROVISIONAL ASSESSMENT INSTRUMENT

Attributes of Practice Guidelines

Types of Attributes

Four attributes identified in the first IOM report on practice guidelines concern the substance of the guidelines—clinical applicability or scope, clinical flexibility, reliability/reproducibility, and validity. Four others— clarity, multidisciplinary process, scheduled review, and documentation— have more to do with process. This instrument explicitly incorporates all attributes but documentation; that attribute is captured in questions directed at the other seven. Each attribute is described in the text of the instrument.

Implicit Weight Accorded to Different Attributes

As discussed below, this instrument has *no* explicit or quantitative scoring system. The attributes are implicitly weighted, however, according to the number of main questions used to cover them. Of a total of 46 questions, validity has 22 questions; clarity, 8; multidisciplinary process, 4; clinical flexibility, 4; reliability and reproducibility, 4; clinical adaptability, 3; and scheduled review, 1. By this rough metric, validity is accorded by far the major emphasis in the document, reflecting the committee's concern for finding a way to judge the soundness of the guidelines themselves rather than just the acceptability of the development process.

Questions and Response Categories

Questions

Most of the seven attributes are dealt with through one or more questions that tap specific "dimensions." For example, validity is divided into five issues: (1) strength of the scientific evidence and professional consensus; (2) qualitative and quantitative statements about health benefits and harms or risks; (3) qualitative and quantitative statements about expected health costs or expenditures; (4) the extent to which specific recommendations are justified by the estimates of benefits, harms, and costs provided in the guidelines *and* the extent to which those estimates are supported by the evidence amassed in the guidelines document; and (5) potential conflicts among existing guidelines, if any.

The instrument has 46 descriptive questions related to the seven attributes. Generally they pertain to the presence of information about the attribute or about a particular dimension of an attribute. Several questions have additional "items" designed to help assessors think about key points implied by the main question and whether a particular dimension of an attribute is satisfactory or not.

Responses to Questions

Responses to each question are typically "yes" or "no" for questions asking about the presence or absence of certain information, features, or development processes. If the answer is "yes," a follow-up question asks about the quality of that information, feature, or development process— essentially whether the information provided is satisfactory or not. If the answer to the main question is "no," the follow-up question probes the significance of the absence of information, a particular feature, or development process and asks whether the omission is important or not.

Satisfactory. Assessors can judge information about a particular attribute as satisfactory if all critical elements have been considered and presented. For example, the discussion or description should be thorough and comprehensive; the guideline developers should have based their work on appropriate and correct information (e.g., from the literature review); and they should have used appropriate methods (e.g., for evaluating the strength of the scientific evidence or reaching professional peer consensus).

Conditionally satisfactory. The description or discussion of an attribute or dimension is conditionally satisfactory if some, but not all, of the critical elements have been considered and presented. For example, the discussion of a particular aspect of an attribute such as scheduled review may be vague or incomplete. Alternatively, guidelines developers may have disregarded important information (about, for instance, likely risks to patients from the use of a technology) in reaching their recommendations, or they may have improperly used certain kinds of methods. These problems with the guideline document may not prevent a clinician from using it or understanding its recommendations, but they may affect its overall usefulness or call certain recommendations into question. Revisions would be presumed to improve the guidelines, but they would not be mandatory.

Unsatisfactory. The description or discussion about a specific attribute is unsatisfactory if most of the critical elements have not been considered or presented. For example, well-known pieces of clinical information (or the views of multiple specialists with an interest in the guideline topic) may have been ignored; methods of analysis may have been misapplied; or recommendations may be based on faulty information or poor logic, or both. In such a case, it would be difficult if not impossible to judge the quality of the process of guideline development or the soundness of the resulting guidelines and recommendations (or both); certainly assessors could not mark those attributes as satisfactory. Serious thought must be given to augmenting or revising the guidelines document before it is promoted further.

Omissions. Omitting a description or discussion about a specific attribute or dimension may be *unimportant* if that omission seems likely to have no demonstrable effect either on the ability of a guideline user to apply the guideline effectively in the clinical decision-making process or on the capacity of the assessor to make an independent assessment of the quality of that attribute. Omitting such a description or discussion is of *minor importance* if it seems likely to affect negatively the ability of a guideline user or of evaluators to apply the guideline effectively or independently to assess its quality. Finally, omitting such a description or discussion is a *major omission* if the absence of such information essentially prevents guideline users or evaluators from applying the guideline effectively or even making an independent evaluation about the soundness of the guidelines document itself (at least on that particular feature).

Special Cases

Special cases may arise in which information appropriately is omitted from the guideline because the question or item is not applicable or is inappropriate (given responses to earlier items, for instance). In such an instance, the assessor is asked to mark the response category most appropriate for the given case (e.g., not applicable). In other situations, assessors may find it difficult to arrive at a single answer to the question, especially if the guidelines document being evaluated is very complex or if necessary background information appears to be missing. "Comments" sections are provided throughout for assessors to record additional remarks or qualifying statements, to highlight areas not well covered by the instrument, and to note special factors that should either be followed up or taken into account in the overall judgment about the guidelines document. Finally, if assessors conclude that the guidelines document is so complex, clinically esoteric, or methodologically sophisticated that it warrants additional, outside expert review, they are asked to note that at the end of the full instrument and also on the summary evaluation sheet.

Alternative Approaches to Responses

The main type of response used in this form is categorical (e.g., satisfactory, conditionally satisfactory, and unsatisfactory). Some reviewers noted that this approach is inherently constraining and requires definitions of the three categories, which may not be interpreted consistently. Furthermore, these categories do not allow assessors to distinguish guidelines that more properly should be characterized as excellent or outstanding. To overcome some of these drawbacks, an approach to responses based on a scale might be tested.

For example, a five- or even seven-point scale might be adopted, with one end of the range described as excellent (exemplary, highly satisfactory, or a similar superlative) and the opposite end described as poor (inferior, or very unsatisfactory). The equivalent approach might also be tried for the responses concerned with omissions of information. The committee believes this change warrants testing at some point in the future development of this form.

Response Scoring

After considerable debate and consideration of reviewers' comments, the committee concluded that this instrument should not be "scored" in any quantitative way. Thus, it does not propose any formal weighting or numerical scoring scheme for the main questions, nor does it suggest a particular threshold, cutpoint, or floor against which current guidelines might be judged acceptable or unacceptable. If most responses to the questions are "satisfactory" (or "unimportant omissions"), however, one might reasonably conclude that such a guidelines document would be sufficient for most clinical situations. Alternatively, if most responses were unsatisfactory (or major omissions), one would probably argue that the guidelines document needed to be revised before it could be used effectively.

The committee was of the view that a defensible scoring system could not be designed *a priori* in any case, regardless of whether scoring would be purely categorical or more quantitative. Review and testing of the assessment instrument itself—with revisions as necessary—will be required before a sensible scoring system can be proposed. Moreover, different users of the assessment instrument may have legitimate reasons to differ on where they would establish such cutpoints. Provision of information on the quality of guidelines documents appears to be more in the public interest than is making "one-size-fits-all" judgments on behalf of others.

In the same vein, no single question is treated as the signal of a "fatal flaw." That is, for no question will a response of "no," "unsatisfactory," or "major omission" *by itself* render the guidelines document unacceptable. Some committee members believed that certain questions, especially those relating to validity, should be so designated. However, the questions that seem to be the most likely candidates for this level of decisiveness[3] were added in response to the external review of the draft document; therefore they have not yet been reviewed or tested further. The committee believes designating these (or other) items as potentially "fatal" is premature.

Response Aggregation and Display

General Comments

Information obtained from applying the instrument might eventually be arrayed in one or more qualitative, summary displays or tables, as might be done, for instance, by a *Consumer Report* article. This might provide a rough indicator of whether the guidelines document could be used effectively in clinical situations. One reviewer, for example, suggested that a report for busy practicing physicians might usefully include "a graphic summary of the degree to which each attribute was successfully achieved, e.g., a bar representing the percent of key items within each attribute that were deemed satisfactory . . . ; and . . . a brief, narrative summary assessment."

Summary Evaluation Sheet

The committee did not pursue the design of such displays, chiefly because such an effort was seen as premature for an instrument that itself warrants additional testing and application. As an intermediate step, however, the instrument does include a "summary evaluation sheet," which is actually a set of pages that condense the findings of the assessment from the primary questions in the instrument. It is filled out only *after* the full instrument has been completed.

---

[3] Two questions that might be candidate "fatal flaw" items, when responses to them were unacceptable (i.e., "no"), are the following from the validity section:

• Generally, the estimates of benefits, harms, and costs are consistent with the evidence presented in the guidelines document. (Yes, completely; yes, partially; or no) (Question 28)

• *Each major recommendation* is consistent with the estimated benefits, harms, and costs of the service or intervention (and thus with the strength of the evidence). (Yes, completely; yes, partially; or no) (Question 31).

In the present version, "better" answers are recorded to the left of the response column, "worse" answers to the right. Thus, a quick scan of this sheet may provide an overall sense of the quality of the guidelines. Put another way, a clinician or other user ought to be able to apply the guideline effectively if all dimensions of the seven attributes (or, at a minimum, all seven attributes) are judged to be "satisfactory" and all omissions of information are considered "unimportant," as those terms were defined earlier. In this (ideal) situation, all notations on the summary sheet would be on the far left. By contrast, if many or most notations are on the right side of the response column, the user might wish to employ the guidelines only selectively or to request clarifications or revisions.

Several reviewers noted that completing the summary evaluation sheet is essentially a clerical task, provided the main part of the assessment instrument has been legibly and fully completed by one or more experts (as discussed earlier). The committee agrees and thus suggests that junior or clerical staff be given this responsibility, and that the instructions on the form indicate that users might wish to do so. Alternatively, the instrument (or at least the recording of responses to its questions) might be computerized. In that case, the summary sheet could be an automatic product of the computer program. The value in pursuing more fully the possibilities of computerization of this form might be considerable.

FINAL CAUTIONS AND CAVEATS

The Ideal: Enemy of the Good

Some commentators noted the IOM's recognition in its 1990 report that most (if not all) guidelines in existence today would "fail" to meet the ideal of this instrument. Reviewers were concerned that "prematurely imposing excessive rigor" would discourage some guideline developers.[4]

---

[4] Comments from the American Nurses Association were particularly to the point: the criteria used to judge the adequacy of guidelines establishes a high standard that likely would seldom be achieved in reality. Several questions need careful consideration prior to accepting the criteria in this instrument:

1. Do the criteria . . . create false expectations of quality which is not achievable with current fiscal restrictions in health care?

2. What are the potential legal and regulatory ramifications of accepting these criteria as representative of quality practice?

3. How would these criteria eventually influence the costs of care through the pursuit of considerable evidence regarding the "best" method of treatment?

4. Are these guidelines intended to weed out bad practice, or is the intention to demonstrate the "best," often misinterpreted as the "only" way of practicing?"

(K. S. O'Connor, Division of Nursing Practice and Economics, American Nurses Association, in a letter to Marilyn Field, IOM study director, dated May 20, 1991.)

At least one reviewer warned that the assessment process should not be used as a "second level expert panel" and cautioned that designing the assessment instrument process itself would take some care. The IOM committee agrees and, in that light, emphasizes that the educational uses of the instrument are more important than its assessment applications (in the near term at least).

Users of the Assessment Instrument

Busy practicing physicians or other clinicians are *not* the intended or anticipated appliers of this assessment instrument. Neither are policymakers, patients, or other nonprofessionals, although all may have some interest in the results. Assessors are expected to have, individually or collectively, expertise in three areas: clinical experience with patient populations covered by the guideline, research experience about the conditions or technologies covered by the guideline, and methodological expertise with techniques and processes of guideline development.

Because no one individual is likely to possess all three kinds of expertise, experience with the instrument may suggest that a "group," "panel," or "study section" approach will be needed to apply it satisfactorily. In this way, different individuals would be responsible for different parts of the assessment (particularly to determine validity). Furthermore, turning the full assessment into a review or evaluation that would be understandable to patients, practitioners, or policymakers will be a separate step, as noted earlier.

This provisional instrument thus proceeds on several assumptions. First, assessors (individually or collectively) are sufficiently schooled either in the methodologic issues inherent in guidelines development or in the clinical issues related to the main topic of the guidelines document that they are able to complete the bulk of the assessment instrument unaided. Second, questions about clinical topics or methods can be referred to appropriate experts when necessary and without undue delay. This kind of referral is particularly important if the AHCPR or some other entity acquires a specific mandate to certify or ratify guidelines from whatever source. Third, in some cases, having a dual or parallel (i.e., simultaneous) review may be a desirable tactic. Fourth, junior staff may well be used to assemble relevant material, perhaps to do an initial check of the document itself, perhaps to evaluate the document for the attribute of clarity, and to complete the summary evaluation sheet. Finally, the experts assembled or asked to apply the instrument (in its current form or any future, modified form) will be carefully trained in its use.

Availability of Supporting Material

Guidelines documents would become unmanageably long and unworkable for busy clinicians if all the information leading to specific recommendations were included in the guideline itself. Nevertheless, the availability of such information *somewhere* is important. Meeting this expectation presents a difficult conflict for guideline developers, and it seriously complicates the task of assessing guidelines.[5]

At this time, the committee takes the position that as much information as possible should be synthesized into a guideline *document*, even if the formal guideline made widely available to practitioners and clinicians is a streamlined version. The assessment process is then to be directed at the complete document (with whatever supporting materials may be submitted with it), not the clinician's version. This stance accords with the committee's general goal of assessing the underlying quality of the guideline itself, not just the process by which it was developed.

For any of the uses to which the present instrument is put, the committee thus assumes that relevant documentation will be in the assessors' hands. This assumption is particularly important when the guidelines to be assessed have been developed by others, and *especially* if those organizations have approached AHCPR or another certifying entity with a specific request for ratification of the guidelines. Hence this instrument assumes that the pertinent information concerning the guidelines document—including information related to the process of development itself—is available for any review effort, with no provision for "later" or "on request" submission of information.

A consequence of this assumption is that this instrument is directed at "guideline documents," however those documents might be construed by the developers. Some guidelines may be contained within a single report, monograph, or other publication. Other guidelines may incorporate related publications by reference, particularly when developers have used a standardized methodology that is described elsewhere. Primary and secondary publications, reports, and records relating to the development of the guideline document being assessed should be assembled before the assessment exercise begins. This might include, for example, reviews and syntheses of

---

[5] For example, the AHCPR Forum panel that has been working on the issue of managing depression in community-based settings started originally with 50,000 citations to the literature, reviewed between 4,000 and 6,000 articles, and based its guidelines document on about 400 relevant articles (J. J. Strain, member of the IOM committee, in a memorandum to Kathleen Lohr and Marilyn Field, dated June 17, 1991). There is no possibility that assessors of the guideline document could replicate that experience or even undertake to review the final set of relevant articles.

the relevant scientific literature, but such a requirement would *not* extend to individual research reports and articles themselves.

Nevertheless, the committee recognizes that published guidelines may be "incomplete" because of limitations placed on the authors by editors and publishers (e.g., space constraints) and that important documentation may not be present. Therefore, if the instrument is applied to published guidelines developed by a group that does not deliberately seek to have its guidelines so assessed (and volunteer the supporting material as assumed above), additional material may need to be gathered from those authors in order to apply this instrument fairly.

Standardized Format Versus Narrative Evaluation

Regardless of what approach to assessing guidelines is finally adopted and what level of expertise the evaluators possess, several basic complexities must be acknowledged. For instance, simply assessing whether guideline developers explain or document a certain piece of information does not allow one to discriminate a comprehensive disclosure from one of poor quality. Similarly, lack of disclosure may have a significant or only a trivial impact on the clinical usefulness and validity of a guideline. No structured instrument of practical length is likely to be able to accommodate these nuances across guideline documents of many different types. Thus, some narrative, global assessment may always be desirable, if not absolutely necessary, if assessments of guidelines are to be useful for a wide set of audiences.

In developing the instrument, the committee asked the first set of reviewers to comment on a "handbook" approach as an alternative to the formal instrument. This approach would provide guidelines assessors with some instructions about the attributes of guidelines to be evaluated and would require them to prepare a narrative evaluation statement, but it would not produce specific responses to specific questions.

Some respondents preferred the "objective, criterion-based" review (i.e., the formal instrument), noting that it might yield "a more standardized evaluation strategy" and "potential benefits such as greater efficiency and reliability, a more readily digested assessment of the strengths and weaknesses of a guideline, and the ability to draw more 'objective' comparisons among a collection of guidelines." Given that no clear preference for the handbook approach emerged, the committee did not pursue this approach further. However, the desire expressed by several reviewers for a narrative, summary statement about a guideline document probably reflects some discomfort with an assessment strategy based solely on the question-and-answer format of the present instrument.

Further Pretesting and Experience with the Instrument

In developing this instrument, the committee recognized the need for more practical experience with it. The present version incorporates revisions suggested by the large number of reviewers, mainly from medical specialty societies, who critiqued an earlier version and in some cases applied it to actual guidelines, as well as changes pursuant to the IOM/NRC review. Nevertheless, the committee takes the view that further application and pretesting of this provisional form should be conducted.

That testing should determine answers to the following questions: Is the instrument too long and too complicated for practical routine use? Does experience applying the instrument as an assessment tool make it easier to use, as several reviewers believed it might? Can shortcuts be found in applying it? For instance, is it useful to have junior staff make an initial check to determine whether all relevant materials appear to be in the guidelines document package or to make a first-assessment pass through the guidelines document itself? Are the results of the assessment consistent with results of any pretests or early evaluations of the guidelines in actual practice?

The present committee takes no stand on how extensive such pre- or pilot-testing might be—for instance, on the number of guidelines that should be assessed to determine the reliability, validity, and practicality of the current form. Two factors are relevant. First, the committee had neither the time nor the resources to pursue these issues further (and certainly not to carry out such activities itself). Second, it considers that such testing might need to be specific to the potential user groups and that setting *a priori* rules risks making them too rigorous or too confining for all purposes.

THE PROVISIONAL ASSESSMENT INSTRUMENT

The form reproduced in the last part of this appendix has three main parts. First is a *general information sheet*, with space for the following items to be briefly described: clinical diagnoses or conditions; health practices, services, or technologies; target populations; primary settings of care; primary types of clinicians targeted; stated purposes of the guideline; source, author, or developer of the guideline document; person to contact for further information about the guideline document; date of issue of the guideline document; and name/affiliation of assessor(s). The second section is the *full instrument* itself, with self-contained instructions. The third section is the *summary evaluation sheet*.

ACKNOWLEDGMENTS

The idea of creating an instrument by which to assess the soundness of clinical practice guidelines can be traced through the work of three Institute of Medicine committees: the Committee to Design a Strategy for Quality Review and Assurance in Medicare, the Committee to Advise the Public Health Service on Clinical Practice Guidelines, and the present Committee on Clinical Practice Guidelines. The present committee wishes, therefore, to acknowledge the groundbreaking efforts of its predecessor panels in this rapidly evolving arena.

Production of this provisional instrument would not have been possible without the assistance of many individuals and organizations. We are indebted to the members of various medical specialty societies who reviewed and in some cases voluntarily applied and tested an earlier draft instrument; we especially thank Betty King, executive director of IMCARE (Internal Medicine Center to Advance Research and Education) for her efforts in organizing a broad review of the instrument by the IMCARE task force on practice guidelines. We thank Anne-Marie Audet of the Health Institute, New England Medical Center Hospitals, for her enthusiastic efforts with the first draft of the instrument.

The project under which this instrument was developed was supported by The John A. Hartford Foundation and by the Agency for Health Care Policy and Research, U.S. Department of Health and Human Services, under Contract No. 282-90-0018. The views presented are those of the Institute of Medicine Committee on Clinical Practice Guidelines and the authors, and are not necessarily those of the funding organizations.

Finally, we extend our appreciation to our Institute of Medicine (IOM) colleagues on this project, Molla Donaldson and Holly Dawkins; to the project's senior secretaries, Theresa Nally and Donna Thompson; and to other members of the IOM staff who provided timely and helpful comments, including Christopher Howson, Michael Stoto, and Malin VanAntwerp.

REFERENCES

AMA (American Medical Association). "Evaluation of a Recently Completed Practice Parameter." Chicago: American Medical Association, 1990.

IOM (Institute of Medicine). *Clinical Practice Guidelines: Directions for a New Program.* M.J. Field and K.N. Lohr, editors. Washington, DC: National Academy Press, 1990.

ASSESSMENT INSTRUMENT

PART ONE. GENERAL INFORMATION SHEET

TO THE ASSESSOR: Please complete this sheet with brief statements about the content of the guideline document you are reviewing. Use whatever information can be found in the document. If you cannot find the relevant information or are uncertain about the appropriate response, indicate "not specified" or "uncertain."

TITLE OF GUIDELINE DOCUMENT _____

1. Clinical diagnoses or conditions

2. Main health practices, services, or technologies considered

3. Target populations (e.g., age, sex, income level, health status)

4. Primary settings of care (e.g., primary or specialty; nursing home)

5. Primary types of clinicians targeted (e.g., profession; specialty)

6. Stated purposes, aims, or goals of the guideline document

7. Source, author, or developer of guideline document

8. Individual to contact for further information about the guideline document (name, organization, phone number)

9. Date of issue of the guideline document

10. Name/affiliation of assessor(s)

PART TWO. ASSESSMENT INSTRUMENT

Background

This instrument itself has seven sections, each corresponding to one of the seven attributes of guidelines to be evaluated. Each section begins with a brief definition of the attribute and then is divided into segments that deal with important dimensions of that attribute.

Instructions: Illustrative Example

Each segment begins with a descriptive question that you should answer yes or no. The responses will then direct you to move to a specific next question. Space is provided for "Comments" throughout the instrument.

For example, in the section on clinical applicability, the first question reads (in part) as shown below, and you are instructed to check "yes" or "no" and then answer the appropriate subquestion:

1. **THE GUIDELINE DOCUMENT DESCRIBES THE PATIENT POPULATIONS TO WHICH THE GUIDELINES ARE MEANT TO APPLY.**

    _____ Yes (Go to 1.1)   _____ No (Go to 1.2)

   1.1. THE DESCRIPTION OF THE PATIENT POPULATIONS IS:

    _____ Satisfactory   _____ Conditionally   _____ Unsatisfactory
                                            satisfactory   (Specify)

Comments:

                                                        >> GO TO QUESTION 2 >>

   1.2. OMISSION OF A DESCRIPTION OF THE PATIENT POPULATIONS IS:

    _____ Unimportant   _____ Minor   _____ Major
                                            omission   omission

In some circumstances you are asked to judge a set of variables—specific elements to consider in evaluating an attribute—and to arrive at a "global" answer to a particular question. When this occurs, you should (1) start with the set of items that are identified alphanumerically (e.g., 1a, 1b, . . .) and answer them directly and then (2) combine those answers into a summary evaluation to determine whether the guideline document has dealt with that particular issue in a satisfactory, conditionally satisfactory, or unsatisfactory manner.

You should then go on to the next question or to the next section, as directed. In the absence of a specific direction, go to the very next question.

Definitions of Terms

The questions in this instrument ask for three different types of responses. The meaning of these response categories is as follows:

Yes and no. Most of the main questions concern the presence of a discussion or piece of information about a particular attribute. Generally, the "yes" and "no" responses direct you to answer follow-up questions. For these items, response choices are "satisfactory," "conditionally satisfactory," and "unsatisfactory," or "unimportant omission," "minor omission," and "major omission." These terms are further defined below.

Satisfactory. You can judge information about a particular attribute as satisfactory if all critical elements have been considered and presented. For example, the discussion or description should be thorough and comprehensive; the guideline developers should have based their work on appropriate and correct information; and they should have used appropriate methods.

Conditionally satisfactory. The description or discussion of an attribute or dimension is conditionally satisfactory if some, but not all, of the critical elements have been considered and presented. For example, the discussion of a particular aspect of the attribute may be vague or incomplete; alternatively, the guidelines developers may have disregarded important information in reaching their recommendations or improperly used certain kinds of methods. These problems with the guideline document may not prevent a clinician from using it or understanding its recommendations, but they may affect its overall usefulness or call certain recommendations into question. Revisions would be presumed to improve the guidelines, but they would not be mandatory or essential.

Unsatisfactory. You can determine the description or discussion about a specific attribute to be unsatisfactory if most of the critical elements have not been considered or presented. For example, well-known pieces of clinical information (or the views of multiple specialists with an interest in the guidelines topic) may have been ignored; methods of analysis may have been misapplied; or recommendations may be based on faulty information, poor logic, or both. In such a case, it would be difficult if not impossible to judge the quality of the process of guideline development or the soundness of the resulting guidelines and recommendations, or both; certainly they could not be assessed as satisfactory, and serious thought must be given to augmenting or revising the guideline document before it is promoted further.

Unimportant omissions. You can regard the omission of a description or discussion about a specific attribute or dimension of an attribute as unimportant if it (1) is likely to have *no meaningful impact* on the ability of a guideline user, such as a practitioner or patient, to apply the guideline effectively in the clinical decision-making process and (2) does not prevent you from easily and independently assessing that aspect of the guideline document.

Minor omissions. The omission of a description or discussion about a specific attribute or dimension is of minor importance if it (1) is likely to have only a *little negative impact* on the ability of a guideline user to apply the guideline effectively in the clinical decision-making process and (2) does not prevent you from assessing that aspect of the guideline document.

Major omissions. You can determine the omission of a description or discussion about a specific attribute or dimension to be a major problem if it (1) is likely to prevent a guideline user from applying the guideline effectively in the clinical decision-making process or (2) prevents you from making an independent assessment about that aspect of the guideline document.

Not applicable or don't know. In some situations, the question may not be applicable to the guideline document you are evaluating. When that occurs, simply mark "NA" for "not applicable" or "DK" for "don't know."

Comments. In other situations, you may find it difficult to arrive at a single answer to the question, especially if the guideline document you are evaluating is very complex or if necessary background information appears to be missing. In these cases, you can record additional remarks or qualifying statements about your response in the "Comments" sections.

Finally, if you believe that the guideline document is so complex, clinically esoteric, or methodologically sophisticated that it warrants additional, outside expert review, please note your comments at the end of the full instrument.

I. CLINICAL APPLICABILITY

Clinical applicability, or the scope of the guideline, means three things in the context of this instrument. First, guidelines should be written to cover as inclusive a patient population as possible, consistent with knowledge about critical clinical and sociodemographic factors relevant for the condition or technology in question. To that end, the patient population(s) covered should be described as accurately and precisely as possible. Second, if patient populations that might be expected to be covered by the guideline are not, then the document discusses why those populations have been excluded; that is, it identifies the patient populations the guidelines are *not* meant to serve or apply to. Third, when the clinical conditions or problems covered by the guideline are likely to be complex, or when the guideline recommendations may be contingent on complex patterns of clinical factors, those points should be explicitly covered in the guideline document.

This attribute requires that two things be true about the guideline document. First, the guideline document accurately and precisely states how broad or narrow the patient population(s) are to which the guidelines are meant to apply, describes the actual population(s) to which statements apply, *and* describes the population(s) to which statements are *not* meant to apply. Population(s) may be described in terms of diagnosis, pathophysiology, severity of primary disease, presence of coexisting diseases, age, sex, race, social support systems, and other characteristics. Second, it notes and discusses any complex clinical issues that may arise for this patient population.

1. **THE GUIDELINE DOCUMENT DESCRIBES THE PATIENT POPULATIONS TO WHICH THE GUIDELINES ARE MEANT TO APPLY.**

    _____ Yes (Go to Question 1.1) _____ No (Go to Question 1.2)

1.1. THE DESCRIPTION OF THE PATIENT POPULATIONS IS:

_____ Satisfactory	_____ Conditionally satisfactory	_____ Unsatisfactory (Specify)

Comments:

>> **GO TO QUESTION 2** >>

1.2. OMISSION OF THE DESCRIPTION OF THE PATIENT POPULATION(S) IS:

_____ Unimportant   _____ Minor   _____ Major
                                   omission   omission

Comments:

2. THE GUIDELINE DOCUMENT DISCUSSES COMPLEX CLINICAL PROBLEMS THAT CAN BE EXPECTED FOR THE POPULATION(S) COVERED BY THE GUIDELINES.

_____ Yes (Go to Question 2.1)

_____ No (Go to Question 2.2)

_____ Not Applicable (Go to Question 3)

2.1. THE DISCUSSION OF EXPECTED COMPLEX CLINICAL PROBLEMS IS:

_____ Satisfactory   _____ Conditionally   _____ Unsatisfactory
                                   satisfactory   (Specify)

Comments:

>> GO TO QUESTION 3 >>

2.2. OMISSION OF THE DISCUSSION OF EXPECTED COMPLEX CLINICAL PROBLEMS IS:

_____ Unimportant   _____ Minor   _____ Major
                                   omission   omission

Comments:

3. **THE GUIDELINE DOCUMENT GIVES A RATIONALE FOR EXCLUDING PATIENT POPULATION(S).**

_____ Yes (Go to Question 3.1)   _____ No (Go to Question 3.2)

3.1. THE RATIONALE FOR EXCLUDING CERTAIN PATIENT POPULATION(S) IS:

_____ Satisfactory   _____ Conditionally satisfactory   _____ Unsatisfactory (Specify)

Comments:

>> GO TO II. CLINICAL FLEXIBILITY >>

3.2. OMISSION OF THE RATIONALE FOR EXCLUDING CERTAIN PATIENT POPULATION(S) IS:

_____ Unimportant   _____ Minor omission   _____ Major omission

Comments:

II. CLINICAL FLEXIBILITY

Clinical flexibility means that two mediating factors should be addressed in the guideline document. First, it should identify major foreseeable exceptions to or options for applying the guidelines, if any exist. Second, it should discuss the role of patient preferences for different courses of health care for those conditions or technologies in which patient values and preferences may be important decision-making factors (for example, being able to choose in an informed way between surgery and watchful waiting).

This attribute requires the guideline document to discuss two topics. First are situations (if any) in which socially relevant factors permit an exception to be made in applying the guidelines. These factors could include the home and family situation of the patient, clinical constraints on the health care delivery setting (e.g., no intensive care beds, no 24-hour anesthesiologist), *non*clinical constraints on the health care delivery setting (e.g., inadequate information systems), or all of these; if no such factors exist, the guideline document should say so. Second is the role of patient preferences for different possible outcomes of care, when the appropriateness of a clinical intervention involves a substantial element of personal choice or values on the part of the patient. For example, this discussion may include information as to major points on which preferences may diverge for the case in hand, specific points to consider in eliciting patient preferences, and means of integrating patient views in the decisionmaking process.

4. **THE GUIDELINE DOCUMENT PROVIDES SPECIFIC INFORMATION ABOUT SITUATIONS IN WHICH CLINICAL EXCEPTIONS MIGHT BE MADE IN APPLYING THE GUIDELINES.**

_____ Yes, the document gives information about *clinical* exceptions (Go to Question 4.1)

_____ No, the document says nothing about *clinical* exceptions (Go to Question 4.2)

4.1. THE INFORMATION OR STATEMENT ABOUT *CLINICAL* EXCEPTIONS IS:

_____ Satisfactory　　_____ Conditionally　　_____ Unsatisfactory
　　　　　　　　　　　　　　　satisfactory　　　　　(Specify)

Comments:

>> GO TO QUESTION 5 >>

4.2. OMISSION OF INFORMATION OR A STATEMENT ABOUT *CLINICAL* EXCEPTIONS IS:

_____ Unimportant   _____ Minor omission   _____ Major omission

Comments:

5. THE GUIDELINE DOCUMENT PROVIDES SPECIFIC INFORMATION ABOUT *NONCLINICAL* SITUATIONS IN WHICH EXCEPTIONS MIGHT BE MADE IN APPLYING THE GUIDELINES.

_____ Yes, the document gives information about *nonclinical* exceptions (Go to Question 5.1)

_____ No, the document says nothing about *nonclinical* exceptions (Go to Question 5.2)

5.1. THE INFORMATION OR STATEMENT ABOUT *NONCLINICAL* EXCEPTIONS IS:

_____ Satisfactory   _____ Conditionally satisfactory   _____ Unsatisfactory (Specify)

Comments:

>> GO TO QUESTION 6 >>

5.2. OMISSION OF INFORMATION OR A STATEMENT ABOUT *NONCLINICAL* EXCEPTIONS IS:

_____ Unimportant   _____ Minor omission   _____ Major omission

Comments:

6. **THE GUIDELINE DOCUMENT DISCUSSES THE ROLE OF PATIENT PREFERENCES, AS THEY RELATE TO HEALTH CARE DECISIONS IN THE PARTICULAR CASE THAT THE GUIDELINES COVER.**

    _____ Yes (Go to Question 6.1)   _____ No (Go to Question 6.2)

    6.1. THE DISCUSSION OF PATIENT PREFERENCES IS:

    _____ Satisfactory   _____ Conditionally   _____ Unsatisfactory
                                      satisfactory   (Specify)

Comments:

                                        >> GO TO QUESTION 7 >>

    6.2. OMISSION OF DISCUSSION OF PATIENT PREFERENCES IS:

    _____ Unimportant   _____ Minor   _____ Major
                                      omission   omission

Comments:

                          >> GO TO III. RELIABILITY/REPRODUCIBILITY >>

7. **THE GUIDELINE DOCUMENT DESCRIBES HOW PATIENT PREFERENCES WERE TAKEN INTO ACCOUNT DURING THE GUIDELINE DEVELOPMENT PROCESS.**

    _____ Yes (Go to Question 7.1)   _____ No (Go to Question 7.2)

7.1. THE DISCUSSION OF HOW PATIENT PREFERENCES WERE CONSIDERED IN DEVELOPING THE GUIDELINE IS:

_____ Satisfactory   _____ Conditionally
satisfactory   _____ Unsatisfactory
(Specify)

Comments:

>> GO TO III. RELIABILITY/REPRODUCIBILITY >>

7.2. OMISSION OF THE DISCUSSION OF PATIENT PREFER-ENCES IN DEVELOPING THE GUIDELINE IS:

_____ Unimportant   _____ Minor
omission   _____ Major
omission

Comments:

III. RELIABILITY/REPRODUCIBILITY

Reliability and reproducibility for the purpose of assessing guidelines means that, given the same circumstances, essentially the same set of guidelines would be developed by a second group; further, the terms mean that, ideally, the guidelines are or would be interpreted and applied consistently by practitioners or other appropriate parties.

Reliability and reproducibility of a guideline document is not likely ever to be assessable empirically. To approach these concepts, therefore, this attribute requires either that guidelines be subjected to some form of explicit, independent review by a group (or groups) other than the original developers, where that group (or groups) is equivalent in expertise and other factors to the original developers, *or* that the guideline recommendations have been pretested in some manner, *or* both. (Pretesting can be done in actual delivery settings or on prototypical cases.) If no such review or pretesting has been done, then the guidelines must explain the reasons.

8. THE GUIDELINES WERE SUBJECTED TO INDEPENDENT REVIEW BY EXPERTS OR OUTSIDE PANELS.

_____ Yes (Go to Question 8.1)   _____ No (Go to Question 9)

8.1. THE DISCUSSION OF INDEPENDENT REVIEW IS:

_____ Satisfactory   _____ Conditionally   _____ Unsatisfactory
                             satisfactory   (Specify)

Comments:

>> GO TO QUESTION 10 >>

9. THE GUIDELINE DOCUMENT EXPLAINS THE LACK OF INDEPENDENT REVIEW.

_____ Yes (Go to Question 9.1)   _____ No (Go to Question 9.2)

9.1. THE EXPLANATION OF THE LACK OF INDEPENDENT REVIEW IS:

_____ Satisfactory   _____ Conditionally satisfactory   _____ Unsatisfactory (Specify)

Comments:

>> GO TO QUESTION 10 >>

9.2. OMISSION OF AN EXPLANATION OF THE LACK OF IN-DEPENDENT REVIEW IS:

_____ Unimportant   _____ Minor omission   _____ Major omission

Comments:

10. THE GUIDELINES WERE PRETESTED IN SOME MANNER.

_____ Yes (Go to Question 10.1)   _____ No (Go to Question 11)

10.1. THE DISCUSSION OF PRETESTING IS:

_____ Satisfactory   _____ Conditionally satisfactory   _____ Unsatisfactory (Specify)

Comments:

>> GO TO IV. VALIDITY >>

11. THE GUIDELINE DOCUMENT EXPLAINS THE LACK OF PRETESTING.

_____ Yes (Go to Question 11.1)   _____ No (Go to Question 11.2)

11.1. THE EXPLANATION OF THE LACK OF PRETESTING IS:

_____ Satisfactory   _____ Conditionally satisfactory   _____ Unsatisfactory (Specify)

Comments:

>> GO TO IV. VALIDITY >>

11.2. OMISSION OF AN EXPLANATION OF THE LACK OF PRETESTING IS:

_____ Unimportant   _____ Minor omission   _____ Major omission

Comments:

IV. VALIDITY: DEFINITION AND EVALUATION QUESTIONS

Validity of practice guidelines means, conceptually, that if they are followed, then they will lead to the health and cost outcomes projected for them. Validity must be judged primarily by reference to the substance and quality of the evidence cited, the means used to evaluate the evidence, and the relationship between the evidence and the recommendations. Validity is the most critical attribute and the most difficult to assess. **Although this section contains 22 questions, questions 28 and 31 are, together, of special importance because they constitute an overall evaluation of this attribute.**

This attribute requires that five things be true for the guideline document. First, the collection, synthesis, and interpretation of scientific evidence must be documented and of satisfactory quality; ideally, each major recommendation will be described as based on "excellent," "acceptable," or "weak" evidence, or with a similar set of descriptive terms.

Second, both qualitative and quantitative statements about health benefits and harms/risks appear in the guideline document, and insofar as possible those estimates are tied to and justified by the evidence amassed as part of the literature review and analysis. For example, a qualitative statement about benefits might read "screening mammography should lead to a decrease in breast cancer mortality"; a similar statement about harms and risks might read "screening mammography can lead to false-positive results and to unnecessary work-up and anxiety." Quantitative statements might read, respectively, "screening mammography in women 50 years of age may reduce mortality from 20 percent to 60 percent" and "among one million women 40 to 50 years of age, radiation from 10 mammography examinations can be expected to cause about 60 new breast cancers." In all cases, such statements should be based on evidentiary information insofar as possible, and appropriate qualifiers or caveats noted when the evidence is weak or conflicting or when the estimates are based on consensus techniques such as expert panels or group judgment methods.

Third, both qualitative and quantitative statements about expected health costs or expenditures appear in the guideline document; the same requirements about the link between the guideline estimates and the data sources should be met, and the same degree of specificity about patient groups should be observed. In addition, the document should be clear as to whether costs referred to are the total for the patient group or the per-patient figure. For example, "use of laparoscopic techniques to treat cholecystitis should reduce the direct and indirect costs associated with using cholecystectomy as the main patient management approach" might be a suitable qualitative statement concerning costs, and "use of laparoscopic techniques in the treatment of cholecystitis may reduce the costs of treatment as much as 75 percent by the end of the decade by reducing hospitalization and time for post-operative (i.e., post-cholecystectomy) morbidity and recovery" might be an appropriate quantitative statement about estimated costs.

Fourth, specific recommendations are clearly tied to and justified by the estimated benefits, harms, and costs provided within the document.

Fifth, conflicts between this set of guidelines and any other independent sets (and their respective recommendations), if any, must be explicitly discussed.

Strength of Scientific Evidence and Professional Consensus

12. THE GUIDELINE DOCUMENT SPECIFICALLY DESCRIBES THE METHOD(S) USED TO COLLECT (I.E., IDENTIFY AND RETRIEVE) THE SCIENTIFIC EVIDENCE ON WHICH RECOMMENDATIONS ARE BASED.

_____ Yes (Go to Question 12.1)   _____ No (Go to Question 12.2)

12.1. ASSESSOR: Respond to Items 12a-d, below, to assess the methods for collecting scientific evidence; then answer Question 12.1, using your best judgment as to the overall rating for this element of validity. Other factors you judge important should be specifically recorded under "Comments or Other Factors."

12a.   The criteria used to include and/or exclude studies are:

_____ Adequate   _____ Inadequate   _____ Not given/described

12b.   The search strategy is:

_____ Adequate   _____ Inadequate   _____ Not given/described

12c.   The sources of information are:

_____ Adequate   _____ Inadequate   _____ Not given/described

12d.   Major studies or other sources of information have been identified.

_____ Yes   _____ No   _____ Don't know
                          (Specify)
Now answer:

12.1. THE METHOD(S) OF COLLECTING SCIENTIFIC EVIDENCE IS:

_____ Satisfactory   _____ Conditionally   _____ Unsatisfactory
                                  satisfactory   (Specify)

Comments or Other Factors:

>> GO TO QUESTION 13 >>

12.2. THE LACK OF A CLEAR METHOD FOR COLLECTING THE SCIENTIFIC EVIDENCE IS:

_____ Unimportant   _____ Minor   _____ Major
                                  omission   omission

Comments:

13. THE GUIDELINE DOCUMENT GIVES ADEQUATE REFERENCES OR CITATIONS TO THE SOURCES OF INFORMATION USED IN DEVELOPING THE GUIDELINES.

_____ Yes   _____ No

Comments:

14. THE GUIDELINE DOCUMENT DISCUSSES IN GENERAL TERMS THE STRENGTH OF THE SCIENTIFIC EVIDENCE ON WHICH RECOMMENDATIONS ARE BASED.

_____ Yes   _____ No

Comments:

15. THE GUIDELINE DOCUMENT EXPLICITLY RATES THE STRENGTH OF THE SCIENTIFIC EVIDENCE.

_____ Yes (Go to Question 15.1)   _____ No (Go to Question 15.2)

15.1 ASSESSOR: Respond to Items 15a-15f, below, to determine whether the method used to rate the strength of the scientific evidence is adequate; then answer Question 15.1 below, using your best judgment as to the overall rating for this element of validity. Other factors you judge important should be specifically recorded under "Comments or Other Factors."

15a. Characteristics of studies used as a basis for guidelines have been described.

_____ Yes   _____ No

15b. Strengths and weaknesses of studies used as a basis for guidelines have been noted.

_____ Yes   _____ No

15c. The way the characteristics, strengths, and weaknesses of studies used as a basis for guidelines have been taken into account (for instance, an explicit weighting scheme) has been clearly described.

_____ Yes   _____ No

15d. The way the characteristics, strengths, and weaknesses of studies used as a basis for guidelines have been taken into account (for instance, an explicit weighting scheme) is:

_____ Adequate _____ Inadequate _____ Not given/described

15e. The discussion in the document of possible *threats to* **internal** *validity and reliability* of studies included in the scientific evidence supporting the guidelines is:

_____ Adequate _____ Inadequate _____ No discussion given

15f. The discussion in the document of possible *threats to* **external** *validity and generalizability* of studies included in the scientific evidence supporting the guidelines is:

_____ Adequate _____ Inadequate _____ No discussion given

Now answer:

15.1. OVERALL, THE METHOD USED TO RATE OR WEIGHT THE SCIENTIFIC EVIDENCE IS:

_____ Satisfactory _____ Conditionally satisfactory _____ Unsatisfactory (Specify)

Comments or Other Factors:

>> GO TO QUESTION 16>>

15.2. THE LACK OF ANY GENERAL DISCUSSION OR EXPLICIT RATING OF THE STRENGTH OF THE SCIENTIFIC EVIDENCE IS:

_____ Unimportant _____ Minor omission _____ Major omission

Comments:

16. *IF A FORMAL METHOD OF SYNTHESIS IS USED TO COM-BINE THE SCIENTIFIC EVIDENCE QUANTITATIVELY OR OTH-ERWISE TO DEVELOP SUMMARY OUTCOME MEASURES THAT REFLECT THE STRENGTH OF THE SCIENTIFIC EVIDENCE,* THEN THE GUIDELINE DOCUMENT EXPLICITLY DESCRIBES THE METHOD.

_____ Yes, method used and described (Go to Question 16.1)

_____ No, method used but not described (Go to Question 16.2)

_____ No, no formal method of synthesis used (Go to Question 18)

16.1. ASSESSOR: Respond to Items 16a-16c, below, to determine whether formal methods for synthesizing scientific evidence are satisfactory; then answer Question 16.1 below, using your best judgment as to the overall rating for this element of validity. Other factors you judge important should be specifically record-ed under "Comments or Other Factors."

16a. The meta-analytic method(s) is:

_____ Adequate   _____ Inadequate   _____ Not applicable/used

16b. The decision-analytic model(s) is:

_____ Adequate   _____ Inadequate   _____ Not applicable/used

16c. Other systematic information synthesis method(s) is:

_____ Adequate   _____ Inadequate   _____ Not applicable/used

Now answer:

16.1 OVERALL, THE FORMAL METHOD(S) USED TO SYN-THESIZE OR COMBINE SCIENTIFIC EVIDENCE IS:

_____ Satisfactory   _____ Conditionally   _____ Unsatisfactory
                                    satisfactory   (Specify)

Comments or Other Factors:

>> GO TO QUESTION 17 >>

16.2. OMISSION OF A DESCRIPTION OF THE METHOD(S) OF SYNTHESIZING THE SCIENTIFIC EVIDENCE IS:

_____ Unimportant   _____ Minor omission   _____ Major omission

Comments:

17. *GIVEN THAT* A FORMAL METHOD OF SYNTHESIS IS USED TO COMBINE THE SCIENTIFIC EVIDENCE QUANTITATIVELY OR OTHERWISE TO DEVELOP SUMMARY OUTCOMES MEASURES, THE GUIDELINE DOCUMENT EXPLICITLY REPORTS THE RESULTS OF THAT SYNTHESIS.

_____ Yes, method used and results reported (Go to Question 17.1)

_____ No, method used but results not reported (Go to Question 17.2)

17.1. RESULTS OF INFORMATION SYNTHESIS ARE:

_____ Satisfactory (e.g., summary outcome measure(s) *with* confidence intervals or discussion of uncertainty)

_____ Conditionally satisfactory (e.g., summary outcome measure(s) *without* confidence intervals or discussion of uncertainty)

_____ Unsatisfactory (e.g., outcome measure(s) are not interpretable, are inconsistent, or are otherwise questionable or erroneous). (Specify)

Comments:

>> GO TO QUESTION 18 >>

17.2. OMISSION OF RESULTS OF SYNTHESIS IS:

_____ Unimportant   _____ Minor   _____ Major
                              omission   omission

Comments:

18. *IF* **FORMAL EXPERT OR GROUP JUDGMENT TECHNIQUES
    ARE USED TO** *REACH PROFESSIONAL CONSENSUS*, **THEN
    THE GUIDELINE DOCUMENT EXPLICITLY DESCRIBES THE
    TECHNIQUES.**

    _____ Yes, techniques used and described (Go to Question 18.1)

    _____ No, techniques used but not described (Go to Question 18.2)

    _____ No, no formal expert or group judgment techniques used
          (Go to Question 19)

18.1. THE EXPERT OR GROUP JUDGMENT TECHNIQUES ARE:

_____ Satisfactory   _____ Conditionally   _____ Unsatisfactory
                            satisfactory   (Specify)

Comments:

>> GO TO QUESTION 19 >>

18.2. OMISSION OF A DESCRIPTION OF THE EXPERT OR GROUP JUDGMENT TECHNIQUES IS:

_____ Unimportant   _____ Minor omission   _____ Major omission

Comments:

19. *GIVEN THAT* EXPERT OR GROUP JUDGMENT. METHOD(S) ARE USED TO REACH PROFESSIONAL CONSENSUS, THE GUIDELINE DOCUMENT EXPLICITLY GIVES *INFORMATION ABOUT THE STRENGTH OF PROFESSIONAL CONSENSUS.*

_____ Yes, techniques used and information given
(Go to Question 19.1)

_____ No, techniques used but information not given
(Go to Question 19.2)

19.1. THE INFORMATION ABOUT THE STRENGTH OF PROFESSIONAL CONSENSUS IS:

_____ Satisfactory (e.g., levels of professional consensus given for all major points in the guidelines)

_____ Conditionally satisfactory (e.g., levels of professional consensus given for some, but not all, major points in the guidelines)

_____ Unsatisfactory (e.g., levels of professional consensus are not interpretable, are inconsistent, or are otherwise questionable or erroneous). (Specify)

Comments:

>> GO TO QUESTION 20 >>

19.2. OMISSION OF EXPLICIT INFORMATION ABOUT THE STRENGTH OF PROFESSIONAL CONSENSUS IS:

_____ Unimportant   _____ Minor   _____ Major
                                  omission   omission

Comments:

Health Benefits and Harms/Risks: Qualitative Descriptions

20. THE GUIDELINE DOCUMENT PROVIDES A *QUALITATIVE DESCRIPTION OF THE HEALTH BENEFITS* THAT ARE EXPECTED FROM A SPECIFIC HEALTH PRACTICE.

_____ Yes (Go to Question 20.1)   _____ No (Go to Question 20.2)

20.1. THE QUALITATIVE DESCRIPTION OF HEALTH BENEFITS IS:

_____ Satisfactory   _____ Conditionally   _____ Unsatisfactory
                             satisfactory   (Specify)

Comments:

>> GO TO QUESTION 21 >>

20.2. OMISSION OF A QUALITATIVE DESCRIPTION OF HEALTH BENEFITS IS:

_____ Unimportant   _____ Minor   _____ Major
                                  omission   omission

Comments:

21. THE GUIDELINE DOCUMENT PROVIDES A *QUALITATIVE DESCRIPTION OF THE POTENTIAL HARMS OR RISKS* THAT MAY OCCUR AS A RESULT OF A SPECIFIC HEALTH PRACTICE.

_____ Yes (Go to Question 21.1)   _____ No (Go to Question 21.2)

21.1. THE QUALITATIVE DESCRIPTION OF POTENTIAL HARMS OR RISKS IS:

_____ Satisfactory   _____ Conditionally satisfactory   _____ Unsatisfactory (Specify)

Comments:

>> **GO TO QUESTION 22** >>

21.2. OMISSION OF A QUALITATIVE DESCRIPTION OF POTENTIAL HARMS OR RISKS IS:

_____ Unimportant   _____ Minor omission   _____ Major omission

Comments:

Health Benefits and Harms/Risks: Quantitative Information

22. THE GUIDELINE DOCUMENT PROVIDES *QUANTITATIVE INFORMATION OR ESTIMATES ABOUT THE HEALTH BENEFITS* TO BE EXPECTED AS A RESULT OF A SPECIFIC HEALTH PRACTICE.

_____ Yes (Go to Question 22.1)   _____ No (Go to Question 22.2)

22.1. THE *QUANTITATIVE INFORMATION* ABOUT THE HEALTH BENEFITS IS:

_____ Satisfactory (e.g., one or more measures of benefits, including accurate summary or composite measures, *with* confidence intervals or discussion of uncertainty)

_____ Conditionally satisfactory (e.g., one or more measures of benefits, *without* confidence intervals or discussion of uncertainty)

_____ Unsatisfactory (e.g., measures are not interpretable, are inconsistent, or are otherwise questionable or erroneous). (Specify)

Comments:

>> GO TO QUESTION 23 >>

22.2. OMISSION OF QUANTITATIVE INFORMATION AND ESTIMATION OF HEALTH BENEFITS IS:

_____ Unimportant   _____ Minor   _____ Major
                                   omission   omission

Comments:

>> GO TO QUESTION 24 >>

23. THE GUIDELINE DOCUMENT PROJECTS HEALTH BENEFITS OR OUTCOMES IN TERMS OF ADDITIONAL LIFE EXPECTANCY OR SIMILAR MEASURES, SUCH AS QUALITY-ADJUSTED LIFE YEARS.

_____ Yes   _____ No   _____ Not applicable/not necessary

Comments:

24. THE GUIDELINE DOCUMENT PROVIDES *QUANTITATIVE IN-FORMATION OR ESTIMATES ABOUT THE POTENTIAL HARMS OR RISKS* OCCURRING AS A RESULT OF A SPECIFIC HEALTH PRACTICE.

_____ Yes (Go to Question 20.1)   _____ No (Go to Question 20.2)

24.1. THE QUANTITATIVE INFORMATION ABOUT POTENTIAL HARMS OR RISKS OCCURRING AS A RESULT OF A SPECIFIC HEALTH PRACTICE IS:

_____ Satisfactory (e.g., one or more measures of harms or risks, in-cluding summary or composite measures, *with* confidence inter-vals or discussion of uncertainty)

_____ Conditionally satisfactory (e.g., one or more measures of harms or risks, *without* confidence intervals or discussion of uncertainty)

_____ Unsatisfactory (e.g., measure(s) are not interpretable, are incon-sistent, or are otherwise questionable or erroneous). (Specify)

Comments:

>> **GO TO QUESTION 25** >>

24.2. OMISSION OF QUANTITATIVE INFORMATION ABOUT POTENTIAL HARMS OR RISKS IS:

_____ Unimportant   _____ Minor omission   _____ Major omission

Comments:

Health Costs: Qualitative Description

25. THE GUIDELINE DOCUMENT PROVIDES A *QUALITATIVE DESCRIPTION OF THE HEALTH COSTS OR EXPENDITURES* THAT ARE EXPECTED FROM A SPECIFIC HEALTH PRACTICE.

_____ Yes (Go to Question 25.1)   _____ No (Go to Question 25.2)

25.1. THE QUALITATIVE DESCRIPTION OF EXPECTED HEALTH COSTS OR EXPENDITURES IS:

_____ Satisfactory   _____ Conditionally satisfactory   _____ Unsatisfactory (Specify)

Comments:

>> GO TO QUESTION 26 >>

25.2. OMISSION OF A QUALITATIVE DESCRIPTION OF EX-PECTED HEALTH COSTS OR EXPENDITURES IS:

_____ Unimportant   _____ Minor omission   _____ Major omission

Comments:

Health Costs: Quantitative Description

26. THE GUIDELINE DOCUMENT PROVIDES *QUANTITATIVE* IN-FORMATION OR ESTIMATES ABOUT THE HEALTH COSTS OR EXPENDITURES THAT ARE EXPECTED AS A RESULT OF A SPECIFIC HEALTH PRACTICE.

_____ Yes (Go to Question 26.1)   _____ No (Go to Question 26.2)

26.1. ASSESSOR: Respond to Items 26a-26e, below, to determine whether potential costs and expenditures have been estimated in a satisfactory manner; then answer Question 26.1, using your best judgment as to the overall rating for this element of validity. Other factors you judge important should be specifically recorded under "Comments or Other Factors."

26a. The cost estimates are done for major subgroups of the patient population, e.g., major risk groups, and for major clinical (diagnostic, therapeutic, etc.) alternatives.

_____ Yes   _____ No

26b. The cost estimates include all the services necessary to achieve the health benefits that are assumed to be achievable.

_____ Yes   _____ No

26c. The cost estimates specify number(s) of services that may be added, substituted, and/or eliminated if the guideline recommendations are followed.

_____ Yes   _____ No

26d. The cost estimates specify charges, production costs, or similar information for the services that may be added, substituted, and/or eliminated if the guideline recommendations are followed.

_____ Yes   _____ No

26e. The quantitative method(s) used to estimate costs is:

_____ Appropriate   _____ Inappropriate

Now answer:

26.1 THE QUANTITATIVE INFORMATION ABOUT EXPECTED HEALTH COSTS OR EXPENDITURES IS:

_____ Satisfactory (e.g., one or more estimates of costs, including accurate summary or composite measures, *with* ranges of uncertainty)

_____ Conditionally satisfactory (e.g., one or more estimates of costs, *without* ranges of uncertainty)

_____ Unsatisfactory (e.g., cost estimates are not interpretable, are inconsistent, or are otherwise questionable or erroneous). (Specify)

Comments or Other Factors:

>> GO TO QUESTION 27 >>

26.2. OMISSION OF QUANTITATIVE INFORMATION ABOUT EXPECTED HEALTH COSTS OR EXPENDITURES IS:

_____ Unimportant	_____ Minor omission	_____ Major omission

Comments:

>> GO TO QUESTION 28 >>

27. *IF* HEALTH BENEFITS ARE PROJECTED IN TERMS OF ADDITIONAL LIFE EXPECTANCY OR SIMILAR MEASURES, SUCH AS QUALITY-ADJUSTED LIFE YEARS, THEN THE COST PER UNIT OF EACH IDENTIFIED BENEFIT IS ESTIMATED.

_____ Yes, benefits projected in such terms and cost per unit estimated

_____ No, benefits projected in such terms but cost per unit not estimated

_____ Not applicable, benefits not so projected and cost per unit not estimated

28. GENERALLY, THE ESTIMATES OF BENEFITS, HARMS, AND COSTS ARE CONSISTENT WITH THE STRENGTH OF THE EVIDENCE PRESENTED IN THE GUIDELINE DOCUMENT.

_____ Yes, completely   _____ Yes, partially   _____ No

Comments:

29. DOES THE GUIDELINE DOCUMENT MAKE MAJOR RECOMMENDATIONS?

_____ Yes (List below, and then go to Question 30)

_____ No (Go to Question 31)

ASSESSOR: Briefly list in the space below the recommendations from the guideline document that the developers consider major. If the developers have not specifically indicated which are their major recommendations, please list those that you have used in answering the questions about the strength of scientific evidence.

30. THE GUIDELINE DOCUMENT EXPLICITLY DISCUSSES THE STRENGTH OF THE SCIENTIFIC EVIDENCE ON WHICH *EACH MAJOR RECOMMENDATION* IS BASED.

_____ Yes (Go to Question 30.1)

_____ No (Go to Question 30.2)

30.1. THE DISCUSSION OF THE STRENGTH OF THE EVIDENCE ON WHICH *EACH MAJOR RECOMMENDATION* IS BASED IS:

_____ Satisfactory for all recommendations

_____ Conditionally satisfactory—i.e., satisfactory for some but not all recommendations

_____ Unsatisfactory—i.e., not satisfactory for most or all recommendations

Comments:

>> GO TO QUESTION 31 >>

30.2. OMISSION OF A DISCUSSION OF THE STRENGTH OF THE SCIENTIFIC EVIDENCE FOR *EACH MAJOR RECOMMENDATION* IS:

_____ Unimportant   _____ Minor omission   _____ Major omission

Comments:

31. *EACH MAJOR RECOMMENDATION* IS CONSISTENT WITH THE ESTIMATED BENEFITS, HARMS, AND COSTS OF THE SERVICE OR INTERVENTION (AND THUS WITH THE STRENGTH OF THE EVIDENCE).

_____ Yes, completely   _____ Yes, partially   _____ No

Comments:

Potential Conflict Among Similar Sets of Guidelines

32. THE GUIDELINE DOCUMENT IDENTIFIES *OTHER SETS OF GUIDELINES* THAT DEAL WITH THE SAME CLINICAL CONDITION, TECHNOLOGY, OR TOPIC.

_____ Yes (Go to Question 33)

_____ No, but similar sets of guidelines are known to exist (Specify below and go to Question 33.2)

_____ Not applicable, no similar sets of guidelines are known to exist (Go to V. CLARITY)

33. THE GUIDELINE DOCUMENT IDENTIFIES *POSSIBLE CONFLICTS AMONG EXISTING GUIDELINES* AND THE REASONS FOR THEM.

_____ Yes (Go to Question 33.1)   _____ No (Go to Question 33.2)

33.1. THE DISCUSSION OF POSSIBLE CONFLICTS AMONG GUIDELINES IS:

_____ Satisfactory   _____ Conditionally satisfactory   _____ Unsatisfactory (Specify)

Comments:

>> GO TO V. CLARITY >>

33.2. OMISSION OF A DISCUSSION OF SIMILAR GUIDELINES, OR OF POSSIBLE CONFLICTS AMONG GUIDELINES, IS:

_____ Unimportant   _____ Minor omission   _____ Major omission

Comments:

V. CLARITY

Clarity means that guidelines are written in unambiguous language and terms, that the logic of the recommendations is clear and straightforward, and that the guideline document has a clear and easy-to-understand structure and format. That is, clarity encompasses the language and the logic with which the guideline document is written and the way it is physically presented. Clarity applies to three content areas of guidelines: (1) a general framework in which health condition(s), health practice(s), patient care goals, and similar topics are defined and discussed; (2) presentation and discussion of the evidence used in developing the guidelines; and (3) recommendations.

More specifically, this attribute requires that, as described below, certain things about language and terms, logic, and structure must be true.

Language and Terms

The guidelines are written in unambiguous language. Vague terms are avoided when describing the patient populations, health conditions, the health interventions, and the recommendations. For example, expressions such as "severe bleeding" are avoided in favor of (or at least qualified by) more precise language, such as a "drop in hematocrit of more than 6 percent in less than 8 hours." Or, for instance, a recommendation such as "thyroid function tests should be obtained whenever appropriate" is replaced by a recommendation that includes the type of test, its frequency, and the specific circumstances under which it should be used, such as "once every 5 years in otherwise healthy adults more than 65 years of age."

34. THE GUIDELINES DESCRIBE THE *HEALTH CONDITION* TO BE PREVENTED, DETECTED, OR TREATED IN UNAMBIGUOUS TERMS.

_____ Yes   _____ No

Comments:

35. THE GUIDELINES DESCRIBE THE *OPTIONS FOR MANAGE-MENT OF THE HEALTH CONDITION* (I.E., THE HEALTH PRACTICE AND ITS ALTERNATIVES) IN UNAMBIGUOUS TERMS.

_____ Yes _____ No

Comments:

36. *IF THE GUIDELINES GIVE MAJOR RECOMMENDATIONS*, EACH IS WRITTEN IN UNAMBIGUOUS TERMS.

ASSESSOR: Refer to the list you developed for Question 29 in answering this question.

_____ Yes _____ No _____ Not applicable, no major recommendations given

Comments:

Logic

The guidelines are as comprehensive as possible in keeping with the attributes "clinical adaptability" and "clinical flexibility." Thus, the logic of the guidelines is such that all clinically important and relevant situations are handled in a consistent, reasonable, and easy-to-follow manner and that situations that are not covered are explained in a logically appropriate place in the guideline statement.

Recommendations are mutually exclusive; that is, they are consistent with each other. For example, a guideline does not recommend "*aortic valvuloplasty* for an 80-year-old man with end stage renal disease" in one place and "*aortic valve replacement* for an 80-year-old man with end stage renal disease" in another.

37. RECOMMENDATIONS ARE COMPREHENSIVE, INSOFAR AS THE EVIDENCE PERMITS, AND RECOMMENDATIONS THAT MIGHT BE EXPECTED ARE GIVEN.
(That is, the recommendations collectively cover all clinically relevant circumstances.)

_____ Yes (Go to Question 38)   _____ No (Go to Question 37.1)

Comments:

37.1 IF EXPECTED RECOMMENDATIONS SEEM TO BE MISSING, THE GUIDELINE DOCUMENT DISCUSSES WHY.

_____ Yes   _____ No

Comments:

38. RECOMMENDATIONS ARE CONSISTENT.
(That is, no two recommendations in the guidelines conflict with each other.)

_____ Yes

_____ No (at least two recommendations appear to conflict with each other)

_____ Not applicable, no recommendations given

Comments:

Structural Clarity

The overall organization and appearance of the guideline document and the mode of presentation of the recommendations are easy for users to understand and follow. A structurally clear guideline is one in which the recommendations are easily accessible to the prospective user. That is, clinicians should not have to read, analyze critically, and distill a detailed manuscript in order to find needed recommendations. Structural clarity may be achieved through the use of a summary, special highlighting techniques, algorithms, or other methods.

39. THE GUIDELINE DOCUMENT USES CLEAR HEADINGS, INDEXES, LISTS, FLOW CHARTS, OR OTHER DEVICES TO IDENTIFY MAJOR TOPICS DISCUSSED.

_____ Yes   _____ No

Comments:

40. THE GUIDELINE DOCUMENT HAS A SUMMARY OR ABSTRACT THAT ACCURATELY REFLECTS THE METHODS, CONTENT, AND RECOMMENDATIONS OF THE ENTIRE DOCUMENT.

_____ Yes   _____ No

Comments:

41. A USER OF THE GUIDELINE DOCUMENT CAN EASILY FIND EACH MAJOR RECOMMENDATION.

ASSESSOR: Refer to the list developed for Question 29 in answering this question.

_____ Yes   _____ No   _____ Not applicable, no major recommendation given

Comments:

VI. SCHEDULED REVIEW

Scheduled review means that a statement specifying a date for review and possible revision of the guideline has been included in the guideline document. Revisions to guidelines should reflect new clinical evidence or changing professional consensus.

This attribute requires that the guideline document either (1) give a specific date for review and possible revision of the guidelines or (2) describe a process by which such a date might be established and the review and possible revision performed.

42. THE GUIDELINE DOCUMENT GIVES A SPECIFIC DATE FOR SCHEDULED REVIEW, GIVES OTHER INFORMATION CONCERNING A PROCEDURE BY WHICH SCHEDULED REVIEW MIGHT BE DONE, OR GIVES A SUNSET OR EXPIRATION DATE.

_____ Yes (Go to Question 42.1)   _____ No (Go to Question 42.2)

42.1. ASSESSOR: Respond to Items 42a-42d, below, to determine whether the scheduled review date information is satisfactory, then answer Question 42.1 below, using your best judgment as to the overall rating for this attribute of scheduled review. Other factors you judge important should be specifically recorded under "Comments or Other Factors."

42a. The target date for review is:

_____ Appropriate   _____ Inappropriate   _____ None given/discussed

42b. The rationale for the target date is:

_____ Adequate   _____ Inadequate   _____ Not applicable

42c. The procedures suggested for determining when the guidelines should be reviewed are:

_____ Appropriate   _____ Inappropriate   _____ None given/discussed

42d. The guideline has a sunset provision that may dictate when a scheduled review should take place or that may indicate when the guideline will expire.

_____ Yes   _____ No

Now answer:

42.1. THE SCHEDULED REVIEW DATE OR PROCEDURE FOR SETTING IT IS:

_____ Satisfactory   _____ Conditionally   _____ Unsatisfactory
                           satisfactory   (Specify)

Comments or Other Factors:

>> Go to VII. MULTI-DISCIPLINARY PROCESS >>

42.2. THE LACK OF A SCHEDULED REVIEW DATE OR PRO-CEDURE FOR SETTING IT IS:

_____ Unimportant   _____ Minor   _____ Major
                               omission   omission

Comments:

VII. MULTI-DISCIPLINARY PROCESS

A *multi-disciplinary process* for practice guidelines means that representatives of a broad range of practitioners, consumers or patients, and other groups likely to be affected by the guidelines have participated in the development process at some stage. These representatives can be individuals who have had direct responsibility for the guideline document or individuals who have reviewed that document or in other ways have contributed to it. This attribute intends that both methodologic and clinical disciplines be involved in the guideline-development process. This document cannot identify in advance all relevant participants, interested parties, or disciplines because each set of guidelines will differ in this respect.

This attribute requires that five things be true. First, some combination of individuals directly responsible for guidelines and those who have otherwise contributed to their development *collectively* represents all the key groups likely to affect or to be affected by the guidelines. Second, the guideline document describes the parties involved (including their credentials and potential biases); "the parties involved" is understood to mean participants in the actual development panel and those in review panels, public hearings, or other review forums. Third, potential biases and conflicts of interests have been discussed or otherwise appropriately taken account of. Fourth, the methods used to solicit panelists' views and arrive at group judgments have been described and are adequate and appropriate to the task of balancing views and potential biases. Fifth, the methods used to solicit outside review comments and present those to panelists have been described and are adequate to the task of making outside views clear to panelists.

43. PERSONS WITH APPROPRIATE CLINICAL AND METHODOLOGIC DISCIPLINES PARTICIPATED IN DEVELOPING THE GUIDELINE DOCUMENT—THAT IS, A MULTI-DISCIPLINARY APPROACH WAS FOLLOWED.

_____ Yes (Go to Question 43.1)

_____ No (Go to Question 43.2)

_____ Don't know or can't tell (Go to Question 43.2)

43.1. ASSESSOR: Respond to Items 43a-43i, below, to determine whether the multi-disciplinary process is satisfactory; then answer Question 43.1 below, using your best judgment as to the overall rating for this element of multi-disciplinary process. Other factors you judge important should be specifically recorded under "Comments or Other Factors."

43a. An explanation, discussion, or rationale for selecting the *guideline panel chairperson* is given.

_____ Yes   _____ No

43b. An explanation, discussion, or rationale for selecting the *members of the guideline panel* is given.

_____ Yes   _____ No

43c. An explanation, discussion, or rationale for *selecting other individuals directly responsible* for the guideline document (such as consultants) is given.

_____ Yes   _____ No

43d. The explanation(s), discussion(s), or rationale(s) for selecting the individuals covered in 43a-c is (are):

_____ Adequate   _____ Inadequate   _____ Not applicable

43e. These individuals reflect all appropriate interest groups and disciplines.

_____ Yes   _____ No   _____ Can't tell

43f. One or more *outside review panel(s)* commented on or reviewed draft guidelines.

_____ Yes   _____ No   _____ Can't tell

43g. One or more *public hearing(s) or similar review mechanism(s)* were held to allow comment or review on draft guidelines.

_____ Yes   _____ No   _____ Can't tell

43h. Collectively, the review panel(s), public hearing(s), or other review mechanisms reflected all appropriate interest groups and disciplines.

_____ Yes   _____ No   _____ Can't tell

43i. If the answer to either question 43e or question 43h is "No" or "Can't tell," please record what groups or disciplines appear to have been omitted.

Now answer:

43.1. THE MULTI-DISCIPLINARY APPROACH TO THE GUIDELINES DEVELOPMENT PROCESS IS:

_____ Satisfactory   _____ Conditionally   _____ Unsatisfactory
                                  satisfactory   (Specify)

Comments or Other Factors:

43.2. THE LACK (OR APPARENT LACK) OF A MULTI-DISCIPLINARY PROCESS IS:

_____ Unimportant   _____ Minor   _____ Major
                                   omission   omission

Comments:

44. THE GUIDELINE DOCUMENT EXPLICITLY NOTES ANY POTENTIAL BIASES AND/OR CONFLICTS OF INTERESTS OF THE PANEL MEMBERS, OR STATES THAT BIASES AND CONFLICTS OF INTEREST WERE DISCUSSED AMONG PANEL MEMBERS OR OTHERWISE TAKEN INTO ACCOUNT.

_____ Yes, potential biases and/or conflicts of interest are noted

_____ Yes, a statement that biases and/or conflicts of interest were discussed is given

_____ No, no note or statement about biases and/or conflicts of interest is given

45. OVERALL, POTENTIAL BIASES AND/OR CONFLICTS OF INTEREST APPEAR TO BE ADEQUATELY BALANCED OR OTHERWISE ACCOUNTED FOR IN THE GUIDELINE DEVELOPMENT PROCESS.

_____ Yes   _____ No   _____ Don't know or can't tell

                                  (Specify)

Comments:

46. THE GUIDELINE DOCUMENT DESCRIBES THE METHODS USED TO SOLICIT VIEWS OF INTERESTED PARTIES NOT ON THE GUIDELINES DEVELOPMENT PANEL AND TO PRESENT THOSE VIEWS TO THE MEMBERS OF PANEL.

_____ Yes (Go to Question 46.1)   _____ No (Go to Question 46.2)

46.1. THE METHODS USED TO SOLICIT VIEWS OF THOSE NOT ON THE PANELS AND PRESENT THOSE VIEWS TO PANELS ARE:

_____ Satisfactory   _____ Conditionally   _____ Unsatisfactory

                                 satisfactory   (Specify)

Comments:

46.2. THE LACK OF A DESCRIPTION OF THE METHODS USED TO SOLICIT VIEWS OF THOSE NOT ON THE PANELS AND TO PRESENT THOSE VIEWS TO PANELS IS:

_____ Unimportant   _____ Minor   _____ Major

                                 omission   omission

Comments:

**PLEASE RECORD ANY SUMMARY JUDGMENTS OR OTHER
COMMENTS YOU MAY HAVE AND ANY RECOMMENDATIONS
FOR ADDITIONAL REVIEW.**

PART THREE. SUMMARY EVALUATION SHEET

Instructions and Key

ASSESSOR: Upon completing the entire assessment instrument, please record answers to the main questions (Questions 1-46) below. Circle the relevant answer, according to the following key:

```
KEY

Y = Yes; YQ = yes, but response qualified;
N = No; NQ = no, but response qualified;
S = Satisfactory, CS = Conditionally satisfactory, US = Unsatisfactory;
UN = Unimportant, MI = Minor omission, MA = Major omission;
NA = Not applicable
DK = Don't know, or can't tell
```

I. CLINICAL APPLICABILITY

Y	N		1.	Description of patient population
S	CS	US		1.1. Quality of description
UN	MI	MA		1.2. Omission of description

Y	N	NA	2.	Discussion of complex clinical problems
S	CS	US		2.1. Quality of discussion
UN	MI	MA		2.2. Omission of discussion

Y	N		3.	Rationale for excluding patient populations
S	CS	US		3.1. Quality of rationale
UN	MI	MA		3.2. Omission of rationale

II. CLINICAL FLEXIBILITY

Y	N		4.	Information about acceptable *clinical* exceptions
S	CS	US		4.1. Quality of information or statement
UN	MI	MA		4.2. Omission of information or statement

Y	N		5.	Information about acceptable *nonclinical* exceptions
S	CS	US		5.1. Quality of information or statement
UN	MI	MA		5.2. Omission of information or statement

Y   N   6.   Discussion of patient preferences in the health care
                               decisions
S   CS   US   6.1.   Quality of discussion
UN   MI   MA   6.2.   Omission of discussion

Y   N   7.   Discussion of patient preferences in guideline
                               development
S   CS   US   7.1.   Quality of discussion
UN   MI   MA   7.2.   Omission of discussion

III. RELIABILITY/REPRODUCIBILITY

Y   N   8.   Independent review by experts or outside panels
S   CS   US   8.1.   Quality of discussion

Y   N   9.   Explanation of lack of independent review
S   CS   US   9.1.   Quality of explanation
UN   MI   MA   9.2.   Omission of explanation

Y   N   10.   Guidelines pretested in some manner
S   CS   US   10.1. Quality of discussion

Y   N   11.   Explanation of lack of pretesting
S   CS   US   11.1. Quality of explanation
UN   MI   MA   11.2. Omission of explanation

IV. VALIDITY

STRENGTH OF THE SCIENTIFIC EVIDENCE AND PROFESSIONAL CONSENSUS

Y   N   12.   Method of collecting (identifying and retrieving)
                               scientific evidence is specifically described
S   CS   US   12.1. Quality of method
UN   MI   MA   12.2. Lack of method

Y   N   13.   Adequate references to sources of scientific evidence

Y   N   14.   General discussion of strength of scientific evidence

Y	N		15.	Explicit rating of the strength of the scientific evidence
S	CS	US		15.1. Quality of rating method
UN	MI	MA		15.2. Lack of general discussion of rating method

Y	N	NQ	16.	If a formal method of synthesis is used, explicit description of the method
S	CS	US		16.1. Quality of formal method
UN	MI	MA		16.2. Omission of description of formal method

Y	N		17.	If applicable, the results of a formal synthesis of scientific evidence are explicitly reported
S	CS	US		17.1. Quality of results of the synthesis
UN	MI	MA		17.2. Omission of results of the synthesis

Y	N	NQ	18.	If applicable, the expert or group judgment techniques used for reaching professional consensus are explicitly described
S	CS	US		18.1. Quality of expert or group judgment techniques
UN	MI	MA		18.2. Omission of description of expert or group judgment techniques

Y	N		19.	If applicable, the strength of professional consensus resulting from use of group judgment techniques is reported
S	CS	US		19.1. Quality of information about strength of professional consensus
UN	MI	MA		19.2. Omission of explicit information about strength of professional consensus

HEALTH BENEFITS AND HARMS/RISKS: QUALITATIVE DESCRIPTION

Y	N		20.	Qualitative description of health benefits
S	CS	US		20.1. Quality of qualitative description
UN	MI	MA		20.2. Omission of qualitative description

Y	N		21.	Qualitative description of potential harms or risks
S	CS	US		21.1. Quality of qualitative description
UN	MI	MA		21.2. Omission of qualitative description

HEALTH BENEFITS AND HARMS/RISKS: QUANTITATIVE
INFORMATION

Y	N		22.	Quantitative information or estimates of health benefits
S	CS	US		22.1. Quality of quantitative information
UN	MI	MA		22.2. Omission of quantitative information
Y	N	NA	23.	Health benefits projected in terms of life expectancy or similar measures
Y	N		24.	Quantitative information or estimates of potential harms or risks
S	CS	US		24.1. Quality of quantitative information
UN	MI	MA		24.2. Omission of quantitative information

HEALTH COSTS: QUALITATIVE DESCRIPTION

Y	N		25.	Qualitative description of health costs or expenditures
S	CS	US		25.1 Quality of qualitative description
UN	MI	MA		25.2. Omission of qualitative description

HEALTH COSTS: QUANTITATIVE DESCRIPTION

Y	N		26.	Quantitative information or estimates of health costs or expenditures
S	CS	US		26.1. Quality of quantitative information
UN	MI	MA		26.2. Omission of quantitative information
Y	N	NA	27.	If health benefits projected in terms of life expectancy or similar measures, costs per unit of each identified benefit also estimated
Y	YQ	N	28.	Generally, estimates of benefits, harms, and costs are consistent with the strength of provided evidence
Y	N		29.	Major recommendations made in the guideline
Y	N		30.	Discussion of strength of the scientific evidence for each major recommendation

S	CS	US		30.1. Quality of discussion
UN	MI	MA		30.2. Omission of discussion
Y	YQ	N	31.	Each major recommendation consistent with strength of scientific evidence

POTENTIAL CONFLICT AMONG SIMILAR SETS OF GUIDELINES

Y	N	NA	32.	Other sets of guidelines identified

Y	N		33.	Possible conflicts among existing guidelines discussed
S	CS	US		33.1. Quality of discussion
UN	MI	MA		33.2. Omission of discussion

V. CLARITY

LANGUAGE AND TERMS

Y	N		34.	Language describing the health condition is unambiguous
Y	N		35.	Language describing the options for management is unambiguous
Y	N	NA	36.	Language for each major recommendation is unambiguous

LOGIC

Y	N		37.	Recommendations are comprehensive and present when expected
Y	N			37.1. Reasons given for lack of expected recommendations
Y	N	NA	38.	Recommendations are consistent

STRUCTURAL CLARITY

Y	N		39.	Guideline document uses clear headings, indexes, etc.
Y	N		40.	Guideline document has accurate summary or abstract
Y	N	NA	41.	Users can find recommendations easily

VI. SCHEDULED REVIEW: DEFINITION AND EVALUATION QUESTIONS

Y	N		42.	Scheduled date for review or a procedure for arriving at such a date is provided
S	CS	US		42.1. Quality of the scheduled review date or procedure for setting one
UN	MI	MA		42.2. Lack of a scheduled review date or procedure for setting one

VII. MULTI-DISCIPLINARY PROCESS

Y	N	DK	43.	Participation of persons in appropriate clinical and methodologic disciplines
S	CS	US		43.1. Quality of the multi-disciplinary approach
UN	MI	MA		43.2. Lack of a multi-disciplinary process
Y	YQ	N	44.	Guideline document notes potential biases or conflicts of interest or indicates they were taken into account
Y	N	DK	45.	Balance of potential biases or conflicts of interest
Y	N		46.	Description of the methods used to solicit views of those not on the guidelines development panel and to present those views to the panel
S	CS	US		46.1. Quality of methods used
UN	MI	MA		46.2. Lack of a description of methods used

SUMMARY JUDGMENT, OTHER COMMENTS, OR NEED FOR ADDITIONAL REVIEW:

C

Institute of Medicine
Committee on Clinical
Practice Guidelines

PUBLIC HEARING PARTICIPANTS

December 3, 1990
Washington, D.C.

John A. Benson, Jr., M.D., President, American Board of Internal Medicine

John Coombs, M.D., Chair, *Ad Hoc* Committee on Physician Practice Guidelines, American Hospital Association

Janet M. Corrigan, Ph.D., Director, Medical Directors Division, Group Health Association of America

William R. Darrow, M.D., Ph.D., Chairman, Medical Section, Pharmaceutical Manufacturers Association

Bruce V. Davis, M.D., Director, Department of Preventive Care, Group Health Cooperative of Puget Sound

Susan Dean-Baar, M.S., R.N., C.R.R.N., Co-Chairperson, Committee on Nursing Practice Standards and Guidelines, American Nurses Association

Donalda Ellek, Ph.D., Manager, Office of Quality Assurance, American Dental Association

Burton S. Epstein, M.D., Chairman, Committee on Standards of Care, American Society of Anesthesiologists

John H. Ferguson, M.D., Director, Office of Medical Applications of Research, National Institutes of Health

Joyce Frieden, *Business and Health*

Ron Geigle, J.D., Geigle and Associates

Barbara Greenberg, Ph.D., Project
Coordinator, Standards, American
College of Radiology

Jerome H. Grossman, M.D.,
Chairman and Chief Executive
Officer, New England Medical
Center

Michael A.W. Hattwick, M.D.,
Practice of Internal Medicine,
Annandale, Virginia

Edward J. Huth, M.D., Member,
Clinical Efficacy Assessment
Subcommittee and Editor Emeritus,
Annals of Internal Medicine,
American College of Physicians

Karen Ignagni, M.B.A., Director,
Employee Benefits, American
Federation of Labor and Congress
of Industrial Organizations
(AFL-CIO)

Alan Kaplan, J.D., Consultant,
American Association of Retired
Persons

Edmund F. Kelly, Ph.D., President,
Employee Benefits Division, Ætna
Life and Casualty

Joyce V. Kelly, Ph.D., Associate
Vice President for Clinical
Services, Association of American
Medical Colleges

Gregory Michael Lenhart, M.S.,
Senior Scientist, Private Healthcare
Systems

Candace L. Littell, Vice President
for Policy, Research, and
Evaluation, Health Industry
Manufacturers Association

Carol A. Lockhart, Ph.D.,
Executive Director, Greater
Phoenix Affordable Health Care
Foundation

Trisha McGillan, R.N., B.S.N.,
J.D., Staff Attorney/Long Term
Care Nurse Specialist, American
Health Care Association

Jane Mulvey, Senior Analyst,
Public Policy Institute, American
Association of Retired Persons

Daniel J. O'Neal, M.A., R.N.,
C.N.A.A., Assistant Director,
Congressional and Agency
Relations, American Nurses
Association

Harold Alan Pincus, M.D., Deputy
Medical Director and Director,
Office of Research, American
Psychiatric Association

Shirley D. Rivers, J.D., Assistant
Director, Office of Quality
Assurance, American Medical
Association

Kenneth B. Roberts, M.D.,
Member, Task Force on Quality of
Care, American Academy of
Pediatrics

James Rosenblum, J.D., Member, Policy Subcommittee, Medicine and Law Committee, American Bar Association

Arnold Rosoff, J.D., Senior Fellow, Leonard Davis Institute of Health Economics, University of Pennsylvania

David B. Siegel, M.D., Medical Director and Vice President for Health and Medical Affairs, Health Alliance Plan of Michigan, Group Health Association of America

Nicole Simmons, Health Care Financing Administration

Sara V. Sinclair, R.N., B.S.N., N.H.A., Administrator, Sunshine Terrace Foundation and Chairman, Long Term Care, Professional-Technical Advisory Panel, JCAHO, American Health Care Association

Edward J. Stemmler, M.D., Executive Vice President, Association of American Medical Colleges

David Tennenbaum, Director, Medical Necessity Program, Blue Cross and Blue Shield Association

Theresa Varner, M.S.W., M.A., Senior Coordinator, Health Team, Public Policy Institute, American Association of Retired Persons

Andrew H. Webber, Executive Vice President, American Medical Peer Review Association

HEALTH CARE LIAISON PANEL

John F. Beary III, M.D., Senior Vice President, Science & Technology, Pharmaceutical Manufacturers Association

Janet M. Corrigan, Ph.D., Director, Medical Directors Division, Group Health Association of America

Carole Cronin, Vice President and Director, Quality Resource Center, Washington Business Group on Health

Donalda Ellek, Ph.D., Manager, Office of Quality Assurance, American Dental Association

Susan Gleeson, Executive Director, Technology Management Department, Blue Cross and Blue Shield Association

Norma M. Lang, Ph.D., R.N., F.A.A.N., President, American Nurses Foundation

Ronald S. Lankford, M.D., (Federation of American Healthcare Systems), Vice President of Medical Affairs, Health Care Division, Humana, Inc.

Candace L. Littell, Vice President for Policy, Research, and Evaluation, Health Industry Manufacturers Association

Daniel R. Longo, Sc.D., President, Hospital Education and Research Trust, American Hospital Association

Robert E. McAfee, M.D., Vice Chair of the Board, American Medical Association

Joel Miller, Deputy Director, Insurance, Managed Care, and Provider Relations Division, Health Insurance Association of America

Malcolm Schoen, M.D., Medical Advisor, Consumers Union

Edward J. Stemmler, M.D., Association of American Medical Colleges

Loring Wood, M.D., U.S. Chamber of Commerce

SPECIALTY LIAISON PROGRAM

Joseph F. Boyle, M.D., Executive Vice President, American Society of Internal Medicine

Betty King, Executive Director, IMCARE, American Society of Internal Medicine

Dr. James N. Cooper, Chair, AGA Committee on Patient Care, American Gastroenterological Association

Pamela M. Cramer, Vice President, Education and Membership Services, College of American Pathologists

LeBaron W. Dennis, M.D., Chair, ASPRS Guidelines Committee, American Society of Plastic and Reconstructive Surgeons

Paul A. Ebert, M.D., Director, American College of Surgeons

James W. Fletcher, M.D., Society of Nuclear Medicine

Lea Gamble, Director, Health Policy Research, American Academy of Ophthalmology

Lee Goldman, M.D., President, Society of General Internal Medicine

Michael Greenberg, M.D.,
American Academy of Neurology

Nancy Peacock Heath, Ph.D.,
Assistant Director for Policy and
Research, American Academy of
Orthopaedic Surgeons

James F. Kelly, D.D.S., American
Association of Oral and
Maxillofacial Surgeons

Donald G. Langsley, M.D.,
Executive Vice President, American
Board of Medical Specialties

Daniel J. Ostergaard, M.D., Vice
President for Education and
Scientific Affairs, American
Academy of Family Physicians

Harold Pincus, M.D., Deputy
Medical Director and Director,
Office of Research, American
Psychiatric Association

Lester Rosen, M.D., Chair,
Standards Task Force of ASCRS,
American Society of Colon and
Rectal Surgeons

Clark C. Watts, M.D., American
Association of Neurological
Surgeons

Richard S. Wilbur, M.D., J.D.,
Executive Vice President, Council
of Medical Specialty Societies

Steven Woolf, M.D., Scientific
Advisor, Expert Panel on
Preventive Services, American
College of Preventive Medicine

Judy Young, Director, Practice
Management, American College of
Emergency Physicians

RELATED ORGANIZATIONS

Frank J. Malouff, M.S.H.A.,
Executive Director, American
Podiatric Medical Association

Russ Newman, Ph.D., J.D.,
Assistant Executive Director,
Practice Directorate, American
Psychological Association

Terry Nickels, D.O., F.A.C.G.P.,
American Osteopathic Association

Index

feedback to practitioners, 16
implementation of practice guidelines for,
37, 41, 205
proposed directions for, 110–111
revision/updating of guidelines, 16
tests of clinical skills, 101
see also Continuous quality improvement
Quality control, in guidelines development, 6
Quality improvement, *see* Continuous quality
improvement; Total quality
management
Quality of care
defined, 100
management commitment to, 103
practice quidelines and, 23, 99, 100

Radiology guidelines, 48, 49, 130
RAND Corporation, 36, 56, 57, 60, 109,
155, 169, 280
Regenstrief Medical Record System, 90
Reimbursement, 74, 89
*Report on Medical Guidelines & Outcomes
Research*, 189
Research agenda
adoption and diffusion of medical
innovations, 21, 35, 216
assessment instrument, 21
conflicts and inconsistencies in guidelines,
181–183, 216
expert panel processes, 176–178, 216
impact of practice guidelines, 21, 35, 104,
216–217
incorporating outcomes information into
guidelines, 179–180
medical liability, 133
methodologies for evaluating scientific
evidence, 178–179, 216
on outcomes and effectiveness of health
care services, 3, 24, 38, 42, 56–57, 104,
215–216
patient preferences, 180–181
testing effectiveness of practice
guidelines, 21, 216
topic selection, 175–176
Retrospective review of care, 17
Risk management
computer applications in, 95
educational strategies and, 87
implementation of practice guidelines in,
17–18, 37, 41, 51, 74–75, 100, 124–125
informed consent and, 147
physician conditions of licensure, 131

see also Medical malpractice
Robert Wood Johnson Foundation, 60, 102

Scientific American Medicine, 62
Selective contracting, 70–71
Society for Medical Decision Making, 50
Society of Nuclear Medicine, 49
Standards for care, 33, 56
Sweden, clinical practice guidelines, 35

Task Force on Assessment of Diagnostic and
Therapeutic Cardiovascular Procedures,
48–49
Terminology, *see* Definitions and terminology
Third-party payers
implementation of practice guidelines by,
5, 16, 22, 27, 41
liability for negligence, 117
Total quality management, 102, 104–105
Triage of injured patients, 145, 264

United HealthCare, 62
Universal precautions, 27–28
Urinary incontinence, 55, 109, 333
U.S. HealthCare, 62
U.S. Preventive Services Task Force,
guidelines, 34, 58–59, 63, 172, 252
U.S. Public Health Service, guidelines
development, 53–57, 143, 172
Utilization review
appropriateness criteria, 57
concurrent review of inpatient care, 115,
117
and cost control, 116
criticisms of, 107–108
by hospitals, 115
implementation of practice guidelines, 116,
206–207
liability, 114 n.9, 117–119
medical review criteria in, 107
by PROs, 57–58, 108, 129
retrospective, 115
role of, 17, 70–71, 101, 123, 207
by third-party payers, 115

Vaccinations for pregnant women, 55, 260
Value Health Sciences, 60
definition of appropriate care, 155
Medical Review System, 109
Visual acuity screening of children, 59, 252

Wishard Memorial Hospital, 90